CARE COORDINATION

Person-Centered Care Across the Continuum

Jayne Josephsen

Boise State University

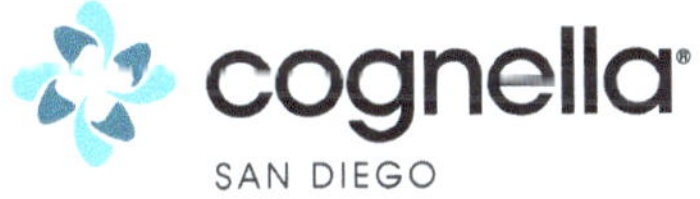

Bassim Hamadeh, CEO and Publisher
Amanda Martin, Executive Publisher
Amy Smith, Associate Editorial Manager
Abbey Hastings, Senior Production Editor
Emely Villavicencio, Senior Graphic Designer
Kylie Bartolome, Licensing Specialist
Natalie Piccotti, Director of Marketing
Kassie Graves, Senior Vice President, Editorial
Alia Bales, Director, Project Editorial and Production

Printed in the United States of America.

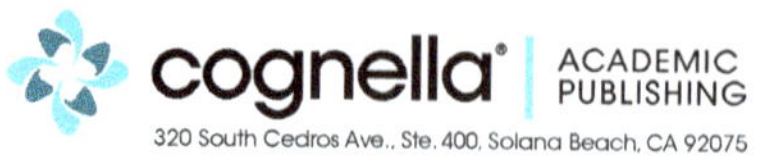

Brief Contents

Detailed Contents

Preface

As the United States health system transitions to value-based healthcare and works to address the multidimensional aspects of health and wellness, the critical necessity of integrating care coordination throughout the health system has been highlighted. Care coordination is essential to the transformation to value-based healthcare and to meeting individual healthcare needs in a relevant and person-centered way. People are multidimensional with various physical, social, emotional, and spiritual needs to be addressed holistically for better outcomes and resource management. Care coordination in nursing practice supports this crucial need in our health system.

In nursing, coordinating care can sometimes be viewed as being provided only by the discharge planner, case manager, or someone with the title of care coordinator. However, with the addition of care coordination to the nursing process, the integration of care coordination in quality measures and legislation, and the critical need for better health outcomes, nurses can no longer view care coordination as someone else's job; it is a core aspect of every nursing role. Unfortunately, few comprehensive resources or textbooks concerning care coordination exist for nurses and nurse educators. This leads many nursing educators and nurses to search for information on implementing care coordination and its connection with better outcomes from various sources and piecemeal content. This book's vision is to provide a comprehensive and relevant resource for all nurses so that they can understand and implement effective person-centered care coordination in their practice.

The need for training and education in care coordination practice is imperative. National nursing organizations have acknowledged this through integrating care coordination into the nursing process and the AACN *Essentials*. Although discussed frequently throughout the health system and nursing organizations, care coordination needs to be more understood. Implementation of care coordination can assist in addressing multiple populations' needs, critical barriers to coordinated care such as health and digital literacy, social determinants and influencers of health, and populations with multiple chronic health conditions. Care coordination is a powerful intervention; solid care coordination practice can reduce readmissions to acute care and duplicative services and address gaps and barriers to care. This requires the ability of the care coordinator to work collaboratively with the interprofessional team, accept accountability for care coordination interventions and actions, utilize health systems thinking, and empower patients and their families or caregivers to be informed, engaged, and activated in their health and well-being.

The book begins by defining care coordination's core elements, competencies, and standards and discussing how these are applied in nursing practice. From this foundation, critical knowledge, skills, and attitudes are considered for effective and quality care coordination practice. A wealth of information and tools are presented, including discussion and application of health technologies, healthcare financing, regulatory issues, quality measures, and continuous quality improvement that assist the nurse in understanding the health system's complexity and how to support coordinated care through the continuum of care.

While the book focuses on nursing students, it is believed to contain critical information that all practicing nurses need to understand and integrate to coordinate care. This book provides an overview of the goals and guiding principles of care coordination practice, giving foundational knowledge to enhance confidence and skills in delivering care coordination in nursing practice. This book offers a central resource for students and nurses alike to go to for foundational care coordination concepts, application to a variety of settings and populations, and a "tool belt" of care coordination interventions and processes. This book differs from previous books on care coordination by discussing the "nuts and bolts," the how and why of care coordination interventions, and pairing the content with explanations, examples, visuals, and case studies to enhance understanding of the concepts and their relation to effective care coordination practice.

Nurses must advocate for and provide effective, person-centered, and relevant care coordination. Advancing better outcomes, managing resources, and addressing critical issues such as health equality and accessibility can be supported through delivering quality care coordination. By educating our students and fellow nurses on the vital yet complex process of coordinating care, we can meet the multidimensional needs of those who enter the health system at various points and support healthcare transformation and a positive healthcare journey.

In addition to this text, instructor resources are available to adopting instructors.

Acknowledgments

The idea for this book emerged from the many comments of students in my care coordination course requesting a textbook that covered the course content. Without these conversations, I would not have considered writing a textbook. I want to acknowledge all the students who struggled with me to find good resources and encouraged me to create a comprehensive resource for their learning. I would also like to thank Brea Shepherd-Crager, Brooke Maynard, and Lorrie Somazzi for their time discussing care coordination practices. I am also extremely thankful to my husband, Mark, who provided continuous support, allowed me to talk through content ideas, and kept me on track and motivated. Lastly, I sincerely thank the reviewers who took the time and effort necessary to review this book.

Reviewers

Pamela W. Baker, PhD, RN, CNE, Pennsylvania College of Technology

Sheila Blank, DNP, RN, LSN, Youngstown State University

Julie S. Fitzwater, PhD, RN, CNRN, CNE, CHSE, Linfield University

Stephanie Gustman, DNP, RN, Ferris State University

Audra Trump, DNP, FNP-C, APRN, Millikin University

Virginia M. White, DNP, Olympic College

Introduction

This book, *Care Coordination: Person-Centered Care Across the Continuum,* is designed for nursing students and practicing nurses as an introductory yet comprehensive text concerning an essential aspect of nursing practice—coordination of care. The beginnings of care coordination can be seen in the acts of Florence Nightingale, who worked to find gaps in care and actively and collaboratively engaged with stakeholders for better health outcomes (Matthews et al., 2020). We can look to Lillian Wald as another pioneer in integrating care coordination into nursing practice, working in interprofessional teams to bring care into homes and communities (Pittman, 2019). Dame Cicely Saunders also contributed to the concept of care coordination by bringing into nursing practice care of the whole person, including physical, emotional, social, and spiritual dimensions (Richmond, 2005). Nursing theorists, such as Betty Neuman, Dorothea Orem, and Hildegard Peplau, also contributed theoretical constructs that support the coordination of care by addressing the multidimensional aspects of health from the foundation of empowerment in health and the nurse–patient relationship (Fawcett, 2005).

The nursing discipline has integrated the framework of care coordination and person-centered care practices from the beginning. Unfortunately, the health system has operated on a disease-focused model of care since the early 20th century. Discovering serious cost and outcome issues with this model did not take long. Disease-based care did not sustain the foundational necessity of meeting the multidimensional needs of patients and coordinate care across settings and systems. Since that time, different care delivery models have been developed, and over 20 years ago, the Institute of Medicine (IOM) created a vision for a new health system for the 21st century (IOM, 2001). Yet the health system continues to struggle to provide care in a coordinated and person-centered way. Regardless of the setting, the discipline of nursing has the duty and potential to support the health system in meeting the health and well-being of patients and their families or support systems in a holistic fashion through person-centered care coordination delivery, which will in turn assist in realizing the vision of a 21st-century health system.

The *Quintuple Aim* signifies this journey in the health system. Beginning in 2007, the Institute for Healthcare Improvement (IHI) began the *Triple Aim,* with the goals of "improving the experience of care, improving the health of populations, and reducing per capita costs of health care" (Whittington et al., 2015, abstract). The *Triple Aim* became a central component of the United States healthcare strategy as it was integrated into the Patient Protection and Affordable Care Act of 2010. The *Quadruple Aim* was introduced in 2014 with the goals of reducing costs and improving population health, patient experience, and team well-being (Arnetz et al., 2020, p. 1). It became apparent that healthcare workers, including nurses, were central in improving outcomes, cost and resource management, and the healthcare experience. So team well-being was added with the goal of improving the performance of the health system.

In 2021, the *Quintuple Aim* was introduced with the goals of "improved patient experience, better outcomes, lower costs, clinician well-being, and health equity" (Itchhaporia, 2021, p. 2263). Health equity was added as a goal for several reasons, one of the main reasons being that 70% of healthcare outcomes are driven by social determinants of health (Itchhaporia, 2021, p. 2262). Without addressing the barriers to health, the gaps in care received, and the siloed nature of the health system, the vision for the IOM's 21st-century health system and the *Quintuple Aim* will not be attainable. Care coordination speaks directly to each aspect of the *Quintuple Aim*, supporting a positive patient experience, managing resources and costs, enhancing satisfaction in the healthcare team, promoting better long-term health outcomes, and meeting the patient in the context of their lived experience, community, and priorities and goals of care. When these goals are met, it will create an equitable and coordinated health system. Throughout the book, we will examine the connection of care coordination to the *Quintuple Aim*, the vision of a 21st-century health system that provides safe, quality, person-centered, equitable, and accessible care, along with the current health system's transformation to value-based healthcare.

The current health system is frequently siloed, offering fragmented care, which results in poor outcomes, duplicative care and services, and patients who need education and support to be active and engaged participants in the self-management of their health. Understanding the care coordination process, its components, and the impact of the health system on the provision of person-centered care coordination is essential for all nurses. This book offers a system-level perspective applied to person-centered care coordination practice and its principles, goals, and outcomes across the continuum of care that address these issues and promote better experiences, outcomes, and management of healthcare resources.

Although care coordination is often discussed in healthcare and is a crucial quality measure in reimbursement and regulatory processes, few comprehensive resources cover the foundational aspects of care coordination practice. This often leaves students and practicing nurses searching for relevant materials to guide their learning or practice in this area. Frequently, the resources found are case examples or pilot projects integrating care coordination into a health system or practice for a particular outcome. This continues to promote a siloed view of the coordination of care in specific settings or for specific populations. However, care coordination is for everyone: all patients, all nurses, and all settings. Understanding the process and impact of person-centered care coordination practices can provide better health outcomes for all and assist in meeting the IOM's vision of a 21st-century health system and the *Quintuple Aim*.

Purpose and Objectives

We know that care coordination is a critical piece of healthcare delivery. Still, we frequently don't understand how to implement it, what tools might work best, how it fits into the health system and meets the *Quintuple Aim*, and how it is part of the nursing code of ethics and scope and standards of practice. The impetus of this book originates from teaching care coordination and resource management to undergraduate and graduate students and finding a lack of a comprehensive resource that practically and understandably presents the complex practice of coordinating care across the continuum. This book aims to provide a comprehensive resource or textbook for nursing students of all levels and practicing nurses to understand the continuum of care and how effective care coordination is critical as the health system transforms into value-based healthcare and a decentralized system of care, offering relevant and accessible care across the continuum.

The reader will obtain a foundational understanding of person-centered care coordination, discover various tools that will prepare them to coordinate care, and explore the multiple aspects of the health system that impact care coordination practice. A synthesis of the knowledge, skills, and attitudes related to care coordination is provided. The book explores evidence-based practices for person-centered care coordination and the needed perspectives of value, quality, and continuous quality improvement in healthcare. It reviews the basics of coordinating care, the variety of ways it may be offered, and various roles that may provide it across the continuum, along with current regulatory and system trends that impact care coordination practices.

The book's content flows from a foundational discussion and analysis of what care coordination is, how it might be integrated into different settings, the competencies needed for effective coordination of care, how care coordination fits into the nursing process, and a review of national nursing standards that support the integration of care coordination into all nursing practice. Once the framework of coordinated care is explored, a detailed review of critical components of care coordination is provided, including a discussion of patient engagement and activation, motivational interviewing, healthcare financing, quality and regulatory requirements, and continuous quality improvement processes. The book ends with a discussion of the health system, current trends, care coordination of special populations, and an assessment of the future of care coordination. The reader will leave with a solid understanding of the importance of coordinating care and how they can integrate it into their nursing practice.

Organization and Coverage

The book is divided into 11 chapters and is organized consistently to aid learning, comprehension, and application of person-centered care coordination. Each chapter begins with listed chapter objectives to orient the reader to the content and how the content connects with care coordination practice. Key terms are also provided, with a glossary of definitions. The chapters begin with an introduction to familiarize the reader with the chapter's content. Each chapter has headings that will alert the reader to how the content and concepts are connected. Text boxes include examples, notable quotations, or additional information that supports the content. Various pictorials are also integrated throughout the chapter to assist the reader in visualizing the care coordination process and how the content fits into the health system and continuum of care. Each chapter ends with a summary that recaps critical points of the content. This format builds upon the content presented, offering examples and care coordination tools to support the content's translation into effective, quality, and person-centered care coordination practice.

Chapter 1 begins with an overview of care coordination and the different types seen in today's health system: population health coordinated care, transition management, case management, and resource and utilization management. The relation of care coordination to the *Quintuple Aim* and selected other roles frequently providing care coordination are presented.

Chapter 1 also reviews national standards for care coordination practice, certification organizations, and requirements. Lastly, the American Nurses Association (ANA) scope and standards of practice and the American Association of Colleges of Nursing (AACN) *Essentials* are examined and applied to the critical need for nurses to understand and integrate care coordination interventions and frameworks into their nursing practice.

Chapter 2 explains the core competencies required for care coordination practice. A review of competency versus skill offers a foundation for discussing the following care coordination competencies: advocacy, assessment and critical analysis, communication, interprofessional practice, connecting community resources, and quality assurance. The connection and dynamic relationship between assessment and critical analysis is explored to deliver person-centered, coordinated care. The competency of communication is presented from various perspectives and needs, including cross-setting communication, challenging conversations, the use of nursing presence, and other considerations. Interprofessional practice is explored with the patient at the team's center and with the integration of collaborative practice. The critical need for competency in connecting the patient to community resources is discussed. Lastly, monitoring and evaluation activities are examined in the context of quality assurance for care coordination practice.

Chapter 3 focuses on the nursing process. All steps of the nursing process are connected to care coordination practices and interventions. A discussion of how to apply ADOPIE (assessment, diagnosis, outcome identification, planning, implementation of coordination of care, health teaching and promotion, and evaluation) is provided in the context of person-centered care coordination across the continuum. There are also three practice focus examples, including assessing for risk in patient populations, preparing for transitions of care, and monitoring care coordination for better outcomes. Examples of assessment tools are provided, the application of gap analysis is reviewed, and the concept of pacing the case is presented and applied to care coordination practice.

Chapter 4 allows for the discovery of the crucial ability of patients to be engaged and activated in the self-management of their health and how care coordination practices can support this. The trajectory framework of health is presented, and the aspects of health are considered. Patient engagement is reviewed with patient activation and tools to assess patient confidence and readiness to become activated in their health. The nurse's and patient's role in supporting patient self-management of health is discussed. Issues such as health literacy, social influencers of health, and shared decision-making are examined, and application examples are given. Chapter 4 ends with exploring motivational interviewing, the stages of change, and how motivational interviewing can be applied to shared decision-making.

Chapter 5 provides an extensive overview of the continuum of care, levels of care, and how these may affect care coordination practices and meet patient needs. Common transitions of care are explored, such as acute care hospitals, long-term acute care hospitals, psychiatric hospitals, rehabilitation centers, home health services, personal care services, and palliative and hospice care. Each level of care is defined and reviewed, and unique care coordination considerations are discussed. The spheres of care and types of care and health services commonly utilized across the continuum of care are presented, and their interconnection is explored. Costs and differences between some types of care are compared as well.

Chapter 6 presents the impact of quality in healthcare and the value of care coordination in ensuring quality healthcare. Care coordination and quality measure sets and their connection to value-based healthcare, scoring, and types are discussed. The role of the care coordination nurse is explored in the context of continuous quality improvement, providing for quality outcomes and decreasing waste or muda in the health system. The critical aspect of documentation of care coordination efforts and interventions is reviewed, and the FACT documentation tool is presented. LEAN's continuous quality improvement processes and its value to care coordination practice are explored.

Chapter 7 explores innovative healthcare delivery models, how each model supports the *Quintuple Aim*, and how care coordination is integrated. Models of integrated care, home-based care, primary care, transitional care, telehealth, those focusing on underserved populations, and community models are examined. Additionally, each model is connected to care coordination practices and the support of person-centered quality, safe, and effective care delivery. The models discussed are all currently present in the health system in some form and offer insight into how person-centered care coordination can be implemented across the continuum to meet rights and principles of care coordination and the *Quintuple Aim*.

Chapter 8 tackles complex healthcare financing and value-based payment models. The myriad of aspects affecting healthcare financing are reviewed, and types of value-based healthcare reimbursement strategies are explored. Connection to quality and care coordination measures is presented, supporting an understanding of how the implementation of person-centered care coordination connects to payment models. Coding and documentation requirements are discussed and connected to the utilization review process. Common third-party payers are reviewed, providing an overview of their framework and matters the care coordinating nurse needs to be aware of. Issues such as premiums, the donut hole, and projected funding sources are explored. Medicare, Medicaid, and commercial third-party payers are discussed in detail so that the complexity and requirements of each type are understood. Those that are uninsured are addressed in the context of care coordination practice. Lastly, the chapter presents current healthcare financing and value-based initiatives.

Chapter 9 delves into health information technology, informatics, and digital health trends. Each is examined for understanding and application to care coordination implementation and practice, and their symbiotic relationship is presented. The connection of knowledge, inquiry, and informatics outcomes in nursing practice is also examined. Regulatory considerations such as HITECH, HIPAA, and CEHRT are discussed, as well as how these can affect care coordination interventions. Data management and pillars are presented, and trade-offs and considerations of health technology are explored. Issues such as digital inclusivity, HIPAA violations, alert fatigue, privacy, and infrastructure concerns are discussed.

Chapter 10 focuses on the need for nurses and those offering care coordination services to have a health science and thinking perspective. The necessity of utilizing a big-picture view and addressing the multidimensionality of health is presented. Legislative trends concerning care coordination are reviewed, and the nurse's essential role in advocacy for person-centered care coordination practices, regulations, and legislation is discussed. Health systems trends of well-being, proactive care coordination, culture, social media, and healthcare technology integration and use are explored. Ethical considerations of autonomy, self-determination, and management of resources are examined. Lastly, the future of care coordination is viewed, including the nurse's role, the need for nursing education to support the integration of care coordination content into curriculum or training, the use of artificial intelligence, and the critical need to advance collaborative and integrated care coordination.

The book ends with chapter 11, in which selected special populations are explored in the context of care coordination practice. The foundation of trauma-informed care is defined and applied to the selected populations: veterans, those with Alzheimer's disease and related dementias (ADRD), those with intellectual or developmental disabilities (IDD), and the unhoused. Each of these special populations has specific needs that care coordinating nurses must be aware of and proactively address, such as the need for trauma-informed care. Each population is discussed, and specific care coordination considerations are presented in the context of promoting better outcomes and providing person-centered care coordination.

Throughout the book, the significant role that nurses have in advocating for and implementing care coordination is highlighted. Care coordination is essential in the health system, and nurses are ethically obligated to ensure that delivery models, legislation, and care coordination regulations maintain a person-centered approach. By utilizing person-centered care coordination practices, nurses can support individualized and relevant care that manages costs and resources while supporting better outcomes and decreasing fragmentation of care. Care coordination is an interprofessional team product; with the patient at the center of the team and care, nurses are in a vital position to advance the integration of coordination of care through the health system for the betterment of all. This book aims to prepare nurses in foundational person-centered care coordination practice so that health outcomes can be improved across the continuum of care.

Features

This book contains several effective aids for learning, comprehension, critical synthesis, and practice application. These include discussion questions, activities, and a Glossary of Acronyms.

Discussion Questions

Each chapter ends with discussion questions. The questions are based on the clinical judgment process, focusing on analyses, outcomes, actions, and solutions. The discussion questions offer the ability to engage in self-reflection, and they support knowledge and meaning integration of the content presented. Concepts can be considered, issues concerning application to nursing practice can be identified and connection of the content presented to the health system, the *Quintuple Aim* and care coordination practice can be accomplished.

Activities

Also found at the end of each chapter are activities that support further knowledge, skill, and attitude development concerning the content presented. The activities are designed to offer active engagement with the content through observation, research, writing, and group activities, supporting the connection of the multidimensional aspects of health and shared knowledge creation. One activity at the end of each chapter is a case study introducing real-world examples of issues, barriers, and gaps in care coordination in the health system. Each case study is followed by various levels of questions that offer the ability to examine and prioritize aspects of the case study, build upon content and previous knowledge, and develop clinical judgment and care coordination practice competency.

Glossary of Acronyms

As the health system, legislation, and healthcare financing use many acronyms, a glossary is provided for reference. Each acronym used in the text is included in the glossary, allowing for ease in the ability to learn pertinent acronyms and connect the acronym to the content provided.

Parting Thoughts

Person-centered care coordination across the continuum of care is part of the code of nursing ethics and the nursing scope and standards of practice. It is a role that every nurse has, no matter the setting or their specialization. This book provides a high-level overview of the foundational aspects of care coordination, why it is critical in today's health system, what person-centered care coordination is, and how to implement care coordination in daily nursing practice. The term *patient* is used throughout the book. instead of terms such as client or consumer, for ease of use and familiarity. While in some settings, terms such as client, consumer, or person may be used by nurses, *patient* is a commonly used term in the health system and is appropriate for the purposes of this book. The following chapters provide the vital knowledge, skills, and attitudes needed for person-centered care coordination and bring attention to different trends and issues that should be considered to deliver person-centered, quality, safe, cost-effective, and coordinated care across the continuum.

REFERENCES

Arnetz, B. B., Goetz, C. M., Arnetz, J. E., Sudan, S., vanSchagen, J., Piersma, K., & Reyelts, F. (2020). Enhancing healthcare efficiency to achieve the Quadruple Aim: An exploratory study. *BMC research notes, 13*(1), 362. https://doi.org/10.1186/s13104-020-05199-8

Fawcett, J. (2005). *Contemporary nursing knowledge: Analysis and evaluation of nursing models and theories* (2nd ed.). F. A. Davis Company.

Institute of Medicine (IOM). (2001). *Crossing the quality chasm: A new health system for the 21st century*. National Academy Press.

Itchhaporia D. (2021). The evolution of the Quintuple Aim: Health equity, health outcomes, and the economy. *Journal of the American College of Cardiology, 78*(22), 2262 2264. https://doi.org/10.1016/j.jacc.2021.10.018

Matthews, J. H., Whitehead, P. B., Ward, C., Kyner, M., & Crowder, T. (2020). Florence Nightingale: Visionary for the role of clinical nurse specialist. *OJIN: The Online Journal of Issues in Nursing*, 25(2), Manuscript 1. https://doi.org/10.3912/OJIN.Vol25No02Man01

Pittman, P. (2019). *Activating nursing to address unmet needs in the 21st century*. Robert Wood Johnson Foundation. https://hsrc.himmelfarb.gwu.edu/sphhs_policy_facpubs/963/

Richmond C. (2005). Dame Cicely Saunders. *BMJ: British Medical Journal, 331*(7510), 238. https://www.ncbi.nlm.nih.gov/pmc/articles/PMC1179787/

CHAPTER 1

Care Coordination

An Overview

LEARNING OBJECTIVES

1. Understand nursing roles involved in delivering care coordination.
2. Define the differences and similarities between types of care coordination.
3. Recognize the need for care coordination in health care.
4. Identify standards for care coordination in nursing practice.

KEY TERMS

- care coordination
- community health worker
- continuity of care
- cultural mediator
- gaps in care
- integrated care coordination
- person-centered care
- population care coordination
- quintuple aim
- risk stratification
- transition management

Introduction

Coordinating patient care is an essential nursing function. No matter what setting, coordinated care is vital for positive patient and system outcomes. When care is coordinated, the patient and their families or support systems are empowered to be engaged and activated in their healthcare plan. Providing coordinated patient care contributes to decreased fragmentation of care, improved teamwork, and effective management of healthcare resources (Ofei & Paarima, 2021).

There are several potential adverse outcomes when there is a lack of coordination and **continuity of care**. Common poor outcomes related to uncoordinated care are medication errors, increased readmission rates, increased healthcare costs, and increased stress and dissatisfaction on the part of the patient and their families or support system. There are many examples of how lack of coordinated care contributes to higher costs, poor outcomes, and lack of patient satisfaction in our healthcare system today. Providing care continuity is associated with increased patient satisfaction, improved health outcomes, increased medication adherence, and decreased hospital use (Pereira Gray et al., 2018, p. 2).

Inadequate care coordination has been shown to account for "between $25 billion and $45 billion in wasteful spending in 2011" (Berwick & Hackwith, 2012, p. e2). Lack of coordinated care with patients for chronic health conditions has also been identified as leading to an increase of over $4,500 in healthcare spending over a 35-month period (Frandsen et al., 2015). A review of root cause analyses by the Veterans Health Administration National Center of Patient Safety found that many medical errors were caused by faulty care coordination, with 27% resulting in death (Aboumrad et al., 2018). Alternately, hospitals with integrated organizational care coordination strategies have been found to have increased overall patient satisfaction ratings and recommendation scores (Figueroa et al., 2018). Care coordination in the community healthcare setting has been associated with increased attainment of clinical quality measures such as cancer screenings, hemoglobin A1C levels, and osteoporosis management (Elliott et al., 2021).

As those experiencing illness, chronic disease, or other health conditions are often more vulnerable and may receive services from various providers and settings to address their healthcare issues, integrated care coordination practice is essential (IOM, 2001). Patients often rely on care coordination nursing activities to ensure that information is transferred to the appropriate providers and settings and that follow-up tests, labs, or appointments are set up or education is provided to the patient concerning these critical follow-up activities. **Integrated care coordination** strategies include transmission of information to and engagement of the interprofessional team across the healthcare system, the community and social services system, and the patient's informal support system (Davie & Rataj, 2018).

Ultimately, when care is not coordinated, the patient may have decreased quality of life or functional ability related to preventable acute care readmissions, long-term care or rehabilitation stays, and the potential inability to remain independent in their own home as they age. Furthermore, the patient may experience increased healthcare costs, potentially leading to the inability to seek healthcare, pay for medications, or cover their living expenses. The nurse may also experience provider fatigue due to what they perceive as a "revolving" door of patients returning to their setting, not following their care plans, or not improving or deteriorating significantly. Care coordination is necessary for all nursing practices to proactively address potential barriers and gaps to patient health and effectively manage healthcare resources.

Care Coordination Overview

Care coordination is a concept often used in healthcare today. It is applied to various settings and situations and may be represented in various titles or job functions. Care coordination may be referred to as care management, case management, clinical resource management, patient navigation, etc. With this variety of terms used, it is critical to understand precisely what care coordination is and why it is so important in healthcare today. Whether you are a case manager, patient navigator, or bedside nurse, care coordination is at the root of your nursing role.

Person-Centered Care

"**Person-centered care** means defining success not just by the resolution of clinical symptoms but also by whether patients achieve their desired outcomes. Some examples of person-centered care include ensuring that patients' preferences, desired outcomes, and experiences of care are integrated into care delivery, integrating patient-generated data in electronic health records, and finding additional ways to involve patients and families in managing their care effectively." (AHRQ, 2016, p. 2)

Care coordination is the primary but critical function of organizing and managing patient care across the continuum of care through information sharing and person-centered care practices. The care coordination process may begin by focusing on preventative and primary care and following the patient through acute care visits, rehabilitation, and back to primary care. The National Quality Forum (NQF) defines care coordination as a "function that helps ensure that the patient's needs and preferences for health services and information sharing across people, functions, and sites are met over time ..." (NQF, 2010, p. 1). The Agency for Healthcare Research and Quality (AHRQ) defines care coordination as "deliberately organizing patient care activities and sharing information among all of the participants concerned with a patient's care to achieve safer and more effective care" (AHRQ, 2018, para. 1). The World Health Organization (WHO) defines care coordination as "a proactive approach to bringing together care professionals and providers to meet the needs of service users, to ensure that they receive integrated, person-focused care across various settings" (WHO, 2018, p. 8). These definitions have common elements of proactive person-centered care and information sharing, leading to integrated, safe, and effective care across settings and providers. This is the foundational goal of care coordination practice.

As patients traverse the continuum of care, from primary care to acute care and back to the community, essential information must be conveyed concerning their medical history, medications prescribed, needs, and care preferences. We can think of care coordination as a compass with the patient at the center and all their healthcare and community providers being drawn to the patient and each other to encompass the patient in person-centered care. See Figure 1.1—Care

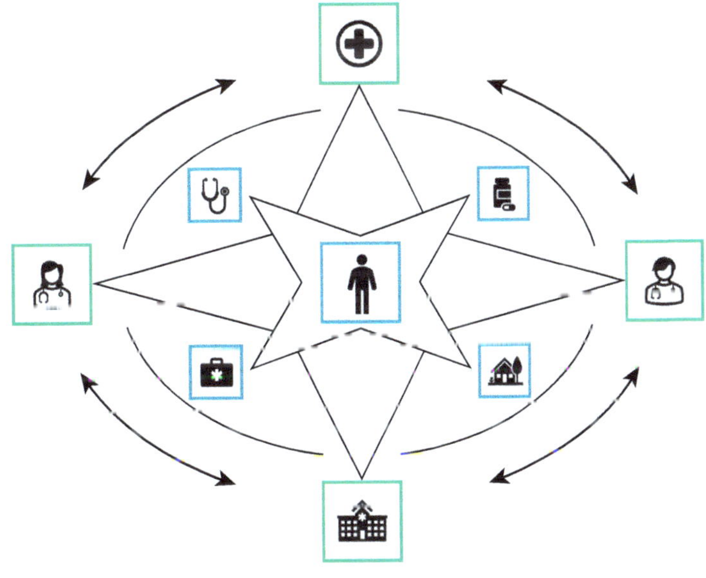

FIGURE 1.1 Care Coordination Compass

Coordination Compass. For the patients' providers to effectively respond to and comprehensively detect patient needs, they must connect and communicate with each other and the patient. Suppose a provider leaves the compass field or remains in the periphery without active collaboration and coordination of care with other providers involved in the patient's care. In that case, there is a high probability that suboptimal and non-person-centered care will be delivered, resulting in poor health outcomes.

Care Coordination Across Settings

Care coordination focusing on continuity of care across settings is needed for good health outcomes, avoiding preventable poor outcomes, and thoughtfully utilizing healthcare resources. Each healthcare provider and service in the care continuum—from preventative care, acute care, rehabilitation, health maintenance, and end-of-life care—may address this goal differently. Nevertheless, the focus is the same: identifying those at risk for poor outcomes or higher healthcare costs, providing patient education, and coordinating and facilitating communication across settings and providers to promote good outcomes.

In the primary care setting, care coordination may focus on identifying those patients at the highest risk for health issues, such as those who smoke or with chronic illnesses. The primary care clinic may offer preventative services, such as smoking cessation classes, to minimize health issues before they arise, preventing poor outcomes and decreasing the use of healthcare resources related to smoking-associated diseases. In a community-based healthcare delivery such as hospice, the care may be coordinated through information sharing and communication with the interprofessional team, the patient, and their family or support system. Collaborative communication and care planning may focus on preventing poor outcomes, such as unmanaged symptoms, and promoting good outcomes, like patient quality of life and decreasing acute care resource use. Care coordination in the acute care setting may target managing healthcare resources through effective discharge planning or preventing readmissions or return emergency room visits. When discharge planning is person-centered and based on a comprehensive assessment of patient needs once they leave the acute care setting, positive outcomes can be achieved, such as increased functional abilities and decreased costs and resource use related to decreased medical incidents. Wherever care coordination is offered, the goal is to promote positive outcomes, provide person-centered care, and appropriately use healthcare services and resources (Sailsman et al., 2018).

A more expansive view of care coordination includes assisting patients and their families/support systems in self-managing their health and health conditions, addressing social determinants of health (SDOH) or psychosocial barriers to self-management of health, coordinating care among multiple providers and settings, bridging gaps in care, and ensuring the patient is receiving the most appropriate level of care (Schraeder & Shelton, 2011, p. 145). SDOH can include economic, educational, environmental, community, and healthcare access and quality factors (Healthy People 2030, n.d.). Psychosocial barriers to health may include depression, distress related to illness, or decreased quality of life (Amankwah-Poku et al., 2021).

For example, a person may have depression for many reasons, such as experiencing an imbalance of neurotransmitters, enduring stressful life events, or carrying a genetic vulnerability

Gaps in Care

"**Gaps in care** are the gulf between the recommended treatment trajectory for a certain patient and the treatment the patient realistically receives. A care gap might refer to a patient who misses her breast cancer screening or a teenager who has not gotten the HPV shot. Care gaps can result in missed or delayed diagnosis and, subsequently, more costly and potentially more invasive treatment down the line" (Heath, 2021, para. 2–3).

to the condition (Harvard Medical School, 2022). Whatever reason depression is present, it is an important factor in health, as those living with depression often develop feelings of fatigue and despair or feel drained. This can interfere with their daily life and their ability to engage in self-care or caring for their health. It can also interfere with basic activities of daily living, such as hygiene, food preparation, and sleeping habits. Symptoms of depression, such as the inability to engage effectively in decision-making or self-care, can be a psychosocial barrier to health.

Including psychosocial aspects of care, SDOH, and addressing gaps in care leads to a more comprehensive view of the patient's life and health experience and the multiple roles involved in coordinating care. Anyone who interacts with a patient can contribute to good care coordination by effectively assessing and communicating patient needs and resources, identifying potential barriers or gaps in care, and offering person-centered care. Coordinating care is not only for nurses, physicians, social workers, or discharge planners; it is a role for everyone who contributes to patient care.

Types of Care Coordination

Several forms of care coordination are offered in the healthcare system today. Some types of care coordination focus on specific patients or where the patient is receiving care. Other varieties of care coordination may focus on short-term care coordination, and others may offer care coordination over the longer term. Care coordination may occur in primary care, inpatient care, or across settings. Widespread types of care coordination in our healthcare system include population-focused care coordination, transition management, care/case management, and resource and utilization management. While this is not an inclusive list of how care coordination may be offered, these care coordination roles are commonly seen in the health system.

Population Care Coordination

Population health focuses on the health outcomes of specific groups or populations and the individual members of that population. These populations can be defined in a variety of ways, such as geographic (e.g., rural), health conditions (e.g., diabetes), or health behaviors (e.g., substance use). However the population is defined, population health examines the link between healthcare interventions, policies, SDOH, and health outcomes (Kindig & Stoddart, 2003). Population health data can be aggregated to inform policy development or healthcare delivery methods. Through assessing the patient in the larger context of SDOH and examining the impacts of national, state, and local policy on the design, delivery, and coordination of healthcare, a connection can be made between the identified population and health trends. Population health and care coordination are intricately connected as they both seek to identify individuals or populations needing support in attaining good health outcomes. Population health and care coordination also focuses on sharing data and information to meet health outcomes and manage unnecessary costs or healthcare services (NACHC, 2016).

Population care coordination includes health promotion as well as disease prevention activities. The population care coordinator may work with the patient and other providers to educate them on their care, conditions, and preventative health options, provide follow-up, and assist with care transitions. When coordinating care with a population focus, the nurse may use data to identify patients at risk for high-cost services or poor outcomes, such as those with chronic illness. In this way, the population care coordinator can prioritize or stratify patients and their health risks to track and provide measures of success, such as improved outcomes, care plan adherence, or specific measures, such as immunization rates (NACHC, 2016).

Population care coordination often begins with the process of **risk stratification**, which categorizes populations of patients based on their health status, other factors, or those with a specific vulnerability (Dom Dera, 2019). By identifying the target population and analyzing the available data, the population care coordinator can predict or stratify which patients are at risk for poor health outcomes. The data utilized in the risk stratification process could be extensive aggregate data from a patient registry, hospital quality measure dataset such as repeat emergency room visits, or specific patient data available in the electronic health record (EHR), such as the number of depression screenings administered (Rushton, 2015). Next, the individuals in the identified population are assessed for health status, potential needs, and gaps in care. This assists with care coordination as resources can be provided to those with the most need, decreasing costs and poor outcomes.

The patient population is often put into high, medium, and low-risk categories, which in turn directs what care coordination interventions may be needed (Dom Dera, 2019). A patient in a high-risk category may need comprehensive chronic disease case management offered. In contrast, someone in the low-risk category may only require reminders sent to ensure that they receive recommended preventative care. Once the risk category information is gathered and assessed, a target intervention is selected for the population. For example, a primary care clinic may identify all patients who have had an emergency room visit in the last 30 days as medium risk and offer follow-up calls or messages in a secure patient portal to ensure timely follow-up care. Then, the planning, implementation, and evaluation stages occur, where the intervention is planned utilizing input from stakeholders and interprofessional team members, delivered to the target population, and evaluated for outcomes (Rushton, 2015).

Throughout population care coordination, there is a system of accountability and tracking patients at risk, monitoring outcomes, and identifying whether health goals are achieved. Population care coordination responds to patients' healthcare needs proactively and relevantly across the continuum of care, from low-risk and healthy people to high-risk or those with chronic conditions (Felt-Lisk & Higgins, 2011). See Figure 1.2—Population Care Coordination Process.

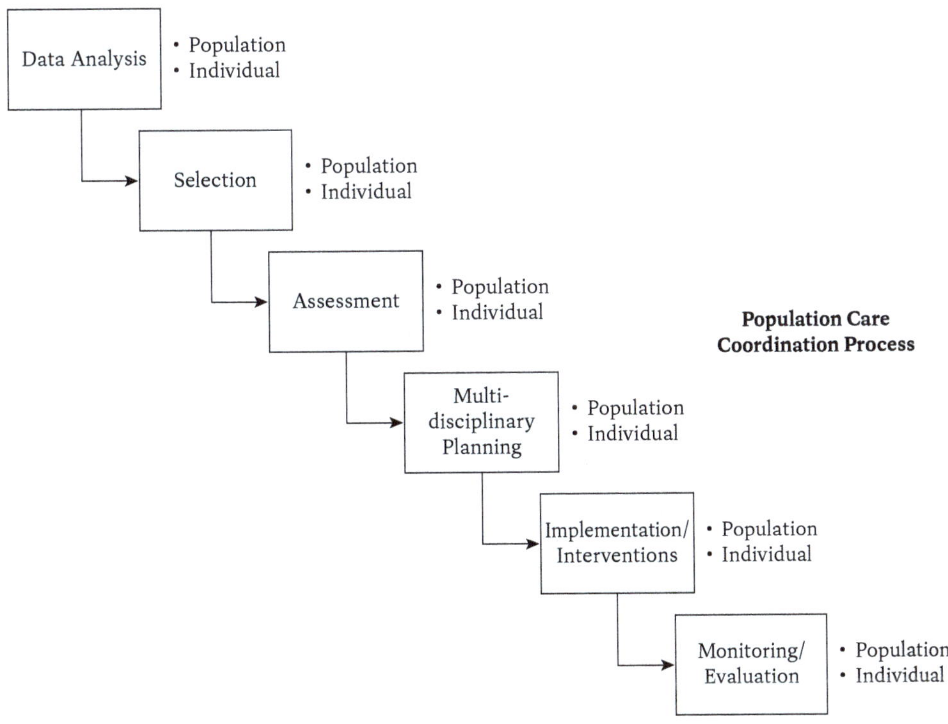

FIGURE 1.2 Population Care Coordination Process

Learn More About Risk Stratification

Explore these websites to learn more about the process of patient risk stratification and the connection with population care coordination.

- https://www.nachc.org/wp-content/uploads/2019/03/Risk-Stratification-Action-Guide-Mar-2019.pdf
- https://healthitanalytics.com/features/howpopulation-health-risk-stratificationsupportvalue-based-care
- https://www.aafp.org/pubs/fpm/issues/2019/0500/p21.html
- https://pubmed.ncbi.nlm.nih.gov/34374573/

Transition Management

Transitions in care usually last a short period and occur at every level and setting where healthcare is delivered. At its most basic function, **transition management** is the patient's movement between healthcare providers and settings. A transition in care may have poor outcomes for a variety of reasons. There may be issues with communication between settings and providers related to differences in EHR systems, or the multiple layers of a transition in care (e.g., medication education, follow-up care, etc.) may need to be completed or need clarification (Sailsman et al., 2018). For example, one study found that 40% of patients had a medication discrepancy at hospital admission or discharge. In another study, out of a total of 1,389 medication discrepancies found, 40.7 % of them potentially contributed to an adverse drug event (Neumiller et al., 2017).

It has also been estimated that patients with five or more chronic conditions may see up to 14 different providers and have up to 50 prescriptions (Warshaw, 2006). In the United States, patients see an average of 18.7 different providers during their lifetime, and for those over 65 years of age, the average increases to 28.4 providers (Practice Fusion, 2010, para. 1). When considering the number of providers, nurses, pharmacists, and other healthcare team members that "touch" a patient, it is evident that care transitions occur almost continuously and could be problematic if excellent communication and care coordination are not provided.

Transition management is not limited to one level of care, setting, or those with chronic conditions. As nurses interact with a patient and their family or support systems, they must consider where the patient will be transitioning to and what will be required to promote a good transition of care. This is not a role only for a nurse titled "transition manager," but for all nurses interacting with a patient in any healthcare setting. Transition management principles serve all patient populations, whether in the acute care setting and transitioning to hospice services, transitioning from a rehabilitation facility to their home with home health services, or transitioning from primary care services to specialist care. As transitions of care occur frequently, their success depends on the integration of a person-centered approach. The patient and their family or support system are the constants in any transition of care. Communication with patients, families or support systems, providers, and organizations is essential. Through person-centered care approaches and effective communication and collaboration, the center of the transition plan is the patient's needs and care priorities.

Transition management is part of any coordination of care, as the patient is being "handed off" to another provider, nurse, or setting. Nurses must proactively address potential communication breakdowns during the care transition. If two different levels of care have alternate views of how the transition will happen or if the patient has a different

Transition Management Standards

- Identify patients at risk for poor transitions.
- Complete a comprehensive transition assessment.
- Perform and communicate a medication reconciliation.
- Establish a care plan that addresses all settings throughout the continuum of care.
- Communicate essential care transition information to key stakeholders across the continuum of care (Transitions of Care, 2019).

expectation, this can lead to an ineffective transition of care. Nurses often rely on verbal handoff processes when transitioning patients between themselves. However, heavy reliance on the verbal transfer of information in a transition of care can lead to communication failures (Ofei & Paarima, 2021). By keeping the person-centered philosophy at the forefront, utilizing standardized procedures and communication tools for "hand-off," such as IPASS-THEBATON, and documenting communication, potential communication breakdowns can be addressed effectively.

IPASSTHEBATON Handoff

This handoff strategy is designed to enhance information exchange during transitions in care.

"I PASS THE BATON"		
I	Introduction	Introduce yourself and your role/job (include patient).
P	Patient	Name, identifiers, age, sex, location.
A	Assessment	Present chief complaint, vital signs, symptoms, and diagnosis.
S	Situation	Current status/circumstances, including code status, level of (un) certainty, recent changes, and response to treatment.
S	Safety	Critical lab values/reports, socioeconomic factors, allergies, and alerts (falls, isolation, etc.).
THE		
B	Background	Comorbidities, previous episodes, current medications, and family history.
A	Actions	Explain what actions were taken or are required. Provide rationale.
T	Timing	Level of urgency and explicit timing and prioritization of actions.
O	Ownership	Identify who is responsible (person/team), including patient/family members.
N	Next	What will happen next? Anticipated changes? What is the plan? Are there contingency plans?

Source. (Pocket Guide: TeamSTEPPS, 2020)

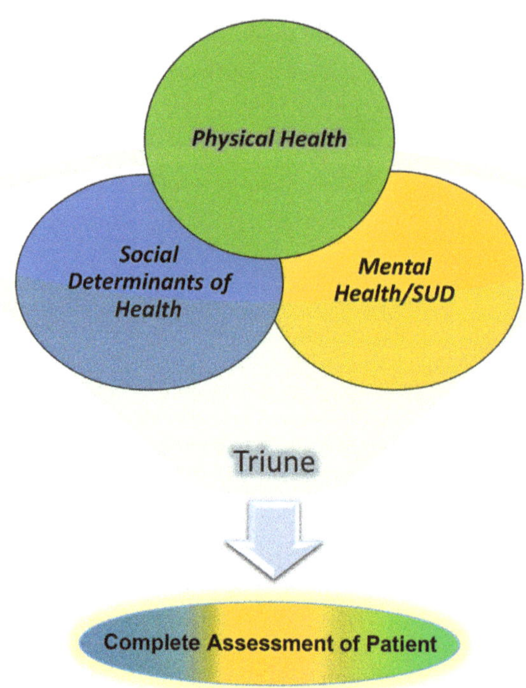

FIGURE 1.3 The Health Triune

Patients and their families/support systems have identified that during transitions of care, they want to feel cared for and cared about by providers involved in their care. They want the providers and systems involved in the transition of care to be accountable for the transition and for themselves to possess the education and tools needed to engage in their care plan (Mitchell et al., 2018). To meet these identified needs, the National Transitions of Care Coalition (NTOCC) developed a *Care Transition Bundle*, which includes medication coordination, transition planning, patient and family/caregiver engagement and education, information transfer, follow-up care, provider engagement and shared accountability, and assessment of the physical health, mental health, and social determinates of health triune (NTOCC, 2022). See Figure 1.3—The Health Triune.

Person-centered care, effective communication, and comprehensive assessment are crucial to any transition management role. Patient navigators, transition managers or coordinators, and patient advocates are roles that may provide transition management as a central duty. Nurses are in a vital position to either fill these roles or assist in successful transition management in the role they hold. Nurses frequently interact with patients and their families or support systems and observe or learn essential information needed for an effective transition. Additionally, nurses can assess for any barriers to the transition plan, such as those that fall in the health triune, and communicate this with the interprofessional team, coordinating the needs and priorities of the patient and family or support system and promoting an effective and efficient transition of care (Camicia & Lutz, 2016).

Care/Case Management

The care/case manager collaboratively coordinates patient care and assists the patient and their family or support system in self-management of health conditions by addressing barriers to health (e.g., SDOH), providing education, and acting as a patient advocate. Care/case management is proactive and comprehensive and focuses on coordinating and integrating the care provided. This is often offered to patients at risk of increased healthcare costs or poor outcomes, such as those with chronic health conditions or requiring ongoing medical interventions. Care/case management aims to assist the patient in obtaining or maintaining optimal functioning through assessment, planning, implementing, coordinating, monitoring, and evaluating care required to meet patient needs (Lyons, 2013). This is beneficial for overall patient health and the healthcare system, while decreasing healthcare costs (Fraser et al., 2018).

Care/case management is offered across various settings. It aims to ensure that care is efficiently and effectively provided through a comprehensive assessment of patient needs and resources and person-centered care planning. The goal is to optimize health outcomes and keep healthcare costs down as much as possible. In acute care settings, the care/case manager may focus on discharge planning and effective transitions out of acute care to the next level of care or the patient's home, ensuring that the acute care setting is appropriately reimbursed for the patient's care and clinical quality measures are met, such as readmission rates.

Health systems and insurance providers may also offer care/case management to those with chronic health conditions such as congestive heart failure or diabetes, or multiple chronic conditions. In this role, the chronic care/case manager focuses on continuity of care through comprehensive assessment and care planning. The chronic care/case manager works with the patient throughout the care continuum by developing a person-centered comprehensive care plan that addresses preventive services, medical care, and functional or psychosocial needs and resources (CMS, 2022). Insurance and chronic care/case management aim to provide the tools and education the patient needs to self-manage their chronic condition and ensure that the patient receives necessary and appropriate care, therefore managing costs and promoting proper outcomes.

Key elements in all types of care/case management are incorporating evidence-based patient education on self-management of health or the disease process, interprofessional team communication and collaboration, person-centered care plan development, while addressing gaps in care to improve patient outcomes and decrease healthcare costs. Central to care/case management is the patient and their families or support systems. The person-centered care plan is collaboratively created through the facilitation of goal setting and prioritization of needs and care with the patient, their families or support systems, and other interprofessional team members as needed. The care/case manager coordinates and evaluates the care provided, communicates with providers and interprofessional team members, and facilitates care transitions. Care/case management works to ensure that all aspects of the seven rights of care coordination are met: (a) the care plan is right for the patient, (b) the right care is received, (c) in the right setting, (d) at the right time, (e) with the right resources, (f) the right transition occurs, and (g) the right education is provided. See Figure 1.4—The Seven Rights of Care Coordination.

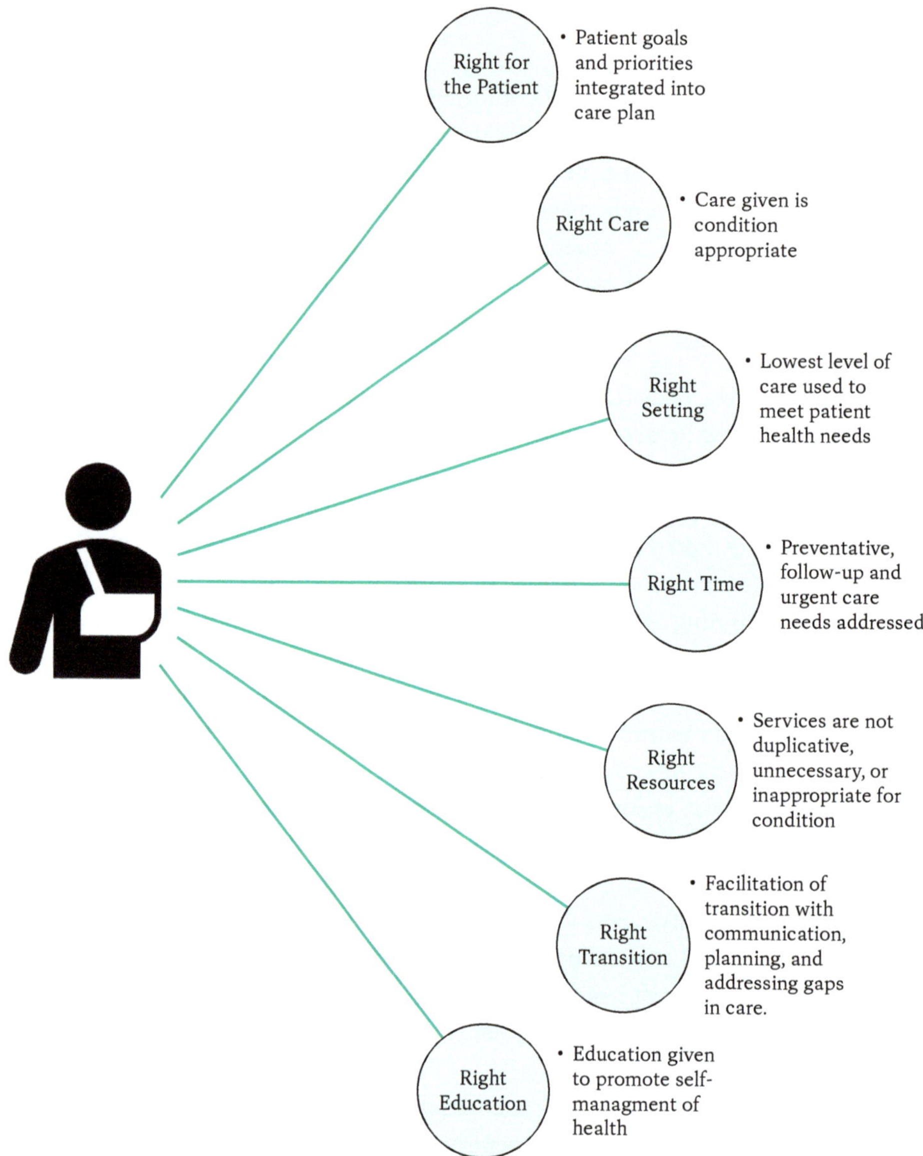

FIGURE 1.4 The Seven Rights of Care Coordination

Resource and Utilization Management

Another aspect of care coordination in practice is resource and utilization management. This area of care coordination focuses on the right care, place, and resources. When engaging in resource management, the goal is to use resources appropriately—in this case, the care a patient receives. Numerous human and nonhuman resources are used to deliver healthcare. Human resources include physicians, nurses, pharmacists, medical technicians, other professionals who have direct contact with the patient, or personnel with an ancillary role in patient care, such as unlicensed roles that can be delegated tasks, housekeeping, maintenance, or billing.

Comparative Effectiveness Research

Comparative effectiveness research (CER) examines which medical intervention will most likely produce desired health outcomes. Patients, providers, policymakers, and healthcare systems can use CER to inform healthcare decisions or policy development. CER includes the following six characteristics:

1. CER aims to inform a specific clinical decision from the patient, health policy, or population perspective.
2. CER compares two or more alternate interventions to determine best practices.
3. CER results are described at the population and subgroup levels.
4. CER measures outcomes, including benefits and harms.
5. CER utilizes appropriate methods and data sources for the decision of interest.
6. CER is conducted in settings similar to where the intervention will be used in practice. (National Academies Press, 2009, pp. 38–39)

Nonhuman resources include physical resources, such as facilities, EHR systems, remote patient monitoring units, hospital beds/rooms, supplies, diagnostic equipment, and utilities needed to provide patient care (Shi & Singh, 2019).

Resource and utilization management focuses on ensuring that health system resources are used judiciously and prudently, as mismanagement of resources can lead to poor patient outcomes, overuse of inappropriate or unnecessary care, duplication of services, and organizational budget shortfalls. The continued use of medical interventions with little benefit to health outcomes can contribute to increased healthcare costs. All nurses have a role in resource and utilization management through planning and delivering nursing care so that it is effective and efficient. Nurses can also manage resources and utilization of those resources through patient education and advocacy. By ensuring patients understand the risks, benefits, and costs of care and supporting patients in obtaining appropriate services, nurses can assist in managing healthcare resources and promoting positive patient outcomes (Haas et al., 2014).

Utilization Management (UM) Role

A nurse may specifically fill the role of utilization manager (UM). In this role, the nurse will work closely with insurance providers, patients, and healthcare providers to ensure the appropriate use and medical necessity of resources. Duties, including utilization review, denial management, and review of quality measures such as readmissions or emergency room use, are key aspects of this role. The UM nurse identifies whether resources are mismanaged by evaluating if the patient's care is in the most appropriate level of care and setting (Shi & Singh, 2019). This can occur at any time or several times throughout the healthcare delivery process, during preadmission screenings/authorizations (prospective review), inpatient stay (concurrent review), or post-discharge review (retrospective review).

Inpatient Versus Outpatient/Observation Status

Inpatient Status: A patient admitted to a hospital for inpatient-identified services usually requiring the patient to stay at least two midnights.

Outpatient/Observation Status: A patient admitted for short-term treatment, assessment, or reassessment. Observation status can be in the emergency room or another hospital area.

Different costs and deductibles apply for inpatient versus outpatient or observation status. Generally, inpatient care falls under Medicare Part A, and outpatient/observation care falls under Medicare Part B for Medicare beneficiaries. Medicare has guidelines on copayments, and although a single outpatient hospital service can't charge more than the inpatient deductible, the total outpatient services copayment could be more, which can be concerning for patients (Medicare.gov, n.d.).

In the prospective review process, the medical necessity of the proposed care is determined before the delivery of the care. This could be a preauthorization process for a specific intervention or the primary care provider determining whether a referral to a specialist is appropriate. The prospective review aims to prevent unnecessary or inappropriate care, such as unnecessary surgeries or inappropriate admissions to inpatient care. Once a patient is admitted to an inpatient setting, a concurrent review occurs, monitoring the length of patient stay, if that stay follows clinical guidelines and patient-specific conditions, and if the patient is appropriately placed in an inpatient or outpatient/observation status, preventing inappropriate use of healthcare services. A retrospective review is based on a review of medical records after a service has been delivered, assessing the appropriateness of the care received (Shi & Singh, 2019). There are processes for a provider-to-provider consultation on cases with questions about necessity or setting and for appealing denials of care coverage.

Interdisciplinary communication, collaborative practice, and clinical knowledge are crucial to successful resource and utilization management (Finkelman, 2016). There are several important outcomes of effective resource and utilization management. The limited resources in the healthcare system are utilized most effectively by managing resources and decreasing waste and duplication of services. Ensuring medical necessity and appropriateness of care promotes optimal patient outcomes. Data indicating a case management or medical social worker referral is often gathered during the utilization review process, proactively addressing gaps and barriers to care. Ultimately, resource and utilization management assist in managing healthcare costs by aiding cost-effective care delivery that is evidence-based, beneficial, and efficient (Giardino & Wadhwa, 2022).

Other Roles that Provide Care Coordination

Those in numerous roles provide coordination and continuity of care. Nurses or the nurse care coordinator may perform care coordination services or work with other interprofessional team members who also provide care coordination functions. Some roles may provide outreach functions, focusing on specific populations or vulnerable groups. Other roles may focus on specific disease processes or health system navigation needs. Each of these roles will have differing educational and training requirements and duties, which is essential for the nurse care coordinator to understand as this may direct what types of tasks the role can provide and the knowledge and skills the worker brings to care coordination efforts. Community health workers, health advisors, and patient navigators are all professions that may offer care coordination or aspects of care coordination. These professions are not all-inclusive of healthcare personnel offering care coordination services but are frequently seen and utilized in today's health system.

Community Health Worker (CHW)

When considering SDOH and health influencers, the **community health worker's** (CHW) role may be integral to a person-centered care coordination care plan. Financial and housing instability, food scarcity, legal status, health insurance, literacy, and the inability to effectively participate in disease self-management can harm health outcomes and increase healthcare resource use. CHWs are community members who partner with a healthcare system or provider. It is a relationship-based model of care where the CHW often shares the same language, ethnicity, and lived experiences as the people they work with. You may see the CHW referred to as a peer advisor, outreach educator, or a *promotora* (National Heart, Lung, and Blood Institute, 2014). Whatever title is used, the CHW offers a link from the healthcare system to patients, assisting them in navigating the healthcare system and educating them on how to access the resources needed (Straughen et al., 2023).

Promotoras in Action

Amigas

Promotoras use CDC training materials to improve cervical cancer screening rates in the Hispanic community. Specifically, the program AMIGAS is used. The acronym stands for "*Ayudando a las Mujeres con Información, Guía y Amor para su Salud,*" which means "Helping Women with Information, Guidance, and Love for Their Health." AMIGAS is a bilingual educational outreach intervention designed to help *promotoras* and other lay health educators increase the following:

- Cervical cancer screening among Hispanic women. The AMIGAS program engaged community health workers, or promotoras, to deliver a multicomponent intervention that doubled the rate of cervical cancer screening among Mexican-American women in Texas and Washington. Community Preventive Services Task Force recommendations were used to inform the selection of program components, which included one-on-one education and small media.
- Cervical cancer screening among Hispanics who have rarely or never had a pap test. A randomized controlled trial recently funded by CDC showed AMIGAS is effective in promoting cervical cancer screening (pap tests) among Hispanics aged 21 to 65 years.

Source: (CDC, 2019)

Most importantly, the CHW is a trusted community member who provides personalized services and allows patients to express their concerns and needs when they feel uncomfortable doing this with a healthcare provider. The CHW can then act as a liaison between the patient and the healthcare provider or assist the patient in directly discussing concerns and needs with the healthcare provider. This type of relationship-based care coordination advocates for populations experiencing a lack of health equity or a history of being underrepresented and supports patient engagement through education, collaboration, and person-centered care.

Patient Navigator or Nurse Navigator

Patient navigators or nurse navigators often specialize in diseases such as cancer or diabetes. They may work in any setting but are most often in hospitals or cancer care centers. As the diagnosis of a serious or chronic illness can be overwhelming, a patient or nurse navigator can provide a central person who offers personalized, person-centered care and guides the patient through the complexities of the healthcare system (National Cancer Institute, n.d.). The navigator focuses on the needs of the patient and their family or support systems and addresses any barriers to care. The patient navigator or nurse navigator is a facilitator and ensures communication between all involved in the patient's care, effectively ensuring the quality of care and patient satisfaction (Perrin, 2017).

Assisting the patient in navigating the healthcare system includes coordinating care, providing education on the disease process and self-management, acting as a liaison with healthcare providers, and being a patient advocate (Nourse & Paauwe-Weust, 2021). By providing person-centered care planning, the navigator may assist the patient with insurance companies or employers, access resources, organize follow-up appointments, or arrange transportation if needed. The patient navigator or nurse navigator is ultimately responsible for providing care coordination, communication, and follow-up to ensure good patient outcomes and decrease healthcare costs.

Origins of Patient Navigation

"The original concept of patient navigation was pioneered in 1990 by Dr. Harold P. Freeman, a surgical oncologist at Harlem Hospital, to eliminate barriers to timely cancer screening, diagnosis, treatment, and supportive care. Many individuals in medically under-served or minority communities were at risk because of financial, communication, healthcare system, and cultural barriers to care ... Over the years, data from Dr. Freeman's programs and others began to prove how valuable navigation could be in improving cancer diagnosis and treatment outcomes. For example, studies found that patient five-year survival rates went from 39% (before the development of the patient navigator program) to 70% for breast cancer patients at Harlem Hospital." (Schuler, 2020)

Health/Care Advisor

The health/care advisor may have a variety of duties, depending on the organization they work for. A key duty of the health/care advisor is to plan person-centered care based on patient needs and mutual goals of care created with the patient, healthcare provider, and interprofessional team. The health/care advisor may also provide initial and ongoing education concerning the patient's disease process or health management, treatment plans, medications, and needed follow-up. The health/care advisor serves as the patient's primary point of contact, providing support for needed resources and referrals, and also acts as a patient advocate when issues arise.

Depending on the setting and organization, the health/care advisor may work to identify patients needing follow-up or those at risk of acute care admission, addressing quality measures such as readmissions or immunization status. They may also be multicultural or multilingual to meet the needs of specific populations (such as those resettling to the United States) and act as a cultural mediator between the healthcare system and a specified population. Ultimately, the goal of the health/care advisor is to act as a patient advocate and educator, addressing barriers to care, assisting with follow-up needs, coordinating care among multiple providers and settings, and helping patients to access and understand resources and services needed to promote good health outcomes.

What Is a Cultural Mediator?

A **cultural mediator** moves beyond language translation to meet the needs of migrants, refugees, survivors of torture or human trafficking, and asylum seekers. Although translation and interpreting services are vital to the cultural mediator, they also assist these populations in navigating the healthcare system, providing health promotion education or other services. Cultural mediators offer more than direct medical translation and also work to help the patient and provider understand the words and concepts being presented, ensuring understanding between the patient and the provider. They are part of the healthcare team, working with the interprofessional team to meet patient needs (Venables et al., 2021).

Care Coordination and the Quintuple Aim

When examining the core components of care coordination practices, it is apparent that care coordination is critical for better health outcomes, improving our healthcare system and addressing the **Quintuple Aim**. Implementing coordinated care across the continuum enhances the patient experience, produces better health outcomes, improves provider well-being, and reduces costs. It also addresses SDOH and, therefore, can enhance health equity (Itchhaporia, 2021). See Figure 1.5—The Evolution of the Quintuple Aim.

Through patient-centered care planning, interdisciplinary communication and collaboration, health education and promotion, and coordination of care, the patient can receive integrated care that is connected and inclusive. By addressing patient needs in a dynamic, strength-based, and advocacy approach, diversity in care coordination practices and more cost-effective care

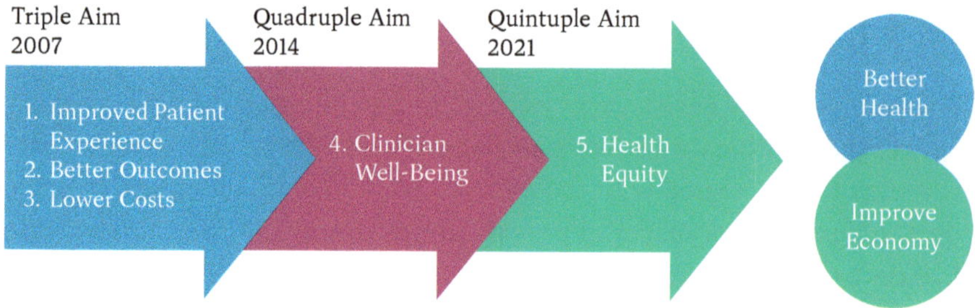

FIGURE 1.5 The Evolution of the Quintuple Aim

with better outcomes will be fostered (National Academies of Practice, 2022). A comparison of various types of care coordination offered across the continuum draws attention to how each contributes to enhancing healthcare delivery and meeting the objectives of the Quintuple Aim. See Table 1.1—Care Coordination Comparison.

TABLE 1.1 Care Coordination Comparison

	Population Care Coordination	Transition Management	Care/Case Management	Resource and Utilization Management
Client	1. Patient populations 2. Individual patients and their family or support systems	1. Individual patients and their family or support systems 2. Healthcare system	1. Individual patients and their family or support systems 2. Healthcare system	1. Healthcare system
Example Services Provided	1. Health promotion 2. Disease prevention 3. Health education 4. Follow-up 5. Linking patient care across providers or settings 6. Targeted interventions 7. Tracking quality measures	1. Linking patient care across providers or settings 2. Communication of essential information for a successful transition 3. Follow-up services	1. Comprehensive Assessment of needs (physical, mental, social determinants of health) 2. Care plan development 3. Coordinating care amongst multiple providers/settings 4. Evidence-Based patient education	1. Appropriate care determination 2. Preauthorization, concurrent and retrospective review 3. Inpatient or outpatient status determination

(Continued)

		4. Compre-hensive Assessment of needs (physical, mental, social determinants of health) 5. Education	5. Patient self-management of health support 6. Managing patient care 7. Patient advocacy 8. Follow-up services	
Time Offered	**Short term to long term**	**Short term**	**Short term to long term**	**Short term**
Care Coordina-tion Focus	1. Population-centered care 2. Any health condition determined a focus (smok-ing, obesity, chronic condition) 3. Prevention of poor health outcomes 4. Continuity of care 5. Appropriate use of health-care resources	1. Person-cen-tered care 2. Transitioning patient care across provid-ers or settings 3. Prevention of poor health outcomes 4. Communi-cation and collaboration 5. Medication coordination 6. Follow-up	1. Person-centered care 2. Chronic and complex health conditions 3. Reducing the need for medical services 4. Promoting cost effective and appropriate care 5. Continuity of care 6. Addressing gaps in care 7. Prevention of poor health outcomes 8. Meeting quality measures	1. Managing healthcare costs 2. Decreasing waste and duplication of services 3. Ensuring med-ical necessity 4. Appropriate use of health-care resources

Coordination of care is a crucial and overarching need in healthcare today. As patients move across settings, systems, and providers and their health needs change, key activities such as person-centered care planning, sending and receiving essential information, and scheduling follow-up services are required. Care coordination supports the Quintuple Aim by providing continuity of care across settings, promoting better health outcomes, providing person-centered care planning, enhancing accessible and quality care, increasing patient satisfaction, and decreasing or managing healthcare costs through the appropriate use of medically necessary and appropriate services. See Figure 1.6—The Coordination of Care Continuum.

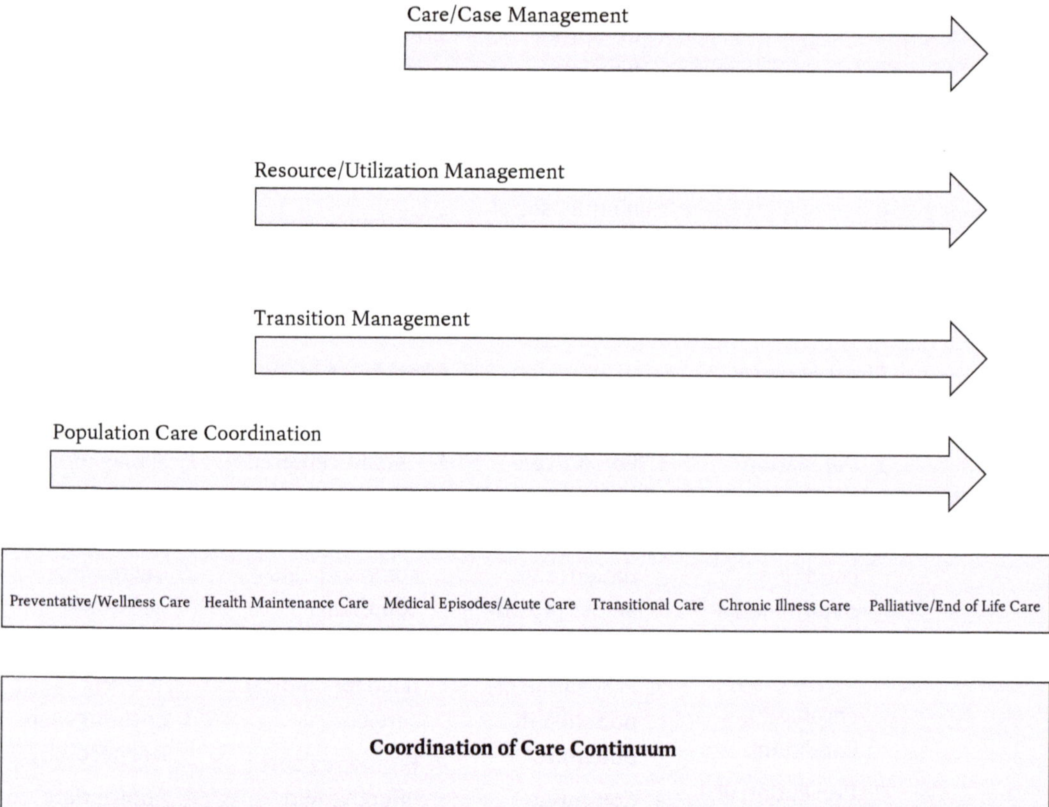

FIGURE 1.6 The Coordination of Care Continuum

Care Coordination Standards

Professional standards are essential to healthcare delivery and define expectations of the role and desired outcomes (Institute of Medicine, 2000). As care coordination becomes more complex across multiple settings, providers, and differing EHR systems, professional standards are essential to direct how nurses can best support the coordinated care of their patients (Yoder, 2017). Several organizations provide professional standards related to care coordination in healthcare, including professional organizations providing certifications that hold care coordination skills as a critical element of their standards. Some nursing organizations also define standards related to foundational skills that all nurses should possess concerning the delivery of care coordination in their nursing practice.

The American Case Management Association

The American Case Management Association (ACMA) provides certification in case management. The ACMA manages the Accredited Case Manager (ACM) certification and is governed by the National Board for Case Management (NBCM). The ACMA focuses on providing mentoring, resources, and education for those providing case management services. The ACMA also works to affect policy and laws that may impact the delivery of case management. The

ACMA provides practice standards, the scope of services for case management, standards of practice, and an implementation guide for care transitions, focusing on healthcare delivery system case managers (ACMA, 2020). The standards of practice endorsed by the ACMA include accountability, professionalism, collaboration, advocacy, resource management, technology use, and certification. The ACM scope of services consists of the following: education, care coordination across settings and time, screening, assessment, plan of care, addressing barriers to the progression of care, transition management, identifying those at risk of adverse health outcomes, implementing the transition plan, building community partnerships, supporting follow-up, ensuring regulation compliance, utilization management, medical necessity, interfacing with payers, managing the length of stay, and managing concurrent denials and reviews (ACMA, 2020).

To become an accredited case manager (ACM) you must be a registered nurse or social worker in good standing, have a valid license, and have at least one year or 2,080 hours of supervised paid case management experience in a health delivery system. The certification test includes a multiple-choice question and a simulation section. The certification exam focuses on the nursing assessment process, planning, implementation of care coordination and transition management interventions, and evaluation (ACMA, 2023).

Case Management Society of America (CMSA) and Commission for Case Manager Certification (CCMC) Collaboration

The Case Management Society of America (CMSA) provides a scope of practice and professional standards for case managers that focuses on interprofessional practice, patient-centered case management, and advocacy throughout the continuum of care. The CMSA philosophy of case management focuses on a strength-based, person-centered approach, promoting patient engagement and self-management of health outcomes. Case management across healthcare settings includes all stakeholders, including the patient, the healthcare provider, the payer, regulatory bodies, and the community. Case management practice adapts to meet the needs of the care setting, the health conditions being addressed, and the reimbursement model. The case manager provides services across the continuum of care and may work for ambulatory care, acute care, rehabilitation centers, population health, insurance providers, etc. CMSA has identified several professional standards for case managers, including those affecting screening, assessment, identification of needs and opportunities, planning, monitoring, outcomes, closure of the client-case manager relationship, facilitation, coordination, collaboration, advocacy, cultural competency, resource management, and legal and ethical areas (CMSA, 2016).

The Commission for Case Manager Certification (CCMC) in collaboration with CMSA certifies individuals as board-certified case managers (CCM). The CCM provides collaborative case management with the patient and their family or support system across various settings. Additionally, the CCM assists in navigating the health care system, engages in person-centered care planning, recognizes patient autonomy, and provides comprehensive and collaborative care addressing resource access and needs, health equity, and SDOH (CCMC, 2022a).

CCMC provides a code of professional conduct and scope of practice for case managers. These standards include the case manager conducting a comprehensive assessment, acting as an advocate, professionalism, protecting confidentiality and privacy, and standards for professional and client relationships (CCMC, 2022b). Five core components of case management are specified: (a) care delivery and reimbursement, (b) psychosocial and support systems, (c) quality, outcomes evaluation and measurements, (d) rehabilitation concepts and strategies, and (e) ethical, legal, and practice standards (CCMC, 2022b, pp. 8–9). CCM applicants must hold a certification or license that allows for conducting independent assessments or possess a baccalaureate or graduate degree that provides supervised field experience in case management, health, or behavioral health. Additionally, the applicant must have at least 12 months of case management experience supervised by a CCM or 24 months of case management experience. If the applicant supervises case managers, they must have 12 months of experience, with at least 20% of their work primarily case management, and perform at least four of the five core case management components (CCMC, 2022b).

American Nursing Association (ANA)

The American Nursing Association (ANA) has developed scope and standards of practice for nursing, which are foundational to nursing practice. The scope and standards apply to all nursing settings and identify essential standards concerning care coordination. The ANA definition of nursing identifies that the nurse "protects, promotes, and optimizes health and human function" (ANA, 2021, p. 2). The ANA also identifies that caring is a crucial aspect of nursing practice and is manifested by viewing the patient as an autonomous individual who should be valued, respected, and understood. These concepts are central to the delivery of person-centered coordination of care.

Patient Autonomy

The nurse has an ethical duty to ensure patient autonomy. The nurse can support the patient's autonomy concerning their healthcare and the patient's right to self-determination in several ways, including the following:

- Enable informed decision-making by providing the patient with accurate, complete, and understandable information and education.
- Support the patient through the decision-making process as they determine the course of their healthcare. This may include assisting the patient with weighing the risks, burdens, and benefits of treatment options.
- Respect the patients' values regarding how they would like to make decisions and with whom, recognizing that there may be cultural differences in beliefs related to privacy, confidentiality, and autonomy.
- Engage in a respectful relationship with the patient that supports independent decision-making without exerting an undue influence (ANA,2015).

The ANA also outlines the nursing process and the need for evidence-based practice in nursing care delivery. The nursing process of assessment, diagnosis, outcomes, planning, implementation, and evaluation (ANA, 2021, p. 12) is the framework for the ACMA and CMSA/CCMC case management standards of practice. Evidence-based practice is also well represented in the ACMA and CMSA/CCMC standards of practice, focusing on health education, support for patient self-management, and resource and utilization management.

The ANA identifies advocacy as a core component in the "how" of nursing. The nurse is to educate the patient so they can engage in self-management and health decision-making. Empowering the patient and their family or support system in obtaining needed resources or support. Advocacy is central to any care coordination provided, ensuring the patient and their family or support system have the education and tools to self-manage health, promote health outcomes, and access resources to address identified needs or barriers to care (ANA, 2021, pp. 34–35).

The ANA scope and standards point to a critical role nursing has in care coordination and healthcare economics. Nurses work in care coordination, transition management, and other areas that directly impact our healthcare system's effective and efficient use of resources. Not only are nurses who fill these specific roles important to cost-effective care delivery, but all nurses also affect the delivery of cost-effective and efficient care. Through person-centered and relationship-based care, the nurse promotes patient satisfaction, which can affect reimbursement in value-based payment models for healthcare. Nurses can also contribute to efficient and effective care delivery by championing innovative ways to deliver healthcare, such as virtual healthcare (ANA, 2021).

Furthermore, the ANA identifies standard 5a Care Coordination as a competency in the scope and standards of practice. To meet this competency, the nurse must collaborate effectively and create a care plan with the interprofessional team, patient, and family or support system. Additionally, the nurse needs to promote patient engagement in the self-management of health, assist with healthcare system navigation, and advocate for person-centered care. Lastly, to meet standard 5a, the nurse should be able to communicate and document care coordination activities and needs effectively to meet a safe and quality transition in care and continuity of care (ANA, 2021, p. 84). Several other ANA standards of practice apply to care coordination, such as health teaching and promotion, advocacy, communication, collaboration, and resource stewardship.

American Association of Colleges of Nursing (AACN): *The Essentials* Core Competencies for Professional Nursing Education

The American Association of Colleges of Nursing (AACN) recently developed a revised set of standards for nursing education. *The Essentials* address the needs of student nurses to be ready to enter nursing practice upon graduation. *The Essentials* have been expanded or changed in many areas and call out the need for graduate nurses to be prepared to coordinate care. Four spheres of care are identified in *The Essentials*, which span the continuum of care, from disease prevention/health promotion, chronic disease care, regenerative or restorative care, and hospice/palliative/supportive care (AACN, 2021, p. 19).

Care coordination is essential across all spheres of care and settings to meet the needs of patients and their families or support systems (AACN, 2021, p. 6). This requires the nurse to understand how nursing practice fits into system-based healthcare delivery, from the inpatient setting to the outpatient or primary care setting. Each setting offers an essential aspect of healthcare needed for optimal patient functioning and health outcomes. It is also important for the nurse to understand the impact of national policies, regulations, and community systems and structures and how these affect healthcare delivery and contribute to population and patient health outcomes (AACN, 2021, p. 7).

The Essentials provides ten domains for nursing. All domains apply to care coordination practice, but five of the ten domains specifically define care coordination competencies in nursing practice: person-centered care, population health, quality and safety, interprofessional partnerships, and system-based practice. Let's consider each of these domains separately.

- Domain 2—Person-centered care: The need to provide individualized care and include families or support systems is recognized in *The Essentials*. Person-centered care calls for care to be coordinated and evidence-based (AACN, 2021, p. 10). Vital aspects of person-centered care coordination standards of practice acknowledge the need for evidence-based health education to promote patient self-management of health and coordinate care across the continuum of care. Specific standards in Domain 2 that apply to care coordination competencies standards are as follows:

  - 2.8 Promote self-care management.
  - 2.9 Provide care coordination (AACN, 2021, p. 32).

- Domain 3—Population health: This domain concentrates on healthcare delivery across the continuum of care, focusing on health promotion, prevention, and disease management of populations to promote health outcomes (AACN, 2021, p. 10). Standards of care coordination practice call for a comprehensive assessment of SDOH, physical and mental health, to determine available needs and resources and address healthcare access and equity. Population care coordination and forms of care/case management are examples of how nursing practice meets this domain. Specific standards in Domain 3 that apply to care coordination competencies standards are as follows:

  - 3.1 Manage population health.
  - 3.2 Engage in effective partnerships (AACN, 2021, pp. 33–34).

- Domain 5—Quality and safety: An integral part of care coordination is ensuring quality and safe care transitions. Effective transition management and care coordination minimize the risk of harm and poor health outcomes (AACN, 2021, p. 11). This benefits the patient and the healthcare system by providing effective, efficient, and appropriate care. Specific standards in Domain 5 that apply to care coordination competencies standards are as follows:
  - 5.1 Apply quality improvement principles in care delivery.
  - 5.2 Contribute to a culture of patient safety (AACN, 2021, p. 39).

Aspects of a Patient Safety Culture

- Open communication: The ability for the nurse to speak up or ask questions when they have a safety concern.
- Error communication: Nurses are informed of errors that have occurred, and feedback is given on changes implemented and how to prevent the error in the future.
- Teamwork: Nurses engage in respectful interprofessional work.
- Nonpunitive response: The organization does not respond to errors in a punitive fashion or record them in personnel files, instead encouraging reporting of errors so that needed changes can be implemented.
- Continuous process learning and improvement: Errors lead to process changes, which are evaluated for effectiveness.
- Managers promote patient safety: Managers support patient safety by addressing safety issues, considering nurse suggestions to improve patient safety, and offering recognition when safety protocols and processes are followed.
- Staffing: There are enough nurses with appropriate hours and workloads to meet patient needs.
- Unit teamwork: Units coordinate with each other to meet patient needs.
- Transitions of care: Hand-off procedures are utilized, and essential information is effectively communicated across settings and providers.
- Organizational patient safety support: There is an organizational climate that supports patient safety and identifies it as a priority.
- Frequency of reports: Errors caught and corrected before affecting the patient, errors that did not harm the patient, and errors that could have harmed the patient but did not are all reported.
- Overall patient safety: Processes and procedures are in place to prevent errors, and there is a lack of patient safety issues (Reis et al., 2018, p. 661).

- Domain 6—Interprofessional partnerships: Collaborative practice is essential to successful care coordination (AACN, 2021, p. 11). Interacting and communicating effectively with the interprofessional team to ensure needs are assessed and met are critical aspects of the coordination of care practice. Follow-up and use of standardized hand-off processes and closed-loop communication are vital for successful care coordination and patient outcomes. Specific standards in Domain 6 that apply to care coordination competencies standards are as follows:
  - 6.1 Communicate in a manner that facilitates a partnership approach to quality care delivery.
  - 6.3 Use knowledge of nursing and other professions to address healthcare needs.
  - 6.4 Work with other professions to maintain a climate of mutual learning, respect, and shared values (AACN, 2021, pp. 42–43).
- Domain 7—Systems-based practice: The healthcare system is complex and challenging to navigate. Effective coordination of care and resource management promotes quality care and outcomes (AACN, 2021, p. 11). Care coordination standards of practice call for efficient use of healthcare resources and knowledge about managing and utilizing healthcare services effectually so equitable care can be provided to all populations. Nurses must understand the healthcare system to provide beneficial care coordination and advocacy and assist the patient and their family or support system in navigating healthcare systems. Specific standards in Domain 7 that apply to care coordination competencies are the following standards:
  - 7.1 Apply knowledge of systems to work effectively across the continuum of care.
  - 7.2 Incorporate consideration of cost effectiveness of care.
  - 7.3 Optimize system effectiveness by applying innovation and evidence-based practice (AACN, 2021, pp. 44–45).

CHAPTER SUMMARY

Coordination of care is vital to ensuring person-centered and quality healthcare. Care coordination is not an add-on to the nursing care provided; it is central to the nursing role in every setting. By using the nursing process and addressing the seven rights of care coordination, nurses can ensure that patients receive integrated, appropriate, and patient-centered care, promoting positive health outcomes and self-management of health.

Although various types of care coordination are offered in the health system, each type focuses on organizing and managing patient care across the continuum of care through person-centered practices and information sharing. All aspects of the health system are integral to health and wellness and must be connected effectively through care coordination interventions. Without effective coordination of care, patients and their families are at risk of untoward health outcomes and increased healthcare costs.

There are many ways that healthcare systems and providers may approach coordinating patient care, including population care coordination, transition management, care/case management, or resource and utilization management. The focus may be health promotion and disease prevention, transitions in care, chronic condition management, or ensuring that healthcare resources are utilized judiciously. Support roles for care coordination practice—such as the community health worker or health advisor—may also be used. Whatever type of care coordination is offered, it is supported by national and nursing standards and educational frameworks.

The result of care coordination where accountability and effective communication are present is quality and safe care, increased patient satisfaction, positive health outcomes, and decreased healthcare resource use. When care is not coordinated with attention to the continuity of care, the healthcare system risks financial penalties, decreased reimbursement rates, and potentially inappropriate or duplicative care delivered. This does not meet patient rights of care coordination or nursing standards of care and practice. Nurses must understand their integral role in providing care coordination in today's health system for quality and safe care delivery.

CHAPTER 1 GLOSSARY

Care Coordination: The primary but critical function of organizing and managing patient care across the continuum of care through information sharing and person-centered care practices.

Community Health Worker: Trusted community members who provide relationship-centered care coordination, act as a liaison between the patient and the healthcare system, and advocate and support the patient through education and personalized services.

Continuity of Care: Coordinated care based on cooperation and collaboration between providers and settings to provide care without disruptions or delays.

Cultural Mediator: Assists populations needing support understanding and navigating the healthcare system, such as refugees or migrants. Provides medical translation and education, ensuring understanding between patient and provider.

Gaps in Care: A recommended or crucial patient care intervention that is not offered, overlooked, or skipped, potentially causing increased healthcare costs and poor patient outcomes.

Integrated Care Coordination: Care coordination that involves an interprofessional team that crosses all systems the patient engages with, such as the patient's support system, community services and resources, and providers across the healthcare system.

Person-Centered Care: Care in which the person is actively involved in managing their care decisions, the person and the provider cocreate the care plan, and the care provided is based upon the person's values, preferences, and care goals.

Population Care Coordination: Care coordination with a health promotion and disease prevention focus for specific groups or populations to manage healthcare resource use and improve health outcomes.

Quintuple Aim: A transformative framework for healthcare improvement focusing on health equity, clinician well-being, pursuing better health, improved outcomes, and lower costs.

Risk Stratification: A process in which populations of patients are categorized based on their health status or other factors, usually in high, medium, and low-risk categories.

Transition Management: Coordinating the patient's movement between one setting or provider and another, requiring effective communication and collaboration between providers and settings.

DISCUSSION QUESTIONS AND ACTIVITIES

Discussion Questions

1. Choose one of the roles identified in the chapter (patient navigator, health/care advisor, care/case manager, etc.) and explore the qualifications, experience, and training needed for this role.
2. Discuss the benefits and challenges of resource and utilization management from the patient's perspective.
3. Choose one of the following ANA (2021) *Standards of Practice* listed below and discuss how this nursing standard of practice could be demonstrated in care coordination.
   - Assessment
   - Diagnosis
   - Outcomes Identification
   - Planning
   - Implementation
   - Evaluation
4. Choose either the American Case Management Association professional standards or the Case Management Society of America professional standards. Review the standards and discuss how one or more standards meet one or more provisions of the ANA *Code of Ethics* (2015). Include which standard(s) and provision(s) you analyze and review.
5. Inadequate care coordination has been shown to cause large amounts of wasteful spending and medical errors in the healthcare system. If the healthcare system continues to deliver inadequate care coordination, what impact could this have on the health of patients, specific populations, communities, and the nation?

Activities

1. Create a Venn diagram identifying the differences and similarities between two roles that provide care coordination or two different types of care coordination described in this chapter.

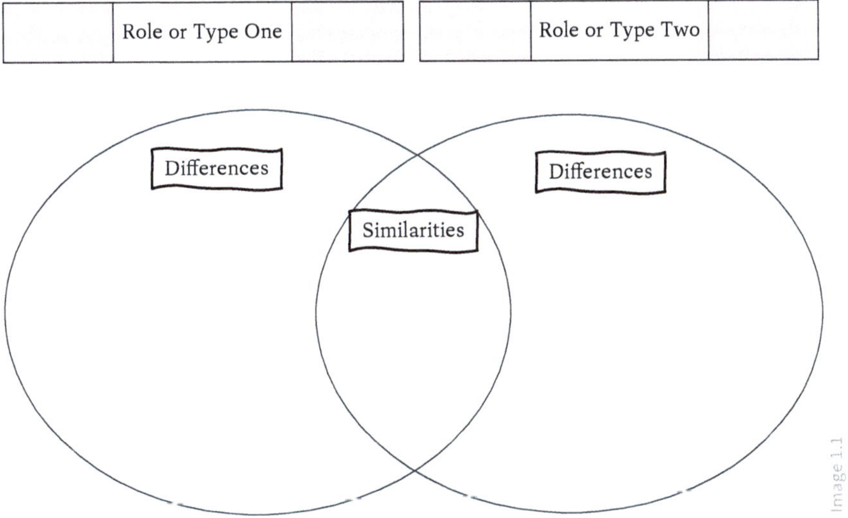

2. Find one article that describes how care coordination improves healthcare delivery and write a short review of the article. Include the following:

    a. Provide the journal reference in APA format.

    b. A summary of the article in your words.

    c. Your opinion as to whether the author's findings are accurate. If so, why? If not, why?

    d. The article review should not be over one page in length.

3. Case Study and Questions

    Mr. R is a 62-year-old male with a 10-year history of chronic obstructive pulmonary disease (COPD) complicated by hypertension and obesity. Mr. R has a BMI of 40 and has been over weight since he was a teenager. Mr. R does not have health insurance and is in the country as an undocumented person. He has tried to get a visa through his embassy but has not been successful. Due to this, Mr. R has not received primary care services for several years.

    Mr. R arrived at the local emergency room with a COPD exacerbation and was admitted for observation overnight. Since he does not have health insurance, the hospital case manager connected Mr. R with the local community health clinic for follow-up and put the appointment date in Mr. R's discharge instructions. Before discharge, the case manager also arranged for a local medical equipment company to deliver a portable oxygen tank to Mr. R's room, and informed him of this.

Mr. R's son arrives to transport Mr. R home, and the oxygen has not arrived. However, Mr. R's son did receive a phone call from the oxygen supplier with the cost. Mr. R's son thought it was expensive and was concerned about paying for the oxygen. Mr. R's son let the bedside nurse know they were ready to go, but the oxygen had not yet arrived, and he was concerned about the cost. The nurse contacted Dr. B, who was following Mr. R in the hospital, and asked Dr. B to talk with the son and Mr. R. Dr. B met with Mr. R and his son and told them not to worry about the oxygen as they could get oxygen at the community health clinic for free because Mr. R does not have insurance. The son takes Mr. R home.

The next day, Mr. R began to have severe respiratory distress. The son contacts the community health clinic and is informed that Mr. R's appointment is not for two weeks and that the community health clinic does not provide durable medical equipment such as oxygen. They are instructed to go to the emergency room.

Upon arrival at the emergency room, Mr. R must be intubated and admitted to the intensive care unit. The case manager learns about the readmission and is distressed about Mr. R's readmission and condition.

1. What would the desired outcomes have been if Mr. R had experienced coordinated care?
2. What were some challenges to Mr. R's care coordination and transitions?
3. Was a person accountable for coordinating Mr. R's care at each interaction with the healthcare system? If yes, who? If not, why not?

NCLEX STYLE QUESTIONS

1. Multiple choice: Care coordination is essential for which of the following reasons? (Select all that apply.)
   a. Patient engagement and activation
   b. Limiting medication adherence
   c. Decreasing fragmentation of care
   d. Increasing healthcare costs
2. Fill in the blank: Care coordination is the primary but critical function of __________ patient care across the __________ through __________ and __________.

3. Multiple choice: Psychosocial barriers to health include which of the following?

    a. Inability to pay for prescribed medications
    b. Food insecurity
    c. Distress related to illness
    d. Lack of transportation

4. Fill in the blank: Population care coordination includes ________ as well as ________ activities.

5. Multiple choice: Throughout population care coordination, there is a system of ________?

    a. Accountability and tracking patients at risk, monitoring outcomes, and identifying whether health goals are achieved
    b. Accountability and tracking patients at risk, intervention delivery, and documenting patient satisfaction
    c. Assessing the population, utilizing the least expensive intervention, and stakeholder engagement
    d. Identifying only high-risk patients with chronic conditions and decreasing health-care costs

6. Multiple choice: What is the movement of patients between health care providers and settings is called?

    a. Patient navigation
    b. Transition management
    c. Utilization management
    d. Population care coordination

7. Multiple choice: How can communication breakdowns be addressed in a transition of care?

    a. Documentation
    b. Using standardized handoff procedures
    c. Using a person-centered philosophy
    d. All of the above

8. Multiple choice: Key care/case management elements include which of the following? (Select all that apply.)

   a. Utilizing evidence-based patient education on self-management of health
   b. Independent creation of the care plan
   c. Addressing gaps in care
   d. Communicating and collaborating with the interprofessional team

9. Fill in the blank: The seven rights of care coordination are:

   a. Right ________
   b. Right ________
   c. Right ________
   d. Right ________
   e. Right ________
   f. Right ________
   g. Right ________

10. Multiple choice: Nurses can contribute to utilization and resource management through which of the following?

    a. Patient education and advocacy
    b. Ensuring patients understand the risks, benefits, and costs of care
    c. Assisting patients in obtaining appropriate services
    d. All of the above

11. Multiple choice: The following outcome was added to the quadruple aim to create the quintuple aim.

    a. Health outcomes
    b. Patient experience
    c. Health equity
    d. Reduced costs

12. Multiple choice: The Case Management Society of America has identified several professional standards for case managers. These include which of the following? Select all that apply.

    a. Closure of the client–case manager relationship
    b. Ensuring the social worker assigned does a screening
    c. Cultural competency
    d. Utilizing a deficit approach in care planning

13. Multiple choice: According to the American Nurses Association, which aspects manifest caring in nursing practice?

    a. Understanding the expertise of the provider
    b. Determining prioritization of care
    c. Providing patient advice concerning healthcare decisions
    d. Recognizing patient autonomy

14. Multiple choice: Which of the American Association of Colleges of Nursing essential domains specifically define care coordination practice competencies in nursing practice?

    a. Person-centered care, population health, quality and safety, interprofessional partnerships, and system-based practice
    b. Knowledge for nursing practice, person-centered care, population health, informatics and healthcare technologies, and professionalism
    c. Personal, professional, and leadership development, population health, quality and safety, interprofessional partnerships, and system-based practice
    d. Systems-based practice, interprofessional partnerships, person-centered care, and population health

15. Multiple choice: The health triune provides a framework for a complete assessment of the patient and includes assessing for which of the following:

    a. Substance use disorder, mental health, physical health
    b. Social determinants of health, environmental factors, behavioral health
    c. Physical health, emotional health, and social support systems
    d. Social determinants of health, physical health, mental health/substance use disorders

REFERENCES

Aboumrad, M., Fuld, A., Soncrant, C., Neily, J., Paull, D., & Watts, B. V. (2018). Root cause analysis of oncology adverse events in the Veterans Health Administration. *Journal of Oncology Practice, 14*(9), e579–e590. https://doi.org/10.1200/JOP.18.00159

Agency for Healthcare Research and Quality (AHRQ). (2016). *National healthcare quality and disparities report chartbook on person- and family-centered treatment.* AHRQ Publication No. 16(17)-0015-9-EF. https://www.ahrq.gov/sites/default/files/wysiwyg/research/findings/nhqrdr/chartbooks/personcentered/qdr2015-chartbook-personcenteredcare.pdf

Agency for Healthcare Research and Quality (AHRQ). (2018). *Care coordination.* https://www.ahrq.gov/ncepcr/care/coordination.html

Amankwah-Poku, M., Akpalu, J., Sefa-Dedah, A., & Amoah, A. G. B. (2021). Psychosocial barriers to well-being and quality of life among type 2 diabetes patients in Ghana. *Lifestyle Medicine, 2*(e33). https://doi.org/10.1002/lim2.33

American Association of Colleges of Nursing. (2021). *The Essentials: Core competencies for professional nursing education.* https://www.aacnnursing.org/Portals/42/AcademicNursing/pdf/Essentials-2021.pdf

American Case Management Association (ACMA). (2020). *Case management standards of practice & scope of services.* http://www.acmaweb.org/forms/Standards%20of%20Care_Brochure_Case%20Management_2020.pdf

American Case Management Association (ACMA). (2023). *Accredited case manager® candidate handbook.* https://www.acmaweb.org/forms/ACMA_ACMhandbook.pdf

American Nurses Association. (2015). *Code of ethics for nurses with interpretive statements.* American Nurses Association.

American Nurses Association. (2021). *Nursing: Scope and standards of practice* (4th ed.). American Nurses Association.

Berwick, D. M., & Hackbarth, A. D. (2012). Eliminating waste in US health care. *JAMA: Journal of the American Medical Association, 307*(14), 1513–1516.

Camicia, M., & Lutz, B. J. (2016). Nursing's role in successful transitions across settings. *Stroke, 47*(11), e246–e249. https://doi.org/10.1161/STROKEAHA.116.012095

Case Management Society of America (CMSA). (2016). *Standards of practice for case management.* https://www.abqaurp.org/DOCS/2016%20CM%20standards%20of%20practice.pdf

Centers for Disease Control and Prevention (CDC). (2019). *Promotores de Salud/Community Health Workers.* https://www.cdc.gov/minorityhealth/promotores/index.html

Centers for Medicare and Medicaid Services (CMS). (2022). *Chronic care management services.* https://www.cms.gov/outreach-and-education/medicare-learning-network-mln/mlnproducts/downloads/chroniccaremanagement.pdf

Commission for Case Management Certification (CCMC). (2022a). *Code of professional conduct for case managers.* https://ccmcertification.org/sites/ccmc/files/docs/2022/CCMC-22-Code-Of-Conduct-Update-Final%20with%20CM%20def%20update.pdf

Commission for Case Management Certification (CCMC). (2022b). *Certification guide to the CCM® examination.* https://ccmcertification.org/sites/ccmc/files/docs/2022/CCMC-22-Certification-Guide-Update-Final%20with%20CM%20def%20update.pdf

Davie, L., & Rataj, A. (2018). *Developing a foundation for integrated care coordination: Part 1.* University of New Hampshire Center on Aging and Community Living and NH Alliance for Healthy Aging. https://chhs.unh.edu/sites/default/files/media/2018/12/care_coordination_part_1.pdf

Dom Dera J. (2019). Risk stratification: A two-step process for identifying your sickest patients. *Family Practice Management, 26*(3), 21–26. https://www.aafp.org/pubs/fpm/issues/2019/0500/p21.html

Elliott, M. N., Adams, J. L., Klein, D. J., Haviland, A. M., Beckett, M. K., Hays, R. D., Gaillot, S., Edwards, C. A., Dembosky, J. W., & Schneider, E. C. (2021). Patient-reported care coordination is associated with better performance on clinical care measures. *JGIM: Journal of General Internal Medicine, 36*(12), 3665–3671. https://link.springer.com/article/10.1007/s11606-021-07122-8

Felt-Lisk, S., & Higgins, T. (2011). Exploring the promise of population health management programs to improve health. *Mathematica Policy Research*, Issue Brief, 1–4. https://www.researchgate.net/publication/254429837_Exploring_the_Promise_of_Population_Health_Management_Programs_to_Improve_Health_Washington_DC_Mathematica_Policy_Research

Figueroa, J. F., Feyman, Y., Zhou, X., & Joynt Maddox, K. (2018). Hospital-level care coordination strategies associated with better patient experience. *BMJ Quality & Safety, 27*(10), 844–851. https://doi.org/10.1136/bmjqs-2017-007597

Finkelman, A. (2016). *Leadership and management for nurses* (3rd ed.) Pearson.

Frandsen, B. R., Joynt, K. E., Rebitzet, J. B., & Jha, A. K. (2015). Care fragmentation, quality, and costs among chronically ill patients. *The American Journal of Managed Care, 21*(5), 335–362. https://www.ajmc.com/view/care-fragmentation-quality-costs-among-chronically-ill-patients

Fraser, K., Lisa, G. B., Laing, D., Lai, J., & Punjani, N. S. (2018). Case manager resource allocation decision-making for adult home care clients: With comparisons to a high needs pediatric home care clients. *Home Health Care Management & Practice, 30*(4),164–174. https://doi.org/10.1177/1084822318779371

Giardino, A. P., & Wadhwa, R. (2022). *Utilization management.* StatPearls Publishing. https://www.ncbi.nlm.nih.gov/books/NBK560806/

Haas, S. A., Swan, B. A., & Haynes, T. S. (2014). *Care coordination and transition management core curriculum.* American Academy of Ambulatory Care Nursing.

Harvard Medical School. (2022). *What causes depression?* Harvard Health Publishing. https://www.health.harvard.edu/mind-and-mood/what-causes-depression

Healthy People 2030. (n.d.) *Healthy People 2030.* U.S. Department of Health and Human Services, Office of Disease Prevention and Health Promotion. https://health.gov/healthypeople/objectives-and-data/social-determinants-health

Heath, S. (2021). *4 patient engagement strategies to close patient care gaps.* https://patientengagementhit.com/news/4-patient-engagement-strategies-to-close-patient-care-gaps

Institute of Medicine (U.S.) Committee on Quality of Health Care in America. (2000). Setting performance standards and expectations for patient safety. In L. T. Kohn, J. M. Corrigan, & M. S. Donaldson (Eds.), *To err is human: Building a safer health system* (Ch. 7). National Academies Press. https://www.ncbi.nlm.nih.gov/books/NBK225181/#_NBK225181_pubdet

Institute of Medicine (IOM). (2001). *Crossing the quality chasm: A new health system for the 21st century.* National Academies Press.

Itchhaporia, D. (2021). The evolution of the Quintuple Aim: Health equity, health outcomes, and the economy. *Journal of the American College of Cardiology, 78*(27), 2262–2264. https://doi.org/10.1016/j.jacc.2021.10.018

Kindig, D., & Stoddart, G. (2003). What is population health? *American Journal of Public Health, 93*(3), 380–383. https://doi.org/10.2105/AJPH.93.3.380.

Lyons, J. (2013). *How case managers help patients navigate the health care maze.* http://hin.com/blog/2013/10/08/infographic-how-case-managers-help-patients-navigate-the-healthcare-maze/

Medicare.gov. (n.d.). *Inpatient or outpatient hospital status affects your costs.* https://www.medicare.gov/what-medicare-covers/what-part-a-covers/inpatient-or-outpatient-hospital-status

Mitchell, S. E., Laurens, V., Weigel, G. M., Hirschman, K. B., Scott, A. M., Nguyen, H. Q., Howard, J. M., Laird, L., Levine, C., Davis, T. C., Gass, B., Shaid, E., Li, J., Williams, M. V., & Jack, B. W. (2018). Care transitions from patient and caregiver perspectives. *Annals of Family Medicine, 16*(3), 225–231. https://doi.org/10.1370/afm.2222

National Academies of Practice. (2022). *National Academies of Practice position paper: Interprofessional collaboration.* https://www.napractice.org/assets/statements/NAP%20Position%20Paper%20on%20IPE%20IPCP%20-%20published%204.26.22.pdf

National Academies Press. (2009). *Initial national priorities for comparative effectiveness research* (Ch. 2). https://nap.nationalacademies.org/read/12648/chapter/4

National Association of Community Health Centers (NACHC). (2016). *Population health management: Care Coordination.* http://www.nachc.org/wp-content/uploads/2015/12/NACHC_carecoord_factsheet_FINAL.pdf

National Cancer Institute (NCI). (n.d.). *Patient navigator.* https://www.cancer.gov/publications/dictionaries/cancer-terms/def/patient-navigator

National Heart, Lung, and Blood Institute . (2014). *Role of community health workers.* https://www.nhlbi.nih.gov/health/educational/healthdisp/role-of-community-health-workers.htm

National Quality Forum (NQF). (2010). *Quality connections: Care coordination.* https://www.qualityforum.org/publications/2010/10/quality_connections__care_coordination.aspx

National Transitions of Care Coalition (NTOCC). (2022). *Care transition bundle seven essential intervention categories.* https://static1.squarespace.com/static/5d48b6eb75823b00016db708/t/625ec7834a90de6335434515/165037862841 4/2022+NTOCC+7+Elements.pdf

Neumiller, J. J., Setter, S. M., White, A. M., Corbet, C. F., Weeks, D. J., Daratha, K. R., & Collins, J. R. (2017). *Advances in patient safety and medical liability: Medication discrepancies and potential adverse drug events during the transfer of care from hospital to home.* Agency for Healthcare Research and Quality. https://www.ahrq.gov/patient-safety/reports/liability/neumiller.html

Nourse, S., & Paauwe-Weust, J. (2021). Patient navigators in the healthcare setting. *MEDSURG Nursing, 30*(1), 48–52.

Ofei, A. M. A., & Paarima, Y. (2021). Perception of nurse managers' care coordination practices among nurses at the unit level. *International Journal of Care Coordination, 24*(1), 17–27. https://doi.org/10.1177/20534345219999

Pereira Gray, D. J., Sidaway-Lee, K., White, E., Thorne, A., & Evans, P. H. (2018). Continuity of care with doctors—a matter of life and death? A systematic review of continuity of care and mortality. *BMJ Open.* https://bmjopen.bmj.com/content/bmjopen/8/6/e021161.full.pdf

Perrin, K. M. (2017). *Principles of health navigation: Understanding roles and career options.* Johns and Bartlett Learning.

Pocket Guide: TeamSTEPPS. (2020). Agency for Healthcare Research and Quality. https://www.ahrq.gov/teamstepps/instructor/essentials/pocketguide.html

Practice Fusion. (2010). *Survey: Patients see 18.7 different doctors on average.* https://www.prnewswire.com/news-releases/survey-patients-see-187-different-doctors-on-average-92171874.html

Reis, C. T., Paiva, S. G., & Sousa, P. (2018). The patient safety culture: A systematic review by characteristics of Hospital Survey on Patient Safety Culture dimensions. *International Journal for Quality in Health Care, 30*(9), 660–667. https://doi.org/10.1093/intqhc/mzy080

Rushton, S. (2015). The population care coordination process. *Professional Case Management, 20*(5), 230–238. DOI: 10.1097/NCM.0000000000000105

Sailsman, A. M., Halley-Boyce, J. A., & Sailsman A. M. (2018). Patient-centered care coordination in population health case management. *Nursing & Care Open Access Journal, 5*(4), 244–247. https://medcraveonline.com/NCOAJ/NCOAJ-05-00155.pdf

Schraeder, C., & Shelton, P. (2011). *Comprehensive care coordination for chronically ill adults.* Wiley-Blackwell.

Schuler, E. (2020). *Patient navigators—who we are and what we do.* https://patientnavigator.com/patient-navigators-who-we-are-and-what-we-do/)

Shi, L., & Singh, D. (2019). *Essentials of the U.S. health care system* (5th ed.). Jones and Bartlett Learning.

Straughen, J. K., Clement, J., Schultz, L., Alexander, G., Hill-Ashford, Y., & Wisdom, K. (2023). Community health workers as change agents in improving equity in birth outcomes in Detroit. *PloS One, 18*(2), e0281450. https://doi.org/10.1371/journal.pone.0281450

Transitions of Care. (2019). *Standards.* https://transitionsofcare.org/standards/guiding-principles/

Venables, E., Whitehouse, K., Spissu, C., Pizzi, L., Al Rousan, A., & di Carlo, S. (2021). Roles and responsibilities of cultural mediators. *Forced Migration Review, 66*, 1–2. https://www.fmreview.org/sites/fmr/files/FMRdownloads/en/issue66/venables-whitehouse-spissu-pizzi-alrousan-dicarlo.pdf

Warshaw, G. (2006). Introduction: Advances and challenges in care of older people with chronic illness. *Generations, 30*(3), 5–10.

World Health Organization (WHO). (2018). *Continuity and coordination of care: A practice brief to support implementation of the WHO Framework on integrated people-centered health services.* https://apps.who.int/iris/bitstream/handle/10665/274628/9789241514033-eng.pdf

Yoder, L. (2017). AMSN president's message: Care coordination and transition management: Critical roles for medical-surgical nurses. *MEDSURG Nursing, 26*(4), 225–228.

Credits

CHAPTER 2

Essential Competencies for Effective Care Coordination

LEARNING OBJECTIVES

1. Identify foundational care coordination competencies.
2. Recognize the importance of interprofessional teamwork, collaboration, and communication in care coordination.
3. Distinguish various knowledge, skills, and attitudes needed for effective care coordination.
4. Comprehend the role of quality assurance in the coordination of care.

KEY TERMS

- competencies
- comprehensive assessment
- cross-setting communication
- empathetic awareness
- functional abilities
- interprofessional care coordination
- interprofessional team
- moral courage
- nursing presence
- quality assurance
- relationship-centered care
- shared mental model
- skills

Introduction

Several nursing organizations have identified and developed competencies for nursing practice. Care coordination has been recognized as one of those competencies for graduating nurses in the *Essentials* (AACN, 2021). Organizations such as The Institute of Medicine (IOM) have also worked to identify and develop competencies for general healthcare professional practice. In 2003, the IOM identified five core competencies for professional practice: (a) patient-centered care, (b) interdisciplinary teamwork, (c) evidence-based practice, (d) quality improvement application, and (d) informatics (p. 4). When considering that care coordination is the primary but critical function of organizing and managing patient care across the continuum of care through information

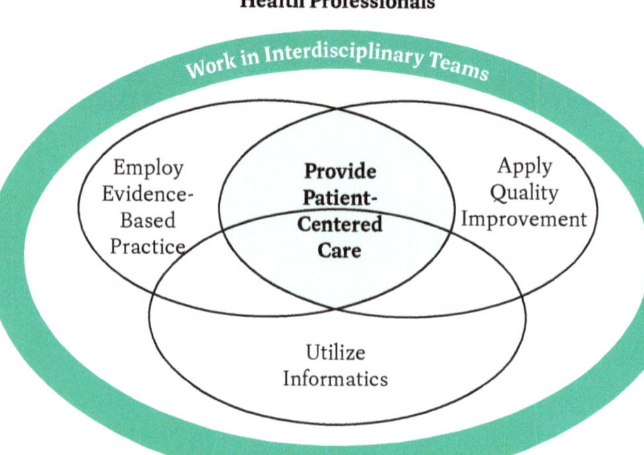

FIGURE 2.1 Relationships Among Core Competencies for Health Professionals

sharing and person-centered care practices, we see the essential need to use evidence-based practices for best patient outcomes, use informatics for transmission of crucial patient information, needs, and preferences, and implement quality improvement processes to ensure that any gap in the coordination of care is addressed and corrected. As seen in Figure 2.1, the IOM professional competencies are not siloed but overlap, with the patient at the center of the care provided.

Competency theory is based on the belief that competence comes from skill development through a domain knowledge base, in this case nursing, and specifically coordination of patient care. Nurses with low skill levels often do not recognize their lack of competence and may overestimate their abilities, leading to poor decision-making. This is thought to be based on the need for ability or competency in critical self-performance assessment (Gross, 2005).

It is important to differentiate between skills and competencies when examining the ability to coordinate care successfully. There are core competencies—such as those identified by the IOM—and other competencies needed to coordinate care effectively. **Competencies** are broad and include knowledge and behaviors such as collaborative practice, knowledge of team functioning, and use of critical analysis and synthesis based upon knowledge attained. **Skills** are abilities learned to perform a job, which may vary by setting or type of care coordination offered. However, nurses in all settings must be able to evaluate their performance and recognize their competency levels. To do this, the nurse needs an awareness of the competencies needed related to care coordination. This will prepare the nurse for lifelong learning opportunities and provide a solid foundation of the knowledge, skills, and attitudes that are critical for efficient and effective care coordination practice.

Competencies for Coordination Care

Many competencies are identified for nursing practice, varying by setting or nursing care provided. In the case of care coordination practice, we can review national standards presented by the Case Management Society of America (CMSA), the American Case Management Association (ACMA), or the *Care Coordination and Transition Management Core Curriculum* sponsored by the American Academy of Ambulatory Care Nursing (AAACN). Each national group focuses slightly differently on competencies developed and their application to care coordination practice. As these national standards for practice are reviewed, a few foundational competencies can be

Person Centered
and Relationship
Centered Care
Quality Assurance
• Evaluation
• Monitoring
Advocacy
Foundational Care
Coordination
Competencies
Interprofessional
Practice
• Collaboration
• Connecting
Community
Resources
Assessment
and Critical
Analysis
Communication
• Cross Setting
• Challenging
Conversations

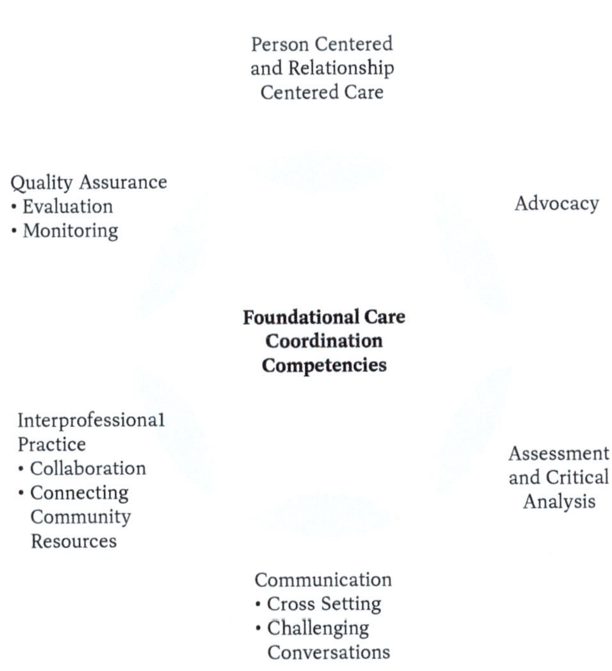

FIGURE 2.2 Foundational Care Coordination Competencies and Sub-Competencies

identified for all care coordination practices, no matter the setting. These core competencies that cross settings and care coordination practice include person and relationship-centered care, advocacy, assessment and critical analysis, communication, interprofessional practice, and quality assurance. See Figure 2.2 for a visual of these competencies and sub-competencies.

Person-Centered Care and Relationship-Centered Care

Traditionally, healthcare has been delivered by a provider "to" a patient. It was a hierarchical relationship with the provider being seen as the "expert" and the patient being viewed as needing to comply with provider directives and what was in the care plan without question. There may have been little to no discussion about patient preferences, lifestyle, or issues with following the care plan developed or communication with other interprofessional team members about what the care plan should include. It was a power hierarchy based on an imbalanced relationship between the provider and the patient (Heath, 2018).

Dr. Berwick exemplifies this power hierarchy in *Escape Fire: Lessons for the Future of Health Care*. As he discussed his experience in the healthcare system when his wife was ill, he wrote, "The experience of patienthood or patient-spousehood, as the case may be, was often one of trying to get the attention of the decision-makers to correct their impressions or their assumptions ... we felt time and again our migration to the edge of the label 'difficult patient'" (2002, p. 25).

Words Matter in Healthcare

There are many words that nurses may use to identify a patient as "difficult," such as non-compliant, challenging, aggressive, etc. Using these terms and the normalization of using these labels when referring to patients defeats the competency of person and relationship-centered care. The following quotations from research studies identify the gravity and potential long-term consequences of using biased and stigmatizing language concerning patients.

> "Patients with stigmatizing conditions such as diabetes, obesity, substance use disorder, and chronic pain are affected by the language of their health care providers. Biased language can worsen feelings of shame, decreasing patients' motivations to complete their treatment plans or engage in treatment at all" (Raney et al., 2021, p. 1).

> "Physicians who use stigmatizing language in their patients' medical records may affect the care those patients get for years to come" (John Hopkins Medicine Newsroom, 2018, para. 1).

Unfortunately, this experience is still occurring in our healthcare system. A survey of intensive care unit (ICU) patients and families found that many respondents did not want to be perceived as "troublemakers," so they were hesitant to voice concerns about goals of care, possible mistakes in care delivery, or not understanding the information given. Many respondents also identified that the healthcare team seemed unavailable to hear their concerns (Bell et al., 2018).

The competency of patient-centered care presented by the IOM in 2003 has expanded over the last 20 years. We have seen this competency transition to include patient-centered, person-centered, and relationship-centered care. All these variations have the patient at the center of care provided. However, the need to see the patient–provider relationship more inclusively has become apparent as our healthcare system has been transforming to address outcome and cost issues. Patients do not live in isolation. They live with caregivers, family members, friends, and in communities. Patients also desire to have a relationship with their healthcare providers where they can voice their concerns and preferences and receive individually tailored healthcare that is relevant to their lifestyle and health goals.

Kuipers et al. (2019, p. 2) define patient-centered care as "providing care that is respectful of and responsive to individual patient preferences, needs, and values and ensuring that patient values guide all clinical decisions." The Centers for Medicare and Medicaid Services (CMS) defines person-centered care as "Integrated health care services delivered in a setting and manner that is responsive to the individual and their goals, values, and preferences, in a system that empowers patients and providers to make effective care plans together" (n.d., para. 1). Beach et al. (2006) define relationship-centered care (RCC) as follows:

> Care in which all participants appreciate the importance of their relationships with one another. RCC is founded upon 4 principles: (1) that relationships in health care ought to include the personhood of the participants, (2) that affect and emotion are important components of these relationships, (3) that all health care relationships occur in the

Reciprocal Determinism and Relationship-Centered Care

Albert Bandura developed the concept of reciprocal determinism, which theorizes that an individual's behavior is influenced by how they think and feel, their environment, and the behaviors exhibited. This, in turn, influences their environment and subsequent behaviors (Bandura, 1978). In relationship-centered care, it is vital to recognize how our own thoughts, feelings, and behaviors influence our work environments, our nursing practice, and the patient care experience.

context of reciprocal influence, and (4) that the formation and maintenance of genuine relationships in health care is morally valuable. (p. S3)

In today's healthcare system, coordinating care effectively requires the nurse to consider all aspects of the patient's values, preferences, goals, lifestyle, community setting, and other stakeholders or participants in the patient's health and care planning to ensure continuity of care. The patient must be seen as a person who has value and is the "expert" on themselves. They must be given the opportunity and tools to engage actively in their care plan development and healthcare decision-making. **Relationship-centered care** involves everyone in the healthcare relationship (e.g., patient, family, interprofessional team, community stakeholders, etc.) to build and enhance relationships and health outcomes. Relationship-centered care values mutual respect, trust, partnership, and understanding the co-constructed nature of relationships. Person- and relationship-centered care competencies are fundamental for successful care coordination and continuity of care. Figure 2.3 differentiates between these different varieties of person-centered models.

Patient Centered Care

Participants: Provider and patient.

Considerations: Patient preferences, needs, and values.

Focus: Clinical decisions that are respectful and responsive to patient preferences, needs, and values.

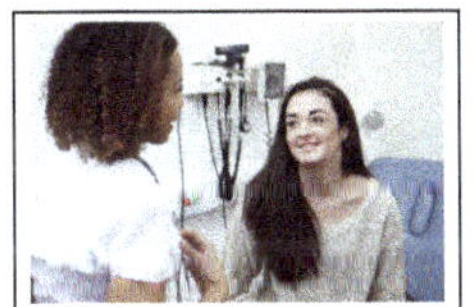

Person Centered Care

Participants: All health care services/providers and patient.

Considerations: Patient goals, values, and preferences.

Focus: Empowering the patient and provider to co-create care plans. Delivery of healthcare that is responsive to patient goals, values, and preferences.

Relationship Centered Care

Participants: All persons involved in a healthcare relationship (patient, provider, family/caregivers, colleagues, community, etc.)

Considerations: The unique nature of each person and relationship. Valuing partnership and understanding relationships are co-constructed between the participants with mutual respect and trust.

Focus: Relationship building to enhance health outcomes, informed decision-making, staff satisfaction, and health of the community.

FIGURE 2.3 Comparison of Patient-Centered Care, Person-Centered Care, and Relationship-Centered Care

An Example of Person-Centered Care

Tyler meets with his doctor about breathing problems and is diagnosed with asthma. In addition to prescribing Tyler a rescue inhaler to treat the symptoms, his doctor follows up with a telehealth visit to identify contributing factors, including smoking and his current living conditions, and develop a treatment plan. Together they come up with a comprehensive plan that considers Tyler's related health, behavioral, and social needs. For example, the plan includes connecting Tyler with a smoking cessation program when he is ready to quit. The plan also leverages community partners and public services that can help him understand what in his apartment might contribute to his asthma and where he can get help to improve his living situation.

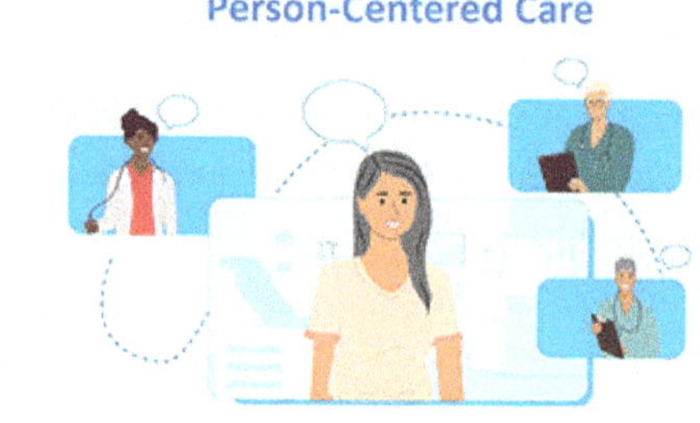

Image 2.1

Source: (CDC, n.d., para. 6)

Advocacy

Competency in advocacy is integral to delivering and coordinating person and relationship-centered care. Advocacy is an ethical principle in Provision 3 of the American Nurses Association (ANA) *Code of Ethics for Nurses* (ANA, 2015). Advocacy is also specified in the ANA *Nursing Scope and Standards of Practice* as a competency in Standard 5A: Coordination of Care (ANA, 2021). Acting as a patient advocate may take on various forms while coordinating care. Advocacy may look like ensuring the patient and family/caregiver have the needed information to make an informed decision and navigate the healthcare system or the nurse collaborating and communicating effectively with other healthcare providers to ensure the patient and family/caregiver are encouraged and empowered in their healthcare.

Advocacy encompasses several ethical principles, including autonomy, beneficence, and fidelity (Haas et al., 2014). As the nurse supports and empowers the patient in their right to engage in autonomous decision-making concerning their care plan and treatment options, they also ensure that the patient is in the "driver's seat" and in control of their healthcare choices. Nurses support patient autonomy by providing education, training, and encouragement for patients to take control of their health through engagement in self-management of their health. Nurses promote beneficence by evaluating the care provided and involving others in the interprofessional team to meet patient healthcare and resource needs. The nurse meets the ethical condition of fidelity by engaging in thoughtful, detailed, and effective coordination and continuity of care, which protects the patient's health and safety (Haas et al., 2014).

Moral Courage in Nursing

When a nurse experiences a dilemma, they may need to use moral courage to speak out and stand up for what they consider to be ethical and moral actions, even when others, colleagues, or the organization would lead the nurse to behave differently (AACN, n.d.).

The acronym CODE can guide nurses in dilemmas requiring moral courage.

Courage to be moral requires:

Obligations to honor (What is the right thing to do?)

Danger management (What do I need to handle my fear?)

Expression and action (What action do I need to take to maintain my integrity?)

(Lachman, 2010, para. 2)

Moreover, to be competent in advocacy, the nurse must also understand health disparities and the connection between poor health outcomes and socioeconomic status, mental health, houselessness, resource scarcity, and access to care issues and how these issues might require advocacy (Haas et al., 2014). Lastly, nurses must engage in **moral courage** in the care coordination process, advocating for the patient's rights, safety, preferences, and needs. This can include engaging in difficult conversations with others on the healthcare team, the patient, or their families/caregivers.

Until 2000, the concept of patient advocacy included characteristics or elements of safeguarding, apprising, valuing, mediating, and championing social justice in healthcare. From 2001 to 2016, the elements of patient privacy, confronting inappropriate policies in healthcare, and identifying and correcting inequalities in healthcare delivery were added to the concept of patient advocacy (Abbasinia et al., 2020). Table 2.1 details advocacy domains and examples of how these may be demonstrated in care coordination practice.

TABLE 2.1 Example Application of Patient Advocacy Domains to Care Coordination Practice

Advocacy Domain	Care Coordination Activities
***Safeguarding*: Protecting the patient**	• Performing comprehensive assessment, identifying risks and gaps in care • Completing medication reconciliation • Documenting care plan • Utilizing evidence-based interventions in care planning • Using quality measures to ensure processes and outcomes are met • Communicating concerns related to safety or hazards

(Continued)

TABLE 2.1 ***(Continued)***

***Apprising*: Informing the patient**	• Addressing patient and family/caregiver questions/concerns • Cross-setting communication and collaboration • Providing health education and information for healthcare decision-making • Identifying and educating the patient on community resources available
***Valuing*: Regarding the patient's personhood and worth**	• Providing tools and resources for self-management of health • Building on strengths to empower patients • Providing person and relationship-centered care planning and practice • Protecting and respecting patient privacy • Engaging in nursing presence with empathetic awareness
***Mediating*: Intervening between parties to bring about continuity and coordination of care**	• Coordinating interprofessional care • Linking patient to needed services, resources, and referrals • Acting as a liaison and facilitator concerning patient goals and values. • Using health information technologies and structured communication tools to ensure continuity and care coordination
***Championing social justice in the provision of healthcare*: Engaging in transforming the healthcare system to address issues of access and equity to care**	• Engaging in policy initiatives concerning social justice issues • Proactively addressing access and equity issues in healthcare delivery • Supporting access to care across settings • Serving as a patient voice in the organization, system, and community

(Abbasinia et al., 2020, p. 145)

Assessment and Critical Analysis

Some may consider assessment and critical analysis to be two different competencies, yet these two nursing actions cannot be siloed in care coordination practice. The nurse must possess competency in assessment as it relates to the coordination of care and be able to integrate the data gathered into the critical analysis of needs, resources, and potential gaps in care. Assessment competency alone is not sufficient. This requires a responsive and dynamic relationship between assessment competency and critical analysis competency. Suppose the nurse cannot proactively assess for and critically analyze potential or real-time patient barriers to coordination and continuity of care. In that case, they cannot develop a quality care plan with the patient and the interprofessional team. They will be unable to identify the areas of the plan that are essential to monitor, evaluate, and collaborate upon. Assessment and critical analysis are dependent upon each other. They should be conducted simultaneously in care coordination practice because critically analyzing data will likely lead to identifying additional assessment or reassessment needs.

Assessment

The competency of assessment is integral to all nursing practice. As with all types of assessment, the information gathered from the assessment process needs to be evaluated and analyzed to promote effective decision-making and care plan development. In coordination of care, assessment is crucial and must be comprehensive, including a holistic assessment and critical analysis of the patient utilizing a person-centered and relationship-centered framework. A comprehensive assessment may need to be conducted over several visits with the patient, considering the patient's energy level, attention span, and health needs. During the comprehensive assessment process, gaps in care may become evident, or risk factors may be identified so that they can be proactively addressed, reducing poor outcomes and added costs. The comprehensive assessment also allows the patient and their family/caregiver to express their goals of care, preferences, needs, and concerns.

The **comprehensive assessment** includes the physical, social (e.g., lifestyle, economic, cultural factors) and psychological domains, and **functional abilities**. It should be repeated if there are changes in the patient's health or physical, social, or psychological condition (Haas et al., 2014; Schraeder & Shelton, 2011). Subjective and objective information is included in the assessment. Objective information is observed directly or indirectly through physical examination of the patient, utilizing the senses of sight, sound, touch, and smell. This could include objective information gathered about the patient through observation of their living environment, their physical appearance, or the manifestation of symptoms. Subjective information is data from verbal or nonverbal communication with the patient and their family/caregiver. This information may include data about feelings, beliefs, care priorities, strengths, barriers to care, and concerns (Haas et al., 2014). Both objective and subjective information is essential to effective coordination and continuity of care.

Functional Abilities

Functional abilities include activities of daily living (ADL) and instrumental activities of daily living (IADL). ADLs, such as eating, dressing, bathing, toileting, etc., affect patients' ability to care for themselves independently. IADLs, such as using the telephone, managing finances, managing medications, etc., affect patients' ability to live independently in their own homes and communities. These abilities run on a continuum of complete independence to entirely dependent. Many patients are in the middle, needing assistance with specific functional areas, such as shopping or food preparation. The patient's physical, social, and psychological domains can affect functional abilities. Often, if a patient has a decline in ADL or IADL, this can signify an area in one of the comprehensive assessment domains that must be assessed and addressed.

Comprehensive assessments are necessary to proactively address risk factors, gaps, or barriers to care and effectively collaborate with the interprofessional team. A comprehensive assessment should be interprofessional (Schraeder & Shelton, 2011), meaning the nurse needs to review and critically analyze assessments and input from all interprofessional team members. For example, a nurse can only ensure a patient is discharged home with all needed assistive devices if they have reviewed therapy recommendations. In addition, if after reviewing therapy recommendations the nurse has information that could benefit the care plan or concerns about assistive device use in the home, they must collaborate with the interprofessional team to address the issue before discharge or transition from their setting.

Person-centered and relationship-centered care is central to conducting a comprehensive assessment, requiring patient and family/caregiver engagement throughout care transitions and the continuum of care (Schraeder & Shelton, 2011). Comprehensive assessment in care coordination practice begins with a review of the patient's physical assessment, vital signs and pain assessment, medical history, and current health status. A comprehensive assessment with a care coordination focus also includes, but is not limited to, the following:

- risk factors such as fall risk, environmental safety, and functional abilities
- medication reconciliation/review
- assistive and care devices used (e.g., glucometer, walker, etc.)
- diet or nutritional concerns
- social assessment (e.g., living situation, financial status, health insurance status, transportation needs, current community services being used, etc.)
- advanced directives status
- specialists and other providers involved in the patient's care (e.g., primary care provider, cardiologist, counselor, when last seen, etc.)
- cultural, language, and communication preferences or needs
- patient engagement, activation, ability to self-manage health conditions, and knowledge of health issues
- patient strengths, resources, and support systems
- psychological assessment (e.g., mental health history or symptoms, substance use disorder, mental status, etc.)
- caregiver assessment (e.g., caregiver strain, need for a caregiver, elder abuse, etc.)
- patient safety concerns (e.g., domestic violence, elder abuse)

While conducting the comprehensive assessment, the nurse must critically analyze the information gathered to determine if additional assessment areas are needed. Identified issues such as food scarcity or lack of insurance can be addressed in the care coordination plan to ensure positive patient and system outcomes. Risk factors may also be identified through a comprehensive assessment (e.g., substance use), and the nurse can proactively manage these risk factors through appropriate referrals and follow-up care facilitation (Haas et al., 2014).

For example, suppose a care coordinator found through their comprehensive assessment that a patient who has received a recent diabetes diagnosis rents a room and only has access to a small refrigerator in their room and a one-burner hot plate for cooking. Furthermore, the care coordinator discovers that the patient is experiencing financial difficulties and does not feel they can afford their medicine or purchase the food the dietician recommends. These issues of financial insecurity and lack of refrigeration and cooking access could potentially lead the patient to not taking their medication as prescribed, not picking up their medications at all, or eating foods that are of low nutritional value and shelf-stable (rather than fresh) and do not need extensive preparation.

All these issues and risks likely would lead to poor outcomes, emergency room visits, and potential readmission to the hospital. In this case, the care coordinator could collaborate with the patient's pharmacy or local diabetes center to see if they have prescription assistance programs. The care coordinator could access community resources such as meal services or food banks, or they could communicate and dialogue with the patient to determine whether they might be able to work with their roommates to have greater access to cooking facilities. Through the comprehensive assessment and analysis process, the care coordinator can determine what resources may be needed, identify if additional interprofessional team members should be consulted (e.g., a diabetic educator or pharmacist), and provide essential referrals, facilitating patient access to required providers and resources and ensuring adequate care coordination.

Critical Analysis

Critical analysis competency is crucial for nursing practice and instrumental when nurses examine assessment data and evidence that informs care coordination interventions. Detailed analysis of patient data to direct care coordination efforts depends on available assessment data and access to this data. Patient data in care coordination efforts are often collected through interviews and reviews of medical records. The competency of critical analysis requires the ability to review and synthesize the available data, cocreate a care plan with the patient, and collaborate with interprofessional team members to address an identified risk factor or gap in care. This necessitates the nurse to determine the relevancy of the available data and view it from various perspectives (Timmins, 2006).

For the nurse to efficiently engage in assessment and critical analysis competencies, they must understand the competency, why it is foundational for successful coordination of care, and be able to rationalize their decisions and how they promote desired outcomes and continuity of care. Furthermore, the nurse must be able to critically analyze and identify organizational or community policies that create barriers to coordination and continuity of care across the continuum to address gaps and inequities in care (Timmins, 2006).

Key Features of Critical Analysis

Critical analysis includes the following four considerations:

- evaluation of knowledge theories, policy, and practice;
- recognition of multiple perspectives;
- different levels of analysis; and
- ongoing inquiry (Timmins, 2006, p. 51).

Comprehensive assessment and critical analysis in care coordination practice are dynamic. The nurse will repeatedly assess and critically analyze assessment findings and patient outcomes. This is fundamental to proactively address potential barriers to continuity of care or gaps in care that may lead to poor outcomes and higher costs. Patients are diverse, and their conditions are ever-changing, so the comprehensive assessment and critical analysis process must be conducted in a responsive, person- and relationship-centered manner. Figure 2.4 shows the dynamic assessment and critical analysis process in care coordination.

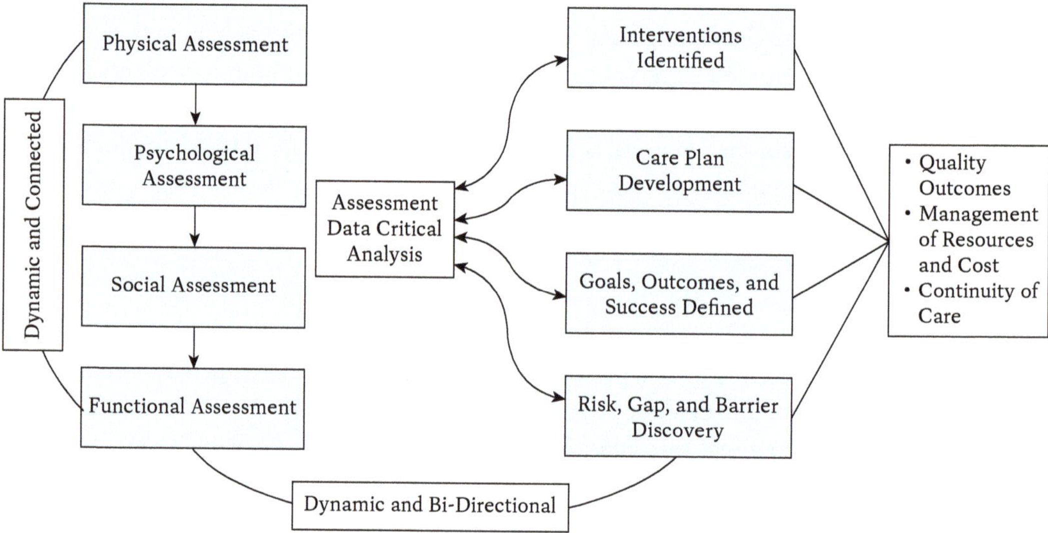

FIGURE 2.4 The Relationship Between Assessment and Critical Analysis in Care Coordination

Communication

While coordinating care, communication is an essential overarching and global competency. The nurse coordinating care must communicate in a person-centered and relationship-centered way with all involved in the patient's care. This could be various members of the interprofessional team (e.g., physicians, therapists, unlicensed personnel), members of the community (e.g., community-based providers and services or resources), members of the insurance groups (e.g., patient insurers such as Medicare), members of the patient's family/caregiver, and of course the patient themselves. This requires the nurse to move beyond simple reflective listening and rudimentary therapeutic communication and be aware of how to communicate best, considering the communication's setting, situation, content, patient goals of care, and privacy considerations. There are two prevalent aspects of communication in care coordination: cross-setting communication and engaging in challenging conversations. These two central components of coordination and continuity of care practices necessitate specific knowledge, skills, and attitudes to meet this competency.

Cross-Setting Communication

Nurses may only consider communication competency relating to patient communication or communication amongst the interprofessional team. However, care coordination is based on the need to ensure continuity of care across settings, from primary care providers to the acute care setting to rehabilitation and back to the community. There are multiple providers, stakeholders, and interprofessional team members in care transitions across the continuum of care, and this requires specific knowledge concerning **cross-setting communication**. This type of communication is big-picture or high-level. It requires timely and relevant communication between various settings so that critical information concerning the patient can be shared and acted upon (Castillo, 2023).

The electronic health record (EHR) or other types of health information technology can assist with cross-setting communication. Unfortunately, not all providers, agencies, or organizations utilize the same EHR system or there may be connectivity problems in rural or frontier areas. Additionally, providers in the same setting or system may use different documentation platforms, limiting real-time access to needed patient data. Because of these issues, cross-setting communication may sometimes rely on traditional faxing of large amounts of paper with patient information or e-faxing. This brings in issues such as patient privacy and ensuring information is sent to the correct fax number. Also, the alternate setting may have to scan the data into the EHR rather than input the information into an easily retrievable electronic patient record. Ultimately, if the relevant and necessary information cannot be communicated effectively, the provider on the other end may not receive the information or may miss critical information. Cross-setting communication systems must be in place so that patients know whom to contact if they have questions and so that timely and accurate patient-related information is available when needed by providers. (IOM, 2001).

If cross-setting communication is ineffective, there can be barriers to needed referrals, duplication of interventions or testing, and disagreement on how to address the patient's care plan (Vargas et al., 2020). Relationship-centered care practice can assist with cross-setting communication and building trust and relationships amongst multiple providers and settings. Fostering a spirit of collaboration based on knowledge of what each setting provides and respect for their role in positive patient outcomes can decrease unnecessary resource use and improve patient and provider satisfaction. When communicating across settings, essential clinical information needed to coordinate care between settings must be shared, as well as the care plan, so that the receiving setting or provider understands the sequence of care and when follow-up is needed.

The discharge summary is often the key component of cross-setting communication, but this is one-way communication. There is no closed-loop communication or follow-up with the

Cross-Setting Communication: A Primary Care Provider (PCP) Perspective

"I was inundated with paper being faxed to my office whenever a patient was discharged from the hospital. The patient information would often take several days to be sorted and entered into the patient's record. Sometimes, due to short staffing or the patient load, it may have been a couple of weeks before I could review the information, and a needed follow-up appointment or test had been missed. Having needed appointments or follow-ups communicated more practically and efficiently would be very helpful."

—Dr. G, PCP

patient or provider to ensure critical aspects of the discharge summary are addressed. There is a need for direct communication methods to close the loop, especially if there are pending or follow-up studies, changes in home medication, several readmissions, or situations where the provider/setting is concerned about the patient (Munchhof et al., 2020). Barriers to direct cross-setting communication can include lack of relationship between providers/settings, lack of time to engage in direct communication, inability to connect with the other provider/setting, and the absence of a process or procedure concerning communication across settings (Munchhof et al., 2020). The nurse must advocate for structure or process improvements and changes if communication barriers are found.

Cross-setting communication can be improved by using structured communication tools with consistent content, including concerns and essential and relevant data, engaging the patient and family/caregiver in care planning (so that they are aware of needed follow-up appointments and whom to contact with questions), directly notifying the PCP or appropriate provider of admissions and discharges in the acute care setting, scheduling follow-up tests/appointments, and providing the patient/caregiver a copy of a dated medication list after medication reconciliation, and sharing accountability for follow-up care and testing with the patient and the providers involved (Haas et al., 2014).

Challenging Conversations

When coordinating care, there may be the need for challenging conversations related to the patient's health, treatment options, insurance coverage, or care plan. These conversations may need to occur with the patient, their family/caregiver, or other interprofessional team members. The nurse must possess various knowledge, skills, and attitudes to meet this aspect of communication competency. Understanding the organizational culture is essential to managing challenging conversations. Many organizational systems support pathways or processes such as the ICARE values (integrity, compassion, accountability, respect, and empathy) integrated into their mission, vision, and core values (Smith, 2008). ICARE values outline a framework for addressing concerns and how to address complex or sensitive issues with patients or colleagues. If the organization has identified a pathway or process for challenging conversations, it should be followed. If nurses need support or training on some aspect of the organizationally supported process, they should seek additional learning opportunities.

ICARE Values

Integrity: The quality of possessing and steadfastly adhering to high moral principles or professional standards.

Compassion: Sympathy for the suffering of others, often including a desire to help.

Accountability: Being responsible to someone else or others.

Respect: A feeling or attitude of admiration and deference toward somebody.

Empathy: The ability to identify with and understand another person's feelings or difficulties.

(Smith, 2008, pp. 26–27).

Nursing Presence

The need for relationship-centered and person-centered care is evident in the ICARE values and care coordination practices. The nurse must be able to coordinate care, completing each task required for continuity of care. Still, they also must be able to develop and support a relationship with the patient, their family/caregiver, interprofessional team members, and other stakeholders in the patient's care. **Nursing presence** is essential when managing difficult conversations and engaging in relationship- and person-centered care. It is not easy to communicate with the person you are having a challenging conversation with if you are not listening, not speaking less than the person you are communicating with, and not communicating caring in your words, attitudes, and behaviors (Whittenberg-Lyles et al., 2013). ICARE values support the foundational use of "presence" in nursing practice and communication. "Nursing presence is a concept experienced in the interaction between the nurse and the patient. It is also a situation known and felt more than what is depicted" (Yesilot & Oz, 2016, p. 95).

Nursing presence involves behaviors such as nonverbal communication, tone of voice, or use of touch. Nursing presence also encompasses attitudes that the nurse holds and expresses, such as the belief that the patient has the power to manage their health and to be autonomous in their decision-making. The nurse may view themselves as a change agent to assist the patient in gaining the knowledge and tools they need to be empowered in their healthcare journey. The nurse must also take conscious actions to attend to and monitor the nursing care provided, ensuring the patient's physical, psychological, social, and functional needs are met (Atashzadeh-Shoorideh et al., 2022). Lastly, to be present with the patient, the nurse must consider the "uniqueness of each patient and, in general, the unconditional acceptance of the patient, including the human dignity" (Atashzadeh-Shoorideh et al., 2022, p. 11).

Nursing presence is required when engaging in challenging conversations, as well as an acknowledgment that the conversation is a two-way experience. Each member of the conversation will influence the communication trajectory and outcome. As nurses communicate with and listen to others, they must recognize that all conversation involves interpreting meaning.

Nursing Presence Scale Dimensions

As a critical element of person- and relationship-centered care, it is essential to understand the conceptual components of nursing presence. Atashzadeh-Shoorideh et al. (2022, pp. 12–13) conducted a study to design an itemized scale related to nursing presence. The final scale included coordination of care as one of the scale's four dimensions.

Nursing Presence Scale Dimensions

Dimension 1: Participation and Assistance

Dimension 2: Conscious Focus and Receptive Encounter

Dimension 3: Monitoring and Accountability

Dimension 4: Coordination in Care

Each person in the conversation brings personal experiences, belief systems, and backgrounds that can affect how they express themselves or interpret what someone else is communicating. As the receiver in communication, the nurse must "decode" or interpret the meaning of what is being communicated. The interpreted meaning can often be validated through simple reflection or clarifying questions. This use of reflection and clarifying questions gives voice to the other participant in the conversation, maintains they are the "expert" on themselves and have been "heard."

Additionally, to effectively navigate challenging conversations, it is crucial to recognize how the setting and situation can affect communication interpretation. Suppose a challenging conversation occurs in the hallway of a busy hospital floor. In that case, there will likely be external noise, such as call lights, carts being moved, other conversations, telephones ringing, etc., which can interfere with presence and effective listening and meaning interpretation. The people involved in the challenging conversation may also have internal noise interfering with their ability to listen or interpret meaning. For example, they may have just received bad news about their health condition and cannot be emotionally present in the conversation. The nurse may need to catch up in seeing patients they are assigned during that shift and be thinking ahead about what they will be doing next rather than being present in the conversation. The setting and the conversation participants' situation are crucial to successfully engaging in a challenging conversation. Ensuring that the appropriate people are present is also vital to an effective challenging conversation. This may include the family/caregiver, the PCP, the insurance representative, or some other interprofessional team member. Lastly, there must be the reassurance that patient or colleague concerns related to the challenge or difficulty will be addressed. See Figure 2.5—Meaning Interpretation in the Listening Process.

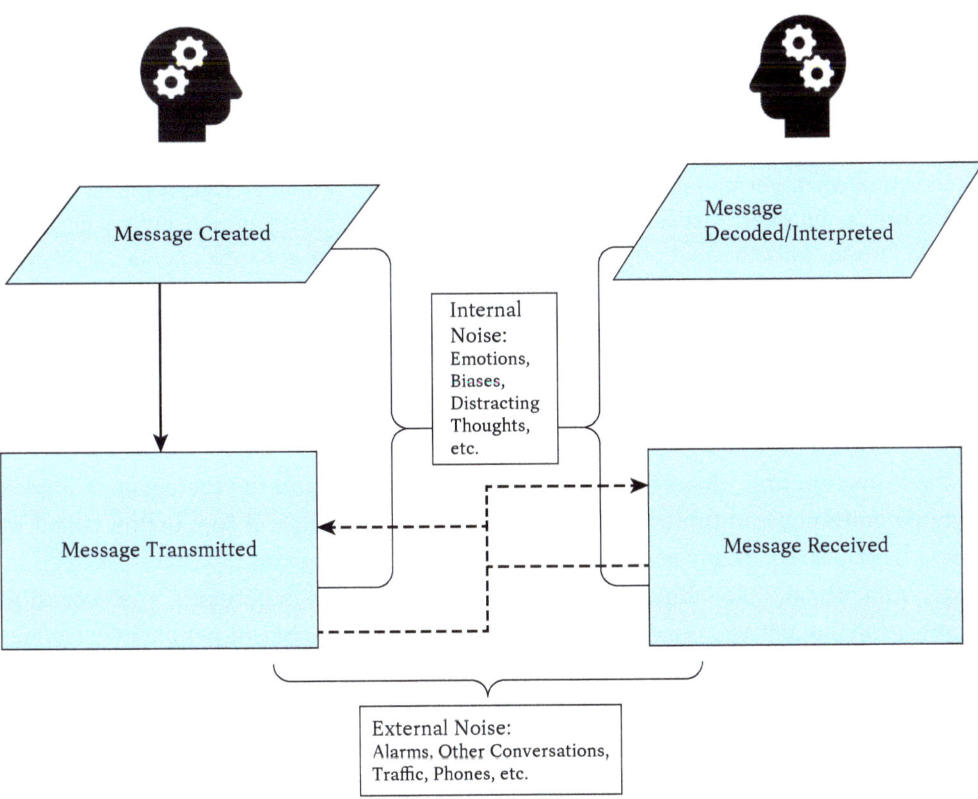

FIGURE 2.5 Meaning Interpretation in the Listening Process

Challenging Conversation Considerations

When engaging in challenging conversations, the nurse must be prepared to have or obtain additional information, actively listen, facilitate emotional reactions, and allow time to process the information. Often, nurses are time-limited and may try to engage in a difficult conversation quickly and then leave, not following up or attending to the patient's or colleague's concerns or emotional reactions. Nurses should utilize **empathetic awareness**, considering how the patient or colleague may process the challenging situation and their emotional responses. For example, the nurse ought to consider whether the other person wanted more information, if follow-up might be needed, or if the issue should be revisited later after the participants have had time to process the information and identify questions or concerns.

Often, challenging conversations elicit emotional responses, and an essential skill in managing these types of conversations may include being present with and witnessing uncomfortable emotions. This includes validating that the other person in the conversation has a right to their emotions and feelings, which are acknowledged. Validating another person's emotions and feelings does not mean the nurse agrees. Instead, it communicates that emotion and feelings exist and are heard and understood.

Empathetic Awareness

Empathy is the ability to recognize emotions and feelings in others. This requires the nurse to be aware of the subtle verbal and nonverbal communication behaviors that signify an emotion or feeling. Additionally, the nurse must be able to take on the other person's perspective, considering how what is being said and what is going on may affect thoughts and feelings. Valuing each other's unique perspectives, acknowledging feelings and thoughts, and approaching the relationship and conversation with openness and respect can enhance a nurse's ability to engage in empathetic awareness.

Interprofessional Practice

With the transition in healthcare models, payment systems, and the increasing complexity of patient conditions and treatments, the days of encouraging and supporting siloed work practices have passed. Today in healthcare, **interprofessional team** practices are seen in all settings, from primary care clinics to hospitals and everywhere in between. The necessity for interprofessional teamwork is evidenced by the increasing number of patients with complex and chronic diseases, the increasing need for healthcare providers to possess specialized skills and knowledge to provide comprehensive care, and the requirement to provide coordinated, quality, continuity of care (Nancarrow et al., 2013). Coordinating care across settings and addressing complex and multiple patients' needs requires effective teamwork (IOM, 2001). This necessitates nurses to be competent in interprofessional care coordination, collaborative practice, and understanding community resources.

Key Tips to Managing Challenging Conversations

1. Utilize organizational communication processes and pathways.
2. Embrace core values such as ICARE values (integrity, compassion, accountability, respect, and empathy).
3. Engage in nursing presence.
4. Acknowledge that communication is a two-way experience.
5. Proactively address any barriers to communication, such as internal or external noise.
6. Recognize the essential role of decoding and constructing meaning in communication.
7. Employ empathetic awareness.
8. Be present and validate emotional responses.

Interprofessional Care Coordination

Interprofessional teamwork has been defined as "A dynamic process involving two or more health professionals with complementary backgrounds and skills, sharing common health goals, and exercising concerted physical and mental effort in assessing, planning, or evaluating patient care" (Xyrichis & Ream, 2008, p. 238). Yet, this definition does not include the patient or their family/caregiver or other members of the team who may not be considered a "health professional" but contribute to the patient care experience through being a key stakeholder, such as an insurance provider, or administrative, support, and ancillary personnel who engage with the patient regularly to promote patient satisfaction and positive outcomes. An interprofessional team is a group of individuals who work together toward a common goal and contribute to the patient's well-being. The interprofessional team includes those directly involved in the patient's care and those who provide support services (Kelly et al., 2018). The team members may include physicians, nurses, social workers, therapists, chaplains, dieticians, pharmacists, community health workers, patient navigators, community liaisons, etc., depending on the patient's needs. Central to the team are the patient and their family/caregiver (Case Management Study Guide, 2023).

The **interprofessional care coordination** offered must be based on care integration. When the interprofessional team needs a high level of collaboration and communication, patient care information is shared to create and implement a comprehensive care plan addressing the patient's physical, psychological, social, and functional needs (American Psychological Association, 2013). For the interprofessional team to work efficiently and constructively to manage the patient's healthcare and needs, shared meanings and processes are required. All interprofessional team members must understand what care coordination is, how continuity of care contributes to positive outcomes, the patient's goals and priorities, and the processes for decision-making and communication (Park et al., 2023).

The care coordinator will consult with other interprofessional team members to address the patient's concerns holistically and in an integrated manner, addressing health and issues such as access to care or social issues that may impact the patient's health. This requires the care coordinator to understand the various roles of the interprofessional team members and when another member with specific expertise or knowledge needs to be added to the team (Fraser et al., 2018). For example, suppose the care coordinator was working with a patient identified as having a risk factor for substance use disorder (SUD). In that case, they may want to engage a clinician specializing in SUD to consult with the team or assess the patient and share assessment findings with the team so that a comprehensive and integrated care plan can be developed.

This model of integrated and interprofessional team practice is often seen in the acute care setting in the form of interprofessional rounds, where the team (physician, nurse practitioner, nurse, pharmacist, physical therapist, social worker, care coordinator, etc.) meets in front of each patient room and discusses the plan of care for the day, addressing any needed changes in treatment, medications, discharge planning, involvement of other professionals, etc. This may also be seen as "huddles" that occur on floors of a hospital or long-term care facility where there is a brief interprofessional team meeting to discuss the day or any specific patient care concerns. In the community, integrated and interprofessional team practice may be seen in

Oregon Wraparound

Oregon has developed a Wraparound process for interprofessional teams to create one care plan for youth and their families involved in multiple systems (Oregon Wraparound, 2023). The Wraparound model involves many aspects of care coordination, including being collaborative, responsive, individualized, and team and outcomes-based.

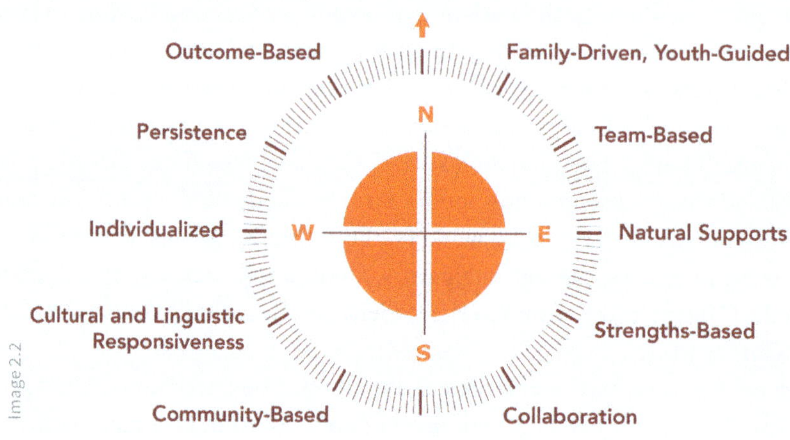

Image 2.2

"wraparound care," where members of a cross-setting interprofessional team meet periodically to review patients that the team members have in common and create or review a comprehensive and individualized care plan. Interprofessional care coordination takes many forms, ensuring that the patient is at the center of care and receives the seven rights of care coordination: (a) right for the patient, (b) right care, (c) right setting, (d) right time, (e) right resources, (f) right transition, and (g) right education.

Interprofessional Collaboration

In the healthcare system, competency in collaboration is essential for interprofessional care coordination practice. Collaborative practice improves health outcomes and encourages optimal healthcare use and delivery. The World Health Organization (WHO) states, "Collaborative practice in health care occurs when multiple health workers from different professional backgrounds provide comprehensive services by working with patients, their families, carers, and communities to deliver the highest quality of care across settings" (2010, p. 13). A direct connection exists between successful interprofessional collaborative practice and the Quintuple Aim. Interprofessional collaborative practice has been shown to positively affect policy development, improve workplace practice, improve patient outcomes, improve patient safety, increase staff satisfaction, and improve access to healthcare services (WHO, 2010).

Sometimes, there may be a misguided idea that collaboration is solely related to working with others as a team. This limited view of collaborative practice does not acknowledge the benefits of shared mental models and expert knowledge in the interprofessional team. A **shared mental model** concerns the common knowledge and understanding that each team member holds related to the team's tasks, skills, organization, processes, expertise, and information and how this knowledge is used to work as a team and meet shared objectives and outcomes (Floren et al., 2018). Shared mental models assist the interprofessional team in working collaboratively, increasing communication and coordination of patient care (Wu, 2018). When considering the interprofessional team in healthcare, shared mental models center on a common understanding of team members' roles and responsibilities, how the team communicates and interacts, and how each member contributes their expertise and knowledge to the global goal of meeting patient needs (Goff-Dupont, 2020). A common understanding or shared mental model of these skills and processes across disciplines improves collaboration. Siloed roles without understanding and respecting each team member's value and contributions will lead to ineffective and dysfunctional interprofessional practice.

Collaboration is broader than the goals of patient care. If an interprofessional team is to work together effectively, they must have a shared purpose and ownership for outcomes. Collaborative practice begins with identifying the team's goals and agreeing to shared accountability for outcomes. Each team member must understand their roles and responsibilities. Each team member, including the patient, brings in expertise, knowledge, and skills that can advance outcomes. To support interprofessional collaborative practice, there must be a foundation of mutual respect for each member's value to the team and respect for their unique contributions and diversity of thought (Babiker et al., 2014). "Collaboration occurs when two or more individuals from different backgrounds with complementary skills interact to create a shared understanding that none had previously possessed or could have come to on their own" (WHO, 2010, p. 36).

Nurses bring tremendous value to the interprofessional collaborative process. Due to the training and education received in nursing programs, nurses are taught to view the patient holistically, seeing the patient and their family/caregivers in the context of their lifestyle, belief systems, and physical, social, and psychological resources and needs. Nurses often create a close connection with the patient and their support system, interacting more frequently with the patient than most interprofessional team members. This allows the nurse to understand the patient and to take on the role of facilitator between interprofessional team members. As nurses often spend a more considerable amount of time with the patient, they also get to know subtle signs or changes in the patient's condition, allowing the nurse to proactively collaborate with the interprofessional team to promote positive outcomes and decrease costs and resource use (Kelly et al., 2018, p. 214).

For example, suppose the nurse care coordinator works with a patient receiving palliative care for a multiple sclerosis (MS) diagnosis. The patient has two children under the age of 10, is married, experiences depression, lives in an older home with three floors with narrow staircases, is very active in their church, and prefers naturopathic approaches to healthcare. The patient is very concerned about financial vulnerability because they have had to quit their job due to the progression of MS and the cost of the medications and care to address symptoms. The patient has multiple needs that cross the health triune, including physical health, mental health, and SDOH factors such as financial insecurity and environment.

In this case, the nurse care coordinator would likely want representation from a social worker (SW), child life specialist, physical therapist (PT), occupational therapist (OT), the PCP and specialist providers, and a chaplain in the interprofessional team. These disciplines have expertise that will contribute to quality care and promote outcomes. The SW may work with the patient and their family on insurance coverage and financial assistance or connect them with support groups. The child life specialist may meet with the children to provide support as they begin to understand the disease process and their mother's prognosis. The PT may assess the home environment to determine if durable medical equipment (DME) or home adaptations are needed. The OT may work with the patient on adaptive tools or techniques for ADLs or IADLs. The PCP and specialist providers may work with the patient and family to find ways to address symptoms through naturopathic methods, and the chaplain may meet with the patient and family to provide spiritual support through the disease process. Moreover, the interprofessional team members can collaborate with each other and contribute their knowledge of the patient's situation and their discipline-specific expertise to the care plan, supporting coordinated care that meets the patient's and their family's holistic needs, promoting patient satisfaction and outcome attainment.

Interprofessional care coordination team collaboration is necessary to ensure care continuity across settings and manage costs and resource use. Nurses are a valuable part of the interprofessional team and must possess competency in collaborative practice to facilitate team functioning and successfully advocate for the patient. Nurses must know the team members' roles and responsibilities and be aware of organizational policies on the interprofessional team and communication practices. Embracing the frameworks of ICARE (integrity, compassion, accountability, respect, and empathy) and person- and relationship-centered care can enhance the interprofessional team's collaborative abilities.

Interprofessional Team Practice Tips

1. Always introduce yourself to the team.
2. Read back/close the communication loop.
3. State the obvious to avoid assumptions.
4. Ask questions, check, and clarify.
5. Delegate tasks to specific people, not to the air.
6. Clarify your role.
7. Use objective (not subjective) language.
8. Learn and use people's names.
9. Be assertive when required.
10. If something doesn't make sense, find out the other person's perspective.
11. Always do a team briefing before starting a team activity, and debrief afterwards.
12. When in conflict, concentrate on "what" is right for the patient, not "who" is right/wrong.

Jayne Josephsen, "Topic: Being an effective team player," *Course: To Err is Human*, p. 5.

Connection with Community Resources

The interprofessional team may include community resource representatives, depending on the patient's needs. When conducting the comprehensive assessment, the psychological and social domains are assessed and critically analyzed for strengths, barriers, and resource needs. Patients often have multiple needs, not only physical health needs. Health is multi-dimensional, and addressing the psychological and social domains and functional abilities is necessary for care coordination and resource management efforts. When conducting the comprehensive assessment, it may become evident that the patient has food scarcity, is at risk for houselessness, has SUD, is experiencing interpersonal violence or abuse, or has financial or health insurance insecurity. These issues could present barriers to implementation or follow-through of care coordination. In care coordination practice, these needs, risks, and gaps in care must be identified, and a proactive plan must be developed to holistically meet the patient's needs (Coyle, 2023).

For example, if the care coordinator were working with a pediatric patient with severe asthma and their family and found they lived in a home without electricity or natural gas, causing the parents to heat the house with kerosene-fueled portable heaters, the child might be at risk for significant exacerbations and poor health outcomes. These types of social needs are actual barriers to health, and even when patients are engaged and motivated to follow the care plan, they may need help. It is essential that when providing care coordination, the nurse is cognizant of community resources available and when to involve representatives of these resources in the interprofessional team.

When engaging community agencies and organizational representatives in the interprofessional team, it is necessary to take a broad view. Community resources may include mental health or substance use clinics, community health clinics, or support groups. They may also include services such as transportation, housing assistance, and food banks. Medicaid, social security, disability, vocational services, and workers' compensation may also need to be involved. Community resources could also include spiritual services from a church, chaplain, or parish. Patients may also have one or more case managers or coordinators in the community related to a disability, mental health issue, or correctional system involvement. Engaging the patient's community-based coordinator or case manager may be essential to creating a comprehensive and appropriate care plan. This may look more like a consultant role on the interprofessional team. Still, as these community roles provide support services to the patient and may have a longer-term involvement with them, it is critical to determine if the patient is receiving these types of services.

Involving community resource representatives in the interprofessional team can assist in creating a more comprehensive care plan that will meet the patient's needs, address socioeconomic status, healthcare access and equity, provide culturally responsive care, and promote positive outcomes while decreasing costs and resource use. As nurses engage with community resource representatives, they learn about the health and needs of their communities, as well as develop relevant and innovative connections, interventions, and solutions to care barriers (Coyle, 2023). Interprofessional teams need to be diverse to meet the patient's holistic needs, and the nurse must educate themselves on the issues and populations in their communities and what resources are available to support patient and community health.

Cultural Application of the Community Resource Connection: A Case Manager's Experience

I had a refugee patient who was a member of the Hmong community. The patient had six children, and during her last pregnancy, the physician became concerned for her health if she had additional children. As a new case manager, I met with the patient with an interpreter and discussed her reproductive health. The patient appeared to agree as the conversation went along, but at the end, refused any pregnancy prevention interventions. The patient, her husband, and the six children lived in a two-bedroom apartment with limited furniture and mattresses. The patient spoke no English, did not drive, and depended on others for transportation and navigating the health and social care system. As the visit occurred, it became evident that the patient's husband was selling drugs from the vehicle parked in front of the residence. The patient shared that one of their children had ingested some "white powder" of the father's and had to be taken to the emergency room for care.

As I left the visit, I was overwhelmed with how to address this patient's issues: overcrowded living conditions, potential poor reproductive health outcomes, lack of ability to navigate the healthcare system, lack of transportation, living amid drug dealing, and potentially severe health and safety outcomes for the children. I contacted the local child protective services agency to report my concerns, and they directed me to contact the Hmong community liaison, who was a lifesaver. I thought I was culturally competent, but I had much to learn about the Hmong community. I also found that the Hmong community has a great support system for its members and provides an invaluable educational service for those who need to know more about the Hmong culture, its strengths, its history, and the resources available to members of the Hmong community.

—J. T., Community Case Manager

Quality Assurance

Assuring quality coordination and continuity of care is a critical competency in care coordination practices. **Quality assurance** focuses on the care coordination process, systematically monitoring the process for gaps or errors and the quality of the care coordination provided (Jevaji, 2016). Ensuring that our care coordination practices promote patient outcomes and that care coordination occurs is integral to the current healthcare climate and payment models. Care coordination has been shown to reduce hospitalizations and emergency room visits. Many payment models provide incentives and penalties related to the length of stay, readmissions, duplicative services, and visits to ambulatory care or the emergency room that are deemed unnecessary (Knickman & Elbel, 2019). Monitoring and evaluating the care coordination provided is critical to ensuring the process meets identified patient and quality outcomes.

Monitoring

Monitoring in care coordination means paying close attention and systematically observing or reviewing the implemented coordination efforts. This could mean following up to ensure that a consult has occurred or communicating updated patient information to an interdisciplinary team member so they can adapt the care provided. Monitoring may also take the form of checking in with the patient or their family/caregiver to ascertain if there have been changes in their needs or care goals (AHRQ, 2018). Monitoring represents proactively reassessing, reanalyzing, and responding to ensure that care coordination interventions effectively address the patient's needs and goals and manage cost and resource use.

The Donabedian model of healthcare quality (structure, process, and outcomes) gives an excellent framework for considering how monitoring fits into quality assurance. "Structures are the setting for care coordination, including physical or organizational aspects; processes are the modes for care coordination; and outcomes include health outcomes or other measurements" (Rural Health Information Hub, 2023a, para. 2). Structural aspects of care coordination practices, such as accessibility to healthcare services, availability of hospitals or primary care providers, financial constraints, and community structure, may affect the quality of healthcare (Lawson & Yazdany, 2012). The care coordinator may implement numerous processes, and these need to be dynamic and responsive to patient and organizational needs. The process can be affected by the experience and training of the nurse providing care coordination and the nurse's knowledge of care coordination-specific quality indicators (Lawson & Yazdany, 2012). The connection between the structure and process of care coordination is directly linked to outcomes. The outcomes may be patient-focused, based on national clinical quality indicators, or organizationally developed outcome goals. Monitoring is central to the process aspect. If there is a lack of monitoring, then care coordination outcomes may not be met. See Figure 2.6 for an example application of the Donabedian model of healthcare quality to monitoring and care coordination practices.

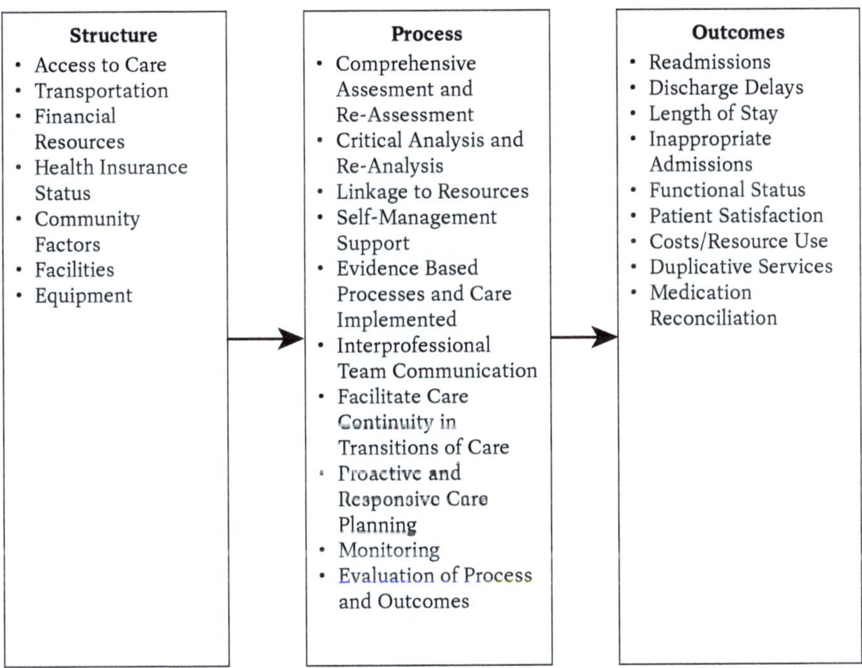

FIGURE 2.6 Example Application of the Donabedian Model to Care Coordination Practice Monitoring

Evaluation

Nurses are often in an ideal position to identify process issues in care coordination practices. As this is the case, they are also in an ideal position to evaluate if their interventions are effective and meet quality indicators and outcomes. Monitoring and evaluation in the quality assurance process are like the pairing of assessment and critical analysis competency. It only assists the patient, outcomes, or the development of evidence-based practice if action is taken after the monitoring process. Suppose the nurse providing care coordination finds that through evaluation of outcomes met or not met, there is a gap in care coordination practice. The gap in process and outcomes attainment needs to be addressed.

Evaluation in care coordination is the critical assessment of the process and interventions and whether they meet identified outcomes (Currie, 2016). The outcomes used for evaluation may vary by setting or type of care coordination offered. An evaluation may examine health outcomes, such as the number of patients with more than one chronic condition, or they may examine costs of care or other measures, such as patient satisfaction, interprofessional team function, or continuity of care delivered. Most quality assurance outcomes evaluated will either focus on the patient or their family or support system's satisfaction or perspectives, how well the interprofessional team functions to meet patient needs, or how the care delivered impacts the organization on a systems level, such as if essential patient information was communicated upon a transition of care (Rural Health Information Hub, 2023b).

Evaluation is the final step in the care coordination process, just as in any nursing care offered. The evaluation phase focuses on the care coordination results and how these have impacted the patient's condition. In the evaluation process, the nurse may consider whether patient goals have been achieved, if gaps in care were addressed, or if other interventions are needed to assist the patient and meet the goals of care. An important aspect of the evaluation process is including the patient and the interprofessional team to ascertain their perspectives and whether they believe outcomes have been met.

Evaluation is an iterative and constant process until patient goals and outcomes are met to the satisfaction of both the patient and the interprofessional team (Haas et al., 2014). Evaluation is a fundamental part of ensuring care coordination interventions provide continuity of care across the continuum and meet patient needs in a relevant and responsive manner. All nursing practice relies on this final aspect of the nursing process to ensure that outcomes are met (Toney-Butler & Thayer, 2022). Like all aspects of the nursing process, evaluation is dynamic, and interventions may need to be reevaluated and adapted frequently to ensure that patient, organizational, and system-level outcomes are met.

What Are Quality Indicators?

"Quality indicators are foundational to quality improvement in health care. They aim to detect how well current systems are working, allow for comparisons between entities that promote shared learning, enable assessments of improvement over time, and improve transparency" (Consortium for Oral Health Systems Integration and Improvement, n.d., para. 1).

CHAPTER SUMMARY

The skills needed to implement care coordination practices and provide continuity of care may vary by setting and type of care coordination offered. However, several foundational competencies exist for care coordination practice across all settings and practice types. Foundational competencies for coordination of care practices include person- and relationship-centered care, advocacy, assessment and critical analysis, communication, interprofessional practice, and quality assurance. Nurses must be aware of their competency levels in these core competency areas related to care coordination and pursue additional learning and training if needed.

Nurses are vital in positively impacting care coordination through competency in person- and relationship-centered care and promoting a partnership in care with the patient and the interprofessional team. Nurses are accountable for engaging in person- and relationship-centered care, realizing that their behaviors are influenced by their thoughts and feelings and influence the behavior of the patient and the interprofessional team. A central competency needed to deliver person- and relationship-centered care is advocacy, which supports the ethical principles of autonomy, beneficence, and fidelity in care coordination practice. As one coordinating care or ensuring continuity of care, the nurse may need to embody moral courage to engage in challenging conversations with respect and empathetic awareness.

Comprehensive assessment and critical analysis competency are central to coordinating care and determining gaps and barriers to care. Addressing the physical, social, and psychological domains and the patient's functional abilities is crucial for a comprehensive assessment. Nurses providing care coordination must take on a global view of the patient and the situation, effectively communicating across settings and collaborating with the patient, their family or support system, the interprofessional team, and community partners.

Valuing individuals' personhood, showing respect, engaging in nursing presence, and being accountable is essential for good care coordination practice. The process of care coordination embraces these values by providing person- and relationship-centered care, advocacy, comprehensive assessment, and critical analysis, communicating across settings and with empathetic awareness, engaging in collaborative interprofessional care coordination, and ultimately engaging in quality assurance of the process and evaluating whether outcomes were met.

CHAPTER 2 GLOSSARY

Competencies: Skill and attitude development through a broad domain knowledge base.

Comprehensive Assessment: Assessment of the physical, social (e.g., lifestyle, economic, cultural factors), psychological domains, and functional abilities of the patient, and includes subjective and objective information.

Cross-Setting Communication: High-level, timely, and relevant communication between settings concerning the patient so that critical information can be shared and acted upon.

Empathetic Awareness: Recognizing and acknowledging others' emotions, feelings, and perspectives with openness and respect.

Functional Abilities: Functional abilities include activities of daily living (ADL) and instrumental activities of daily living (IADL). ADLs, such as eating, dressing, bathing, toileting, etc., affect patients' ability to care for themselves independently. IADLs, such as using the telephone, managing finances, managing medications, etc., affect patients' ability to live independently in their own homes and communities.

Interprofessional Care Coordination: The creation and implementation of a comprehensive care plan addressing physical, psychological, social, and functional needs based upon interprofessional team care integration, collaboration, and communication.

Interprofessional Team: A group working collaboratively, sharing goals, information, and identifying needs to create and implement integrated care and to support patient and resource outcomes.

Moral Courage: When the nurse speaks out and stands up for what they consider ethical and moral actions, even when others or the organization encourage the nurse to conduct themselves differently.

Nursing Presence: The conscious, receptive, and participatory interaction between a nurse and another person, which involves behaviors, attitudes, and actions that support the dignity, value, and unconditional acceptance of the other person.

Quality Assurance: Systematically monitoring processes for quality, gaps, or errors and evaluating if identified patient and quality outcomes are met.

Relationship-Centered Care: Involvement of all persons affiliated with the healthcare experience to build and enhance relationships and health outcomes. Valuing partnership and understanding relationships are co-constructed between the participants with mutual respect and trust.

Shared Mental Model: The common knowledge and understanding each team member holds related to the team's tasks, skills, organization, processes, expertise, and information and how this knowledge is used to work as a team and meet shared objectives and outcomes.

Skills: Abilities and behaviors learned to perform a job that may vary by setting.

DISCUSSION QUESTIONS AND ACTIVITIES

Discussion Questions

1. In your care coordination practice, you may need to discuss challenging or uncomfortable issues with patients concerning their health behaviors or life circumstances. What questions would you ask to illicit essential information and promote dialogue concerning the physical, psychological, and social domains of health? What things might you need to be aware of before addressing a challenging or uncomfortable issue with a patient?

2. Consider a time that you had a challenging conversation and answer the following questions:

    a. What was the situation?

    b. What were you thinking and feeling at the time?

    c. Would you consider the experience bad or good and why?

    d. If you had this conversation again, would you have done anything differently? If so, what would you have done differently and why?

3. Monitoring the care coordination process is an essential component of quality assurance competency. How might you approach monitoring in your care coordination practice? How would you know if your process is effective or ineffective? If you found the process was ineffective, what would you do to address this process issue?

4. Nursing presence involves attitudes and beliefs the nurse holds and expresses. What attitudes and beliefs do you hold that would enhance your ability to engage in nursing presence with your patients? What attitudes and beliefs do you have that might inhibit you from being fully engaged in nursing presence with the patients you care for?

5. After reviewing the competencies for care coordination presented in this chapter, how would you rate your competency level in patient and relationship-centered care, advocacy, assessment and critical analysis, communication, interprofessional practice, and quality assurance? Identify one competency for which you need additional learning/support. What three things can you personally do to enhance your development in this competency?

Activities

1. Consider interprofessional team members you have worked with in your clinical time or workplace. Identify one team member's profession you are unfamiliar with or would like to learn more about. Please write a short essay describing the team members' profession, educational preparation, and expertise they bring to the interprofessional team.

2. Consider the Wraparound model of care. This model is typically used in the community setting for youth involved in multiple systems. How might this model be applied to our healthcare system? Create a concept map applying the Wraparound model to healthcare.

3. Case Study:

As a home health care manager, you have just arrived at your patient's home and find multiple family members in the home. One family member is the patient's daughter, who has just arrived from another state and has not seen the patient in the last year. The daughter is shocked by the patient's condition and demands to know what you are doing to assist the patient. She also wants to know the patient's treatment plan and current medications and tells you that the patient should recover more quickly. The patient's grandson lives in the area and helps care for the patient. He overhears the conversation, becomes agitated, and tells his aunt to leave because he has been taking care of the patient for the last year when no one else would and the recommendations are none of her business. You notice the patient looking down at their lap, fidgeting with their hands, and looking uncomfortable with the conversation.

1. What internal noise may be occurring that might affect this situation?
2. How could nursing presence be used in this situation?
3. What are ways to manage this challenging conversation?

NCLEX STYLE QUESTIONS

Bonnie Smith, a 64-year-old patient hospitalized with diabetic ketoacidosis, is being discharged home from the hospital. The care coordinator has identified that Ms. Smith is at risk for readmission and needs to coordinate the patient's continuity of care with Ms. Smith's primary care provider. (Questions 1 and 3 related to this scenario)

1. What **critical** information should the care coordinator include when communicating with the primary care provider?

   a. Specialist providers, pharmacies, and community support services that the patient has received care from in the last 12 months

   b. The discharge plan, including discharge location

   c. A narrative of why the patient was admitted and what led to the diabetic ketoacidosis event

   d. Discharge summary, including medication reconciliation, follow-up appointments, labs and tests, and discharge instructions

2. During a post-discharge follow-up call with Ms. Smith, the care coordinator finds that Ms. Smith is confused about whom she is supposed to contact concerning her Medicaid application. Ms. Smith indicates that the hospital social worker and the financial advocate discussed this with her before leaving the hospital, but she cannot remember what was said concerning what she was to do once she got home. The care coordinator begins reviewing the patient chart and cannot find notes from the hospital social worker or

financial advocate. Upon further investigation, the care coordinator discovers that those notes are charted on a different system that the care coordinator cannot access. What is the best solution to prevent this information barrier in care coordination?

a. Advocate for the social worker and financial advocate to handwrite or type notes and then have them scanned into the Electronic Health Record (EHR).

b. Advocate for all interprofessional team members to utilize and have access to the same documentation system in the EHR.

c. Advocate for a structured handoff communication system in which the social worker and financial advocate verbally update the care coordinator.

d. Advocate for the patient to contact the social worker and financial advocate directly to clarify any questions.

3. The care coordinator has identified that Ms. Smith needs help with transportation to medical appointments, which has contributed to Ms. Smith missing some follow-up appointments. What is the best action for the care coordinator to take for Ms. Smith to address this issue?

a. Let Ms. Smith know that if she continues to miss follow-up appointments, her provider may "fire" her and refuse to see her again.

b. Give Ms. Smith brochures on transportation options in the community with her discharge information.

c. Mail Ms. Smith information on transportation services to her home address as a follow-up.

d. Link Ms. Smith to community transportation resources and provide a handoff to the community resource to support Ms. Smith in accessing transportation to follow-up appointments.

4. Which of the following best describes person-centered care?

a. The care encourages each interprofessional team member to contribute only to goals in their area of expertise.

b. The care supports having family or caregivers speak for patients concerning their healthcare if they take narcotics or medications that may cause drowsiness.

c. The care integrates and responds to the patient's values, preferences, and goals.

d. The care ensures that the patient's preferences guide the provider's clinical decision-making.

5. During the morning huddle, the team discusses patients' care plans and needs for the day. The care coordinator present knows that these types of huddles are good representations of which type of practice:

   a. Clinical practice

   b. Nursing practice

   c. Interprofessional practice

   d. Patient-centered care practice

6. Which of the following ethical principles does advocacy encompass? (Select all that apply.)

   a. Veracity

   b. Beneficence

   c. Fidelity

   d. Nonmaleficence

7. Moral courage can be required in nursing practice. Which acronym can guide nurses as they navigate dilemmas requiring moral courage?

   a. STAT

   b. ICARE

   c. IPE

   d. CODE

8. What are the outcomes of a comprehensive assessment?

   a. Care plan development

   b. Discovery of gaps in care

   c. Interventions identified

   d. All of these

9. When conducting a comprehensive assessment, the patient reports that their son purchased a new cellular phone for them. However, they prefer to avoid using it because they cannot see the keys very well, they need help remembering how to use the phone, and when they try, it does not seem to work. This patient is having difficulty with which of the following?

a. Instrumental activities of daily living

b. Activities of daily living

c. Decision-making capacity

d. Sensory decline

10. Mr. Roach was admitted for a right hip open reduction internal fixation (ORIF) surgery after an unwitnessed fall in his home. The physical therapist recommends that Mr. Roach be discharged to a rehabilitation center. When the care coordinator discusses which rehabilitation center he would like to go to, he indicates he will only go to Sunnyside Rehabilitation and is not interested in considering any other place. The care coordinator discovers that Mr. Roach's insurance has not contracted with Sunnyside Rehabilitation, and he will need to go to an alternate facility. Which communication technique would be most helpful as the care coordinator approaches this potentially difficult conversation?

    a. Inform Mr. Roach that he has no choice as he needs rehabilitation and must go to a different facility contracted by his insurance.

    b. Discuss the situation with Mr. Roach after he has completed physical therapy, as he will be tired and less likely to be argumentative.

    c. Present Mr. Roach the insurance company's response, acknowledging his disappointment at the inability to discharge to his first facility choice.

    d. Request that the care coordinator you are training let Mr. Roach know the insurance company's response because this will be good experience for them in managing difficult conversations.

11. The care coordinator is working with the family of a patient who has advanced Parkinson's disease and is now exhibiting hallucinations. The patient's spouse/caregiver appears exhausted and states "I cannot deal with this anymore," becoming visibly upset. The patient's adult children live out of state, except for one son who has a substance use disorder. The patient's spouse states they cannot rely on their son as they do not always know how to contact him. Which care coordination intervention would be the most helpful for this family?

    a. Set up a family meeting, including the son in town, and let him know that he must assist his parents.

    b. Recommend that the spouse place the patient in a long-term care facility so they do not have to provide care any longer.

    c. Connect the spouse with support groups and community services for caregivers and those with Parkinson's.

    d. Recommend a therapist for the spouse to see the value of caregiving.

12. Effective interprofessional collaboration requires the interprofessional team to have which of the following? (Select all that apply.)

    a. Shared accountability for outcomes

    b. Mutual respect for each other's value and expertise

    c. Understanding of roles and responsibilities

    d. Similar skills and backgrounds

13. Which of the following are examples of the "structure" component of the Donabedian model applied to care coordination practice?

    a. Readmission rates

    b. Interprofessional team communication

    c. Access to healthcare

    d. None of the above

14. The care coordinator explains to a new care coordinator "evaluation" as it applies to quality assurance. Which is the best explanation of "evaluation"?

    a. Evaluation occurs at the end of the care coordination, examining the process and looking for areas of improvement.

    b. Evaluation is an iterative and constant process ensuring patient goals and outcomes are met.

    c. Evaluation occurs when gaps in care are identified.

    d. Evaluation considers only system-level outcomes.

15. Fundamental care coordination competencies include which of the following? (Select all that apply.)

    a. Diagnosis

    b. Advocacy

    c. Communication

    d. Patient-centered care

REFERENCES

Abbasinia, M., Ahmadi, F., & Kazemnejad, A. (2020). Patient advocacy in nursing: A concept analysis. *Nursing Ethics, 27*(1), 141–151. https://doi.org/10.1177/0969733019832950

Agency for Healthcare Research and Quality (AHRQ), (2014). *Care coordination measures atlas update: Chapter 3 care coordination measurement framework*. https://www.ahrq.gov/ncepcr/care/coordination/atlas/chapter3.html

Agency for Healthcare Research and Quality (AHRQ). (2018). *Care coordination*. https://www.ahrq.gov/ncepcr/care/coordination.html

American Association of Colleges of Nursing (AACN). (n.d.). *Moral courage*. https://www.aacnnursing.org/5b-tool-kit/themes/moral-courage

American Association of Colleges of Nursing (AACN). (2021). *The Essentials: Core competencies for professional nursing education*. https://www.aacnnursing.org/Portals/42/AcademicNursing/pdf/Essentials-2021.pdf

American Nurses Association (ANA). (2015). *Code of ethics for nurses with interpretive statements*. American Nurses Association.

American Nurses Association (ANA). (2021). *Nursing: Scope and standards of practice* (4th ed.). American Nurses Association.

American Psychological Association. (2013). *Integrated health care*. https://www.apa.org/health/integrated-health-care

Atashzadeh-Shoorideh, F., Parvizy, S., Hosseini, M., Raziani, Y., & Mohammadipour, F. (2022). Developing and validating the nursing presence scale for hospitalized patients. *BMC Nursing, 21*(1), 1–16. DOI: 10.1186/s12912-022-00896-0

Babiker, A., El Husseini, M., Al Nemri, A., Al Frayh, A., Al Juryyan, N., Faki, M. O., Assiri, A., Al Saadi, M., Shaikh, F., & Al Zamil, F. (2014). Health care professional development: Working as a team to improve patient care. *Sudanese Journal of Paediatrics, 14*(2), 9–16. https://www.ncbi.nlm.nih.gov/pmc/articles/PMC4949805/

Bandura, A. (1978). The self system in reciprocal determinism. *American Psychologist, 33*(4), 344–358. https://doi.org/10.1037/0003-066X.33.4.344

Beach, M. C., Inui, T., & Relationship-Centered Care Research Network (2006). Relationship-centered care. A constructive reframing. *Journal of General Internal Medicine, 21,* (Suppl 1), S3–S8. https://doi.org/10.1111/j.1525-1497.2006.00302.x

Bell, S. K., Roche, S. D., Mueller A., O'Reilly, K., Sarnoff, B., Sands, K., Talmor, D., & Brown, S. M. (2018). Speaking up about care concerns in the ICU: Patient and family experiences, attitudes and perceived barriers. *BMJ Quality & Safety, 27*(11), 928–936. DOI:10.1136/bmjqs-2017-007525

Berwick, D. M. (2002). *Escape fire: Lessons for the future of health care*. The Commonwealth Fund. https://www.commonwealthfund.org/sites/default/files/documents/___media_files_publications_other_2002_nov_escape_fire__lessons_for_the_future_of_health_care_berwick_escapefire_563_pdf.pdf

Case Management Study Guide. (2023). *Interdisciplinary care team (ICT)*. https://casemanagementstudyguide.com/ccm-knowledge-domains/healthcare-management-delivery/interdisciplinary-care-team-ict/

Castillo, L. (2023). The three C's of cross-continuum care coordination. *HIT Leaders and News*. https://us.hitleaders.news/the-three-cs-of-cross-continuum-care-coordination/

Centers for Medicare & Medicaid Services (CMS). (n.d.). *Person-centered care*. https://innovation.cms.gov/key-concept/person-centered-care#main-content

Consortium for Oral Health Systems Integration and Improvement. (n.d.). Oral health quality indicators for the maternal and child health (MCH) population. *National Maternal and Child Oral Health Resource Center Georgetown University*. https://www.mchoralhealth.org/cohsii/indicators/purpose.php

Coyle, S. (2023). Interprofessional practice in community outreach—health crisis creates new challenges. *Social Work Today, 20*(3), 12. https://www.socialworktoday.com/archive/MJ20p12.shtml

Currie, C. (2016). Study design for assessing effectiveness, efficiency and acceptability of services including measures of structure, process, service quality, and outcome of health care. *HealthKnowledge*. https://www.healthknowledge.org.uk/public-health-textbook/research-methods/1c-health-care-evaluation-health-care-assessment/study-design-assessing-effectiveness

Floren, L. C., Donesky, D., Whitaker, E., Irby, D., ten Cate, O., & O'Brien, B. C. (2018). Are we on the same page? Shared mental models to support clinical teamwork among health professions learners: A scoping review. *Academic Medicine 93*(3), 498–509. https://doi.org/10.1097/ACM.0000000000002019

Fraser, K., Lisa, G. B., Laing, D., Lai, J., & Punjani, N. S. (2018). Case manager resource allocation decision-making for adult home care clients: With comparisons to a high needs pediatric home care clients. *Home Health Care Management & Practice, 30*(4), 164–174. https://doi.org/10.1177/1084822318779371

Goff-Dupont, S. (2020). How to boost your team's success with shared mental models. *Work Life.* https://www.atlassian.com/blog/teamwork/shared-mental-models-improve-team-performance

Gross, M. (2005). The impact of low-level skills on information-seeking behavior: Implications of competency theory for research and practice. *Reference & User Services Quarterly, 45*(2), 155–162. https://www.researchgate.net/publication/289559530_The_impact_of_low-level_skills_on_information-seeking_behavior

Haas, S. A., Swan, B. A., & Haynes, T. S. (2014). *Care coordination and transition management core curriculum.* American Academy of Ambulatory Care Nursing.

Heath, S. (2018, July 23). Understanding the power hierarchy in patient-provider relationships. *PatientEngagementHIT.* https://patientengagementhit.com/news/understanding-the-power-hierarchy-in-patient-provider-relationships

Institute of Medicine (IOM). (2001). *Crossing the quality chasm: A new health system for the 21st century.* National Academy Press.

Institute of Medicine (US) Committee on the Health Professions Education Summit (IOM) (2003). The Core Competencies Needed for Health Care Professionals. In Greiner, A. C. & Knebel, E. (Eds.) *Health Professions Education: A bridge to quality.* National Academies Press. https://www.ncbi.nlm.nih.gov/books/NBK221519/

Jevaji, S. (2016). *The Q series: What is health care quality assurance?* National Committee for Quality Assurance. https://www.ncqa.org/blog/the-q-series-what-is-health-care-quality-assurance/

John Hopkins Medicine Newsroom (2018, May 18). *Words matter: Stigmatizing language in medical records may affect the care a patient receives.* https://www.hopkinsmedicine.org/news/newsroom/news-releases/words-matter-stigmatizing-language-in-medical-records-may-affect-the-care-a-patient-receives

Kelly, P., Vottero, B. A., & Christie-McAuliffe, C. A. (2018). *Introduction to quality and safety education for nurses: Core competencies for nursing leadership and management* (2nd ed.). Springer Publishing Company.

Knickman, J. R., & Elbel, B. (Eds.). (2019). *Jonas & Kovner's health care delivery in the United States* (12th ed.). Springer Publishing Company.

Kuipers, S. J., Cramm, J. M., & Nieboer, A. P. (2019). The importance of patient-centered care and co-creation of care for satisfaction with care and physical and social well-being of patients with multi-morbidity in the primary care setting. *BMC Health Services Research, 19*(13), 1–9. https://doi.org/10.1186/s12913-018-3818-y

Lachman, V. D. (2010, Sept. 30). Strategies necessary for moral courage. *OJIN: The Online Journal of Issues in Nursing, 15*(3), 1–12. DOI:10.3912/OJIN.Vol15No03Man03

Lawson, E. F., & Yazdany, J. (2012). Healthcare quality in systemic lupus erythematosus: Using Donabedian's conceptual framework to understand what we know. *International Journal of Clinical Rheumatology, 7*(1), 95–107. https://doi.org/10.2217/ijr.11.65

Munchhof, A., Gruber, R., Lane, K. A., Bo, N., & Rattray, N. A. (2020). Beyond discharge summaries: Communication preferences in care transitions between hospitalists and primary care providers using electronic medical records. *Journal of General Internal Medicine, 35,* 1789–1796. https://doi.org/10.1007/s11606-020-05786-2

Nancarrow, S. A., Booth, A., Ariss, S., Smith, T., Enderby, P., & Roots, A. (2013). Ten principles of good interdisciplinary team work. *Human Resources for Health, 11*(19), 1–11. https://doi.org/10.1186/1478-4491-11-19

Oregon Wraparound. (2023). *About Oregon wraparound.* https://oregonwraparound.org/about/

Park, A. I., Lansigan, F., Kong, L., O'Brien, J. G., Lastrilla, P. C., & Nagle, J. (2023). Nurse-driven interprofessional rounds: Improving care coordination and length of stay. *Clinical Journal of Oncology Nursing, 27*(1), 40–46. https://doi.org/10.1188/23.CJON.40-46

Raney, J., Pal, R., Lee, T., Saenz, S. R., Bhushan, D., Leahy, P., Johnson, C., Kapphahn, C., Gisondi, M. A., & Hoang, K. (2021). Words matter: An antibias workshop for health care professionals to reduce stigmatizing language. *MedEdPORTAL 17*(11115), 1–6. https://doi.org/10.15766/mep_2374-8265.11115

Rural Health Information Hub. (2023a). *Evaluation frameworks.* https://www.ruralhealthinfo.org/toolkits/care-coordination/5/evaluation-frameworks

Rural Health Information Hub. (2023b). *Evaluation measures.* https://www.ruralhealthinfo.org/toolkits/care-coordination/5/evaluation-measures

Schraeder, C. & Shelton, P. (2011). *Comprehensive care coordination for chronically ill adults.* Wiley-Blackwell.

Smith, M. (2008). *Back to ICARE: Extending the reach of the ICARE philosophy.* http://www.icarevalues.org/December%202008%20EMS%20Mag%20Article.pdf

Timmins F. (2006). Critical practice in nursing care: Analysis, action and reflexivity. *Nursing Standard, 20*(39), 49–54. https://doi.org/10.7748/ns2006.06.20.39.49.c4172

Toney-Butler, T. J., & Thayer, J. M. (2022). *Nursing process.* StatPearls Publishing https://www.ncbi.nlm.nih.gov/books/NBK499937/

Vargas, I., Eguiguren, P., Mogollón-Pérez, A. S., Samico, I., Bertolotto, F., López-Vázquez, J., & Vázquez, M. L. (2020). Can care coordination across levels be improved through the implementation of participatory action research interventions? Outcomes and conditions for sustaining changes in five Latin American countries. *BMC Health Services Research, 20*(941), 1–16. https://doi.org/10.1186/s12913-020-05781-7

Whittenberg-Lyles, E., Goldsmith, J., Ferrell, B., & Ragan, S. L. (2013). *Communication in palliative nursing.* Oxford.

World Health Organization (WHO). (2010). *Framework for action on interprofessional education & collaborative practice.* https://www.who.int/publications/i/item/framework-for-action-on-interprofessional-education-collaborative-practice

World Health Organization (WHO). (2012). *Being an effective team player.* https://cdn.who.int/media/docs/default-source/patient-safety/curriculum-guide/resources/ps-curr-handouts/course04_handout_being-an-effective-team-player-.pdf?sfvrsn=50aecf5a_9&download=true

Wu, A. W. (2018). Reaching common ground: The role of shared mental models in patient safety. *Journal of Patient Safety and Risk Management, 23*(5), 183–184. https://doi.org/10.1177/251604351880532

Xyrichis, A., & Ream, E. (2008). Teamwork: A concept analysis. *Journal of Advanced Nursing, 61*(2), 232–241. https://doi.org/10.1111/j.1365-2648.2007.04496.x

Yesilot, S. B., & Oz, F. (2016). Nursing presence: A theoretical overview. *Journal of Psychiatric Nursing, 7*(2), 94–99. https://jag.journalagent.com/phd/pdfs/PHD_7_2_94_99%5BA%5D.pdf

Credits

Fig. 2.1: Source: https://www.ncbi.nlm.nih.gov/books/NBK221519.

Fig. 2.3a: Copyright © 2016 Depositphotos/monkeybusiness.

IMG 2.1: CMS.gov, https://www.cms.gov/priorities/innovation/key-concepts/person-centered-care, 2022.

Fig. 2.5a: Source: Copyright © by Microsoft.

IMG 2.2: Source: https://oregonwraparound.org/about/.

Fig. 2.6: Adapted from Erica F. Lawson and Jinoos Yazdany, "Healthcare Quality in Systemic Lupus Erythematosus: Using Donabedian's Conceptual Framework to Understand What We Know," *International Journal of Clinical Rheumatology*, vol. 7, no. 1, 2012.

CHAPTER 3

Care Coordination in Nursing Practice

LEARNING OBJECTIVES

1. Compare care coordination principles to the nursing standards of practice.
2. Apply the nursing process to care coordination practice.
3. Examine care coordination practice from initial assessment to evaluation.
4. Explore the health and regulatory system's impact on care coordination practice.

KEY TERMS

- anticipatory guidance
- care coordination care plan
- community paramedicine
- disease model of healthcare
- evidence-based practice
- fragmented care
- guiding principles
- muda
- multidimensional healthcare model
- pace the case
- regulatory and quality measures
- strength-based diagnosis
- unlicensed personnel

Introduction

The nursing process has developed to integrate the role expansion of nurses who work to their full licensure and training. It has also begun transitioning away from the **disease model of healthcare** that has been so prevalent. The disease model of healthcare is characterized by focusing on signs, symptoms, and diagnosis of the disease and then treatment. The emphasis has been on illness and typically did not address patient strengths, resources, or preventative healthcare and wellness. This traditional healthcare model worked for patients with acute conditions that resolved with treatment (Agusti, 2018). But today's patient population often has multidimensional needs, rather than one specific disease-based condition.

These needs frequently involve health issues, symptom management, mental health, and socioeconomic conditions. To address these multidimensional aspects of health, the nurse must have insight into the patient's strengths and resources. Information such as what has worked for the patient before, what sort of support systems are in place, what resources the community has, and which resources the patient already has accessed is essential to coordinate care effectively. A **multidimensional healthcare model** is strength-based and meets the multidimensional aspects of health, including physical health—preventative, acute, and chronic health—mental health—substance use and emotional health—and social determinants of health (SDOH)—healthcare quality, access, and equity. A variety of nursing theories support a multidimensional healthcare model, such as Neuman's systems theory and Peplau's theory of interpersonal relations. The intersection of nursing theory, care coordination guiding principles, and the nursing process provides a solid foundation for the advancement of care coordination practice, which, in turn, provides for multidimensional healthcare needs.

The classic nursing process taught in the past—assessment, diagnosis, planning, implementation, and evaluation or ADPIE—has transformed in the latest version of the American Nurses Association (ANA) *Scope and Standards of Practice* (4th ed.). The five-step nursing process has now advanced to a six-step process with two sub-steps in the implementation phase (2021). The standards of practice for the nursing process reflect the transformation of our healthcare system, the need for person-centered care to address healthcare accessibility, equity, and outcomes, and the expanding role of the nurse in meeting the needs of the patient in a multidimensional and holistic manner.

The ANA's standards for professional nursing practice now include assessment, diagnosis, outcomes identification, planning, implementation (with coordination of care and health teaching and health promotion as sub-steps), and evaluation or ADOPIE (ANA, 2021). Integrating the nursing process is foundational for care coordination practice. Each nursing process step must be performed to achieve identified outcomes and deliver person-centered care. As the care coordinating nurse begins the assessment step, they will collect pertinent data and information about the patient, their support system, and their life situation from various sources. Critical analysis of the assessment data assists in clinical judgment and the development of strength-based nursing diagnoses, which direct care planning and outcomes identification. A solid assessment and diagnosis foundation helps establish a care plan with person-centered and relevant outcomes.

Diagnosis, outcomes identification, and care planning in care coordination are collaborative and involve the interprofessional team, patient, and support system. The collaborative care planning process focuses on the best way to promote outcomes attainment and implementation of the plan of care. Through the implementation process, person- and relationship-centered actions are taken to coordinate care, provide health teaching and health promotion, troubleshoot barriers to transitions in care, and manage resources. The care coordination plan of care may be adjusted to ensure continuity of care and outcomes achievement by analyzing and evaluating the nursing process and attainment of identified patient outcomes, measures, and benchmarks. See Table 3.1 for an example of nursing standards of practice applied to care coordination practice.

TABLE 3.1 Nursing Standards of Practice Applied to Care Coordination Practice

Standard	Care Coordination Application
Standard 1: Assessment	Collection of pertinent data and information concerning the patient, their support system, or situation.
Standard 2: Diagnosis	Critical analysis of assessment and other available data leading to clinical judgment and strength-based care planning and nursing diagnoses.
Standard 3: Outcomes Identification	Identification and development of care outcomes that are person-centered, individualized, and relevant to the patient, their support system, and the situation.
Standard 4: Planning	Engagement in collaborative interprofessional care planning, strategizing, and coordination of care so that identified outcomes can be achieved
Standard 5: Implementation	Actions taken to implement the plan of care, address patient and support system preferences, troubleshoot barriers to transitions, and manage resources, ensuring identified outcomes are met.
Standard 5a: Coordination of Care	Care is coordinated with the interprofessional team, community providers, the patient, and their support system to ensure a successful transition in care and that health system and regulatory requirements and measures are met.
Standard 5b: Health Teaching and Health Promotion	Person-centered health teaching is provided to promote patient engagement and activation in self-management of health and promotion of proactive health and wellness practices.
Standard 6: Evaluation	Identified patient outcomes, regulatory and quality measures, and benchmarks data is collected and analyzed to determine attainment. Quality improvement processes or plan of care adjustments are enacted as needed to ensure continuity of patient care and outcome attainment.

(ANA, 2021, pp. 75–107)

Adding the outcomes identification step and the sub-steps of coordination of care, health teaching, and health promotion are critical for addressing the Quintuple Aim, health system, and regulatory measures. By applying the nursing process of ADOPIE, nurses can provide person-centered care that meets identified outcomes, delivers effective health teaching and health promotion, and safeguards the patient through effective coordination and continuity of care, ensuring costs are managed and resources are utilized thoughtfully. As care coordination processes are applied to the standards of nursing practice, we can see that nurses universally have a role and duty to implement a comprehensive nursing process that addresses these additional steps in the nursing standards of practice.

Nursing Theory Application to Care Coordination

The primary function of managing patient care through person-centered care and information sharing is to deliver integrated, quality, safe, and cost-effective care. This requires a broad view of care coordination and the application of a variety of nursing theories in conjunction with the nursing process. Care coordination is based on structure and processes across the continuum of care and a collaborative and relational approach, which are also essential to nursing practice (Hynes & Thomas, 2023). Because of this, several nursing theories support care coordination practice. Three nursing theories directly apply to person-centered care and address barriers to successful transitions of care and self-management of health. These are Neuman's systems theory, Orem's self-care framework, and Peplau's interpersonal theory. These theories are not an all-inclusive list of nursing theory applications, but they offer insight into the complementary nature of nursing theory and care coordination practice.

Neuman's systems theory is very relevant when considering the care coordination foundation of person-centered care and the multidimensional aspects of health. Neuman's systems model is based on a belief in wholism and the dynamic interrelationship of health and wellness with the patient's physiological, psychological, sociocultural, developmental, and spiritual systems (Fawcett, 2005). Neuman's model calls for nurses to engage in person-centered care by partnering with the patient to determine priorities, goals, and care outcomes. The nurse's role is to identify factors that affect health and then collaborate with the patient concerning health management to achieve optimal wellness (Fawcett, 2005). This points to the importance of the nurse–patient relationship for integrated care delivery and ensures that the patient is receiving the right care for them.

Orem's self-care framework also has significant application in care coordination. One fundamental right of care coordination is that of education to support the self-management of health. This also contributes to using the right resources, offering healthcare at the right time, and ensuring the right care is given. Central aspects of Orem's self-care framework are the beliefs that patients may need support from social or healthcare services and resources to promote self-care and that adult patients have the right and responsibility to care for themselves (Fawcett, 2005). However, what may be the most essential aspect of the self-care framework is the connection of care coordination with the health system, the appropriate use of resources, and the need to minimize psychological and physical stress for patients (Fawcett, 2005). Through the integration of care coordination in all nursing practices, self-management of health can be supported by addressing needed resource connections and supporting well-being.

Peplau's theory of interpersonal relations creates a foundation for care coordination practice in relationship-centered care and the dynamic interaction between the care coordination nurse and the patient. This theory also acknowledges that the nurse cannot change the patient but can create a respectful and educational relationship that supports problem solving and relationship-based care (Fawcett, 2005). Research has shown that implementing Peplau's interpersonal theory in communication systems and skills and working through the phases of the nurse–patient relationship from building a trusting relationship to developing a care plan, and then delivering education, support, and follow-up, patient satisfaction and quality of care can be increased (Fathidokht et al., 2023).

It is evident that care coordination is a critical need in the health system and can decrease fragmented care and adverse patient outcomes. It is also clear that there are many aspects of health and wellness that nurses can positively impact. Many nursing theories can be applied to care coordination practice, depending on the patient population, goals, and needed outcomes. Nurses are integral to implementing responsive and effective care coordination across the continuum of care and within nursing theoretical frameworks.

Guiding Principles of Care Coordination

Nurses must also base their care coordination interventions on principles that guide care coordination practice. Even with excellent care planning that addresses patient preferences and supports interpersonal and relational practice and self-management of health, circumstances, barriers, and communication challenges can affect coordination and continuity of care. In these situations, the nurse must revisit foundational guiding principles of care coordination to provide direction and determine appropriate changes to their practice.

Guiding principles are expressions of core care coordination values, such as the seven rights of care coordination: (a) the care plan is right for the patient, (b) the right care is received, (c) in the right setting, (d) at the right time, (e) with the right resources, (f) the right transition occurs, and (g) the right education is provided. They are standards of how care coordination should be implemented or a lens through which the nurse can examine the situation and guide judgment regarding care coordination. Several ethical elements underlie these guiding principles, such as advocacy, patient autonomy, and collaborative practice.

The provision of advocacy, which nurtures patient autonomy and person and relationship-centered care, is central to all guiding principles and is the basis for ensuring that the care coordination provided supports interpersonal, accessible, evidence-based, and appropriate care offered in the least restrictive and resource-intensive environment. Through proactive and responsive care coordination, barriers to care can be addressed, integrated care delivered, and education and support offered to enhance patient engagement and activation in their healthcare. See Table 3.2 for an example of care coordination rights paired with care coordination guiding principles.

TABLE 3.2 Care Coordination Rights and Guiding Principles

Core Value/Care Coordination Right	Guiding Principle
Right for the patient	Proactive advocacy and care planning are provided nurturing patient autonomy and a person and relationship-centered model involving the interprofessional team.
Right care received	Interventions, coordination, and education offered are evidence-based and care is provided in the least restrictive environment, respecting patient preferences and goals of care.
Right setting	Interventions are appropriately offered in the least resource-intensive level of care and setting.

Right time	Accessible care is provided in a timely manner, proactively addressing healthcare issues, and offering health promotion and wellness activities and education. Accountability for outcomes and delivery of care is shared amongst the interprofessional team.
Right resources	Dynamic coordinated care planning, which addresses gaps/barriers to care, and patient needs is provided, monitored, and follow-up is offered to improve outcomes and appropriately utilize resources and manage costs.
Right transition	Integrated care is sustained based on collegial collaboration and communication of essential information to the patient/support system, interprofessional team, and community resources/providers, ensuring transitions in care meet identified patient needs, preferences, and outcomes.
Right education	Proactive identification of options and care goals is provided through health self-management strategies and education that promote autonomous decision-making and patient engagement and activation.

(Agency for Healthcare Research and Quality (AHRQ), 2018; Finkelman (2016); Johns Hopkins Medicine Alliance for Patients, 2023)

For example, consider the following situation: The attending provider contacts a care coordinator nurse to facilitate a patient's discharge to a skilled nursing facility (SNF). The nurse knows the patient has Medicaid, so they will need a Preadmission Screening and Resident Review (PASRR) by the state's health and welfare office before being admitted to the SNF. The nurse care coordinator tells the provider that the patient cannot be discharged that day; they will begin working on discharge planning, but it may be a couple days before the patient can be discharged. The provider disagrees with this assessment, calls the SNF for direct admission, and is told by the nurse on call at the facility that it is okay to send the patient. The provider then calls the care coordinating nurse and says they have arranged for the patient to be accepted by the SNF, and the patient will be leaving for the facility later that afternoon. Where in this situation did the guiding principle of "Integrated care is sustained based on collegial collaboration and communication of essential information ..." go wrong?

Challenges to coordination and continuity of care should be met by reviewing the guiding principles, determining if any gaps in care are causing the guiding principle be unmet, and engaging with the interprofessional team for solution development. This may be an ongoing process that will need revisiting regularly with the interprofessional team, the patient, and their support system to find solutions for significant challenges to coordination and continuity of care. In the situation described, the care coordinating nurse would then need to explain and educate the provider on the regulatory guidelines for skilled nursing admissions and PASRRs in their state and, in the future, make sure that this essential information is communicated early in the care transition process.

If the care coordinating nurse had passed this vital information to the provider early on, community resources such as the skilled nursing facility would not have been prematurely involved in the transition process. Consider if the patient had been sent to the skilled nursing facility for admission, where the admitting facility nurse discovered they could not accept the

Preadmission Screening and Resident Review (PASRR)

The Preadmission Screening and Resident Review (PASRR) is a federal requirement for Medicaid-certified nursing facilities to ensure that patients are not placed inappropriately in skilled nursing facilities for long-term care. There are two levels of the PASRR. Level 1 PASRR evaluates whether the patient has a serious mental illness or intellectual disability. Level 2 PASRR determines the need and appropriate setting and offers plan of care recommendations. The purpose of the PASRR is to ensure that those with a serious mental illness or intellectual disability are in the most appropriate care setting and receiving needed specialized services. The PASRR includes questions concerning diagnoses, symptoms, functional level, and psychiatric or dementia-related medications (Medicaid.gov, n.d.).

patient due to the lack of a PASRR. This likely would lead to the patient being sent back to the discharging acute care facility and what might be considered an all-cause 30-day readmission for regulatory and quality measures purposes.

ADOPIE and Care Coordination Practice

Care coordination is central to today's nursing practice standards and our transforming healthcare system, and essential for meeting the Quintuple Aim. Yet nurses may not see how care coordination translates into their daily nursing practice. Nurses may wonder what they are assessing for in the coordination of care, what nursing diagnosis would be appropriate, and how they will know if their care coordination interventions meet identified outcomes. When examining the nursing process in care coordination, it becomes apparent that its stepwise, yet responsive nature lends itself to the coordination of care practices. Integrating all the steps of the nursing process into care coordination practice produces effective, efficient, and successful coordination and continuity of care. Let's consider each step separately.

Assessment

Assessment in care coordination refers to collecting pertinent data and information concerning the patient, their support system, or their situation. This could be done during an in-person, telephone, or video interview, through an electronic health record (EHR) review, or by examination of other relevant information. Assessment is crucial in meeting the seven rights of care coordination and several guiding principles. The assessment is not only needs-based, it is comprehensive. Care coordination needs are determined using a global framework, such as the health triune, health and safety risks, functional status, health self-management knowledge and skills, including patient strengths and resources (AHRQ, 2014). Assessment in care coordination provides the framework for the delivery of evidence-based interventions, coordination, education, and healthcare, respecting patient preferences and goals of care.

Several assessment tools can assist the nurse in coordinating patient care, and many EHR programs have embedded care coordination assessment tools. These programs may require the nurse to populate questions concerning the current primary provider, patient choice of post-acute care placement, and tracking referrals to post-acute care facilities. The nurse may also be required to document assessments concerning support systems, financial resources, issues such as food scarcity, home medications, patient understanding and education offered, and follow-up appointments scheduled. All these EHR features assist in coordinating and communicating the care assessment process and promoting continuity of care.

Several assessment tools outside the EHR may also be utilized in care coordination practice. Most times these tools focus on one specific area to identify risks or gaps in care, such as the PHQ-9 (Patient Health Questionnaire version 9), which assesses for signs and symptoms of depression. Other assessment tools may be more comprehensive, such as the PRAPARE®: Protocol for Responding to and Assessing Patient Assets, Risks, and Experiences, which asks questions concerning finances, housing, social and emotional health, etc., to give a more multidimensional picture of the patient situation and health needs. See Table 3.3 for common assessment tools that may inform care coordination practice. The nurse can effectively move on to the diagnosis step of ADOPIE by assessing healthcare needs and determining resource gaps and strengths.

TABLE 3.3 Example Assessment Tools Used in Care Coordination

Example Assessment Tool	Purpose
PHQ-9	Assessment of signs and symptoms of depression
Katz Index of Independence in Activities of Daily Living	Assessment of functional status
CAGE-AID	Assessment of drug or alcohol use
Mini-Cog©	Assessment of mental status in older adults
Modified Caregiver Strain Index	Assessment of the caregivers' experience and needs
Patient Activation Measure (PAM®)	Assessment of the patient's knowledge, skills, and confidence concerning self-management of health
Elder Assessment Instrument	Assessment for elder mistreatment
LACE Index	Risk assessment for 30-day readmission or death in acute care settings
BOOST	Risk assessment tool for readmission to acute care
Prapare®: Protocol for Responding to and Assessing Patient Assets, Risks, and Experiences	Risk assessment tool addressing social determinants of health and personal characteristics
Integrated Case Management Complexity Assessment Grid	Comprehensive assessment tool of strengths and risks, used with complex patients

(Haas et al., 2014, pp. 47–50; Fraser et al., 2018, pp. 55–57; Fulmer & Chernof, 2019)

Diagnosis

"Diagnosis" in care coordination is the critical analysis of assessment and other available data, leading to clinical judgment, strength-based care planning, and nursing diagnoses. NANDA (North American Nursing Diagnosis Association) divides nursing diagnoses into problem-focused, health promotion, risk, or syndrome diagnoses (NANDA International, 2023). In care coordination practice, although problems and needs are identified, the goal of the care plan is strength-based, building upon patient and support system strengths and resources. The transition from disease or deficit-driven diagnoses to proactive, preventative, and health-promoting diagnoses requires a change in focus from what is "wrong" with the patient to what resources, abilities, and strengths the patient possesses to address potential issues in outcome attainment.

Nursing diagnoses typically have three parts: the problem, the disease or health condition, and symptoms or risk factors. **Strength-based diagnoses** also have these components but are based upon recognizing that the patient is the expert on their needs, priorities, and care goals. The core tenets of the strength-based approach include the belief that all patients have strength, resiliency, and capability. The nurse's role may include assisting in discovering or developing these qualities (Gottlieb & Gottlieb, 2017). The nurse may need further or continual focused assessments to assist in this process.

Types of Nursing Diagnosis

Problem-Focused Nursing Diagnosis

The diagnosis is related to an undesirable response to a health condition or life process with an etiology and a defining characteristic (e.g., symptoms).

Health-Promotion Nursing Diagnosis

The diagnosis is related to increasing well-being and readiness to engage in specific health behaviors, often beginning with the phrase "expresses the desire to ..."

Risk Nursing Diagnosis

The diagnosis is related to the potential for developing an undesirable response to a health condition or life process, supported by identified risk factors.

Syndrome

The diagnosis is related to a cluster of diagnoses that occur together and are typically addressed through similar nursing interventions. Related factors may also be included in the diagnosis.

(NANDA International, 2023)

Example: Strength-Based Diagnoses

Strength-based diagnoses begin with person-centered and person-first language, which means that the patient is viewed in their personhood, not as the disease or condition they may possess. Additionally, the nurse takes the time to discover the strengths and resiliency of the patient so that the limitations or effects of their health condition or situation are not how the patient is identified (Yale University School of Medicine Program for Recovery and Community Health, 2007). When considering vulnerabilities and barriers to effective coordination and continuity of care, a "possible" diagnosis may also be appropriate for proactive care planning and coordination of care. Examples of strength-based diagnoses include the following:

Problem-Focused Diagnosis

- Experiencing symptoms of anxiety; opportunity to develop and apply coping skills.
- Patient with congestive health failure; symptoms interfere with the ability to perform activities of daily living (ADLs).

Risk

- Maximize using a walker for ambulation, decreasing the risk of falls.
- Patient chooses not to take medications as prescribed, increasing the risk of COPD exacerbation.

Health Promotion

- Empower self-management of health through promoting health literacy.
- Reinforce patient ability to use specialist care and community resources to support their health.

Syndrome

- Patient diagnosed with chronic fatigue syndrome and experiences joint pain, dizziness, and exhaustion.
- Patient's chronic pain symptoms interfere with their ability to maintain employment.

Possible

- Possible barrier to transition in care due to patient preferred placement options not being available.
- Patient prefers to use alternative medicine to treat nausea and vomiting related to chemotherapy received, reoccurrence of symptoms possible.

The nurse can ask questions such as the following when considering a strength-based nursing diagnosis:

1. What supports are needed to optimize outcomes and goals of care?
2. What is working well for the patient? What brings them enjoyment?
3. What connections or supports are present (family, friends, resources)?

4. What is needed to minimize gaps or barriers?
5. What is required to strengthen what is already working?
6. What new skills, connections, or resources need to be developed?
7. What is the patient's vision for themselves?
8. What are the patient's goals and priorities of care? (Gottlieb & Gottlieb, 2017, p. 325).

The nurse will want to conclude these types of questions with one of these questions: Is there anything else you would like to share? or What did we not talk about yet that is important to you?

This allows the patient to engage in the assessment and diagnosis process actively, enabling them to be in the driver's seat of their health. Once the nurse understands the patient's situation, lifestyle, goals, and care priorities, they can develop relevant strength-based diagnoses in collaboration with the patient and other interprofessional team members.

Outcomes Identification

The focus in care coordination outcomes is providing person-centered care, ensuring seamless transitions in care, and managing resource use and costs. These central outcomes are met through clear communication and information sharing concerning the transition between both sides of the transition so that the care delivered meets the patient's goals and manages resource use and costs (Healthstream, 2021). Key to these overarching goals is the need for the nurse to engage with the interprofessional team to ensure that identified outcomes are comprehensive and meet the patient's needs holistically.

This step focuses on identifying and developing person-centered, individualized, and relevant outcomes based on assessment information gathered, potential strength-based diagnoses, evidence-based practice, and system or regulatory parameters (ANA, 2021). Several national guidelines have been identified that can direct care coordination practice and outcomes identification, such as HEDIS (Healthcare Effectiveness Data and Information Sets), the AHRQ (Agency for Healthcare Research and Quality) *Care Coordination Measures Atlas*, or the CMS (Centers for Medicare and Medicaid Services) HCAHPS (Hospital Consumer Assessment of Healthcare Providers and Systems) survey measures to name a few. With so many **regulatory and quality measures** focusing on care coordination practice, the outcomes identified may appear to focus solely on outcomes such as 30-day all-cause readmissions, length of stay (LOS), or primary care provider (PCP) notification of acute care admissions. It is important to realize that all these regulatory and quality measures also promote good patient health outcomes and resource/cost management through effective transitions and continuity of care.

Other care coordination outcomes may include ensuring patients have a PCP for follow-up care or referring them to a community paramedicine program to enhance preventative and proactive care. This type of outcome allows the patient to become engaged in their healthcare and develop support and resources to self-manage their health, and also provides a connection or bridge for the patient to their community. This somewhat simple-sounding outcome of ensuring your patient has a referral to a PCP (if they do not have one), providing education to

HCAHPS and Communication

The Hospital Consumer Assessment of Healthcare Providers and Systems (HCAHPS) measures patient satisfaction with their healthcare and is an integral part of reimbursement related to the quality of healthcare provided. HCAHPS asks questions about care and communication from nurses, care and communication from doctors, the hospital environment, the hospital experience, care after discharge, the likelihood of recommending the hospital, and patient education and communication. Care transitions and communication are key areas of the survey; low scores often indicate the need for the healthcare system to improve communication and patient education. "Patient satisfaction is about making the patient feel safe and cared for during the hospital stay ... signaling why nurse communication is of such high value" (Heath, 2022, para. 27).

the patient as to the importance and benefits of having a PCP, and facilitating appointment scheduling can improve the patient experience, reduce barriers to care, and promote good health outcomes for the patient. In addition, this promotes good communication amongst the levels of care, meets organizationally identified outcomes, and helps to manage resource use and costs (Singer & Porta, 2022).

Community Paramedicine

Services offered in the community by emergency medical services (EMS) can be referred to in various ways. Sometimes, the service may be called "Community Paramedicine," "Community EMS," or "Community Health Emergency Medical Services (CHEMS)." Whatever it is called in the community, it can provide a bridge between the healthcare system and community residents. **Community paramedicine** utilizes paramedics and emergency medical technicians (EMTs) to assist with public health, primary healthcare, and preventive services to improve care access and avoid duplicative services (Rural Health Information Hub, 2023).

In these programs, paramedics and EMTs serve the public in care models other than emergency medicine, often broadening their scope of practice (Brydges et al., 2016). The paramedic or EMT may act as a patient advocate, provide health education and health promotion interventions, assist with community resource connection, or act as a liaison with the person's PCP or the local hospital to proactively address medical and social needs. Community paramedicine programs often focus on underserved or vulnerable members of the community, such as seniors living alone, people with multiple comorbidities, or frequent visitors to the emergency department (Agarwal et al. 2017).

Planning

Planning involves engagement and collaborative care planning, strategizing, and coordination to achieve identified outcomes. This occurs with the patient and their support system if appropriate. "Care coordination plans are essential for ensuring that all a patient's care needs, from medical care to social services and long-term care planning, are addressed in an organized and effective manner" (Coon, n.d., para. 1). It is a mutually agreed upon and developed plan, between the patient and the interprofessional team. The patient is the expert on themselves and often will take a leading role in plan development, indicating what barriers or needs they are experiencing that affect their health outcomes or ability to self-manage their health. The multidimensional and holistic care plan addresses global health impact areas, such as mental health, substance use, socioeconomic issues, transportation, health literacy and educational needs, strengths, available resources, etc.

When engaging in care coordination care planning, it is essential to maintain a person- and relationship-centered approach. The nurse will want to engage in dialogue to ensure the patient has adequate knowledge concerning their health condition(s) and overall health so that their goals and values of care can be elicited and developed with a realistic understanding of potential treatments, interventions, and outcomes (Fulmer & Chernof, 2019). Care planning begins with an assessment that ascertains the patient's needs, values, and preferences. Once this information is gathered, it is critically analyzed in the context of the patient's health history, medical assessments, and other ancillary assessments. Having a holistic view of the patient's conditions, history, and preferences will assist the nurse in supporting the patient to identify their care goals and formulate them in specific and measurable ways (Fulmer & Chernof, 2019).

It is essential to understand that the **care coordination care plan** is dynamic and flexible, being updated and revised as needed to guide the successful attainment of identified outcomes. The nurse should take the time to understand the patient's long-term and short-term vision of their health, support people available to aid with care plan implementation if needed, and how the patient sees the care plan goals contributing to their health, needs, and preferences (Fulmer & Chernof, 2019). Once care plan goals are developed that support identified outcomes, they should be shared with the interprofessional team and revisited if there is a change in the patient's medical condition or functional abilities, preferences, level of care, or situation.

A shared care coordination care plan is a person-centered health record that facilitates interprofessional team communication and supports integrated care. Through the patient's active role in developing the shared care plan, the nurse–patient relationship is transformed and assists in the nurse's understanding of the patient's values, goals, and care priorities. Ultimately, the care plan should be agreeable and understandable to the patient, reflect patient-driven and centered goals of care—not provider-focused or centered goals—and be responsive to patient needs and identified outcomes.

Implementation

Implementing actions that address patient preferences and transition barriers and manage resources depends upon the partnership between the patient and the interprofessional team. For the plan to be implemented in a timely, accessible, and equitable manner that meets the patient's preferences and values, the nurse must consistently engage in collaborative practice and utilize effective communication methods (ANA, 2021). The care coordinating nurse must ensure receipt of essential information and address patient, support system, or interprofessional team questions or requests for additional information to ensure continuity of care and outcome attainment (ACMA, 2020). When communication and collaboration are ineffective in implementation, it can lead to **fragmented care** rather than integrated care delivery and increase costs and resource use, while decreasing outcome attainment (CMS, n.d.). Collegial collaboration and communication is essential for integrated care and ensuring transitions in care meet identified patient needs, preferences, and outcomes.

Implementation strategies should be evidenced-based, relevant, and meet the patient's situational and contextual needs and support system (Dickson et al., 2022). **Evidence-based practice** (EBP) is a process that reviews, analyzes, and interprets research information with the goal of timely integration into clinical practice in combination with the nurse's clinical experience and the patient's goals and priorities of care to direct care decisions (Finkelman & Kenner, 2007). Several agencies provide guidelines for care coordination evidence-based practices, such as the Centers for Disease Control, The Agency for Healthcare Research and Quality, The Institute for Healthcare Improvement, and the American Nurses Association. These agencies utilized data-driven research that has been shown to improve patient outcomes and manage resource use and costs to develop evidence-based care coordination practice guidelines. Nurses are obligated to participate in self-directed learning to keep up-to-date on best practices for care coordination implementation (Haas et al., 2014).

EXAMPLE: Care Coordination Evidence-Based Practice Guidelines

1. Timely and accurate information exchange and communication among all members involved in care plan outcomes.
2. Use of standardized information exchange systems to promote complete and up-to-date information exchange.
3. Integrated and interprofessional care delivery.
4. Ongoing relationship-building and resource development.
5. Ongoing active patient participation and adjustment of the care plan to meet patient preferences and goals as appropriate.
6. Delivery of evidence-based patient education to enhance self-management of health and autonomous decision making.
7. Encouragement of patient confidence, empowerment, and engagement in managing their health outcomes.
8. Role clarity and accountability amongst the interprofessional team.
9. Barriers and challenges to care transitions proactively addressed across the continuum of care.

(Clinical Solutions, 2019)

Also critical to consider when implementing the care coordination care plan is the training and knowledge of the nurse or **unlicensed personnel** delivering the care coordination interventions. Care coordination requires the nurse to be knowledgeable about the patient's medical conditions, socioeconomic issues, health insurance coverage, community resources, needs, values, and preferences (Williams et al., 2019). The healthcare organization may provide unlicensed personnel to assist the nurse or to conduct many care coordination interventions. The nurse's role in these situations is to ensure that the implementation of tasks delegated to unlicensed personnel is appropriate to that person's training and scope of practice and follows any Nurse Practice Act guidelines in the state where they work (ANA, 2021).

As with all nursing interventions, the implementation of the care coordination care plan needs to be documented. This is critical for a variety of reasons. Documentation of care coordination implementation is often linked to financial reimbursement and utilized to pull data from the EHR to identify if regulatory and quality benchmarks have been met or to evaluate processes and services provided. Furthermore, other members of the interprofessional team and providers throughout the continuum of care may need access to timely and accurate information concerning interventions offered, successes and barriers, education provided, etc., to develop their own relevant person-centered care plan in the next level of care.

It is essential when documenting the implementation of the care coordination plan of care that standardized terminology and data elements are used so that all members of the interprofessional team can understand what was implemented and data can be easily retrieved (Lamb & Newhouse, 2018). Often, the EHR will provide the framework for care coordination documentation, allowing for clear documentation and data retrieval concerning the status of system-identified patient outcomes (such as 30-day all-cause readmissions), essential patient health information (such as PCP or comorbidities), and whether evidence-based health promotion and education were offered.

Why Document Care Coordination Implementation?

1. Communication: Documentation is used by the interprofessional team, and if it "is not timely, accurate, accessible, complete, legible, readable, and standardized," it may interfere with their ability to provide quality person-centered care (ANA, 2010, p. 6).
2. Reimbursement: Documentation is used to determine patient admission status, intensity of service needed, and if quality care was provided.
3. Regulatory and Quality Measures: Documentation is used to measure performance and quality benchmarks and outcomes. This data is used to determine published ratings of the health system, measure whether clinical quality indicators are met, and for financial purposes (reimbursement rates vs. fines).

(ANA, 2010)

Coordination of Care

Care is coordinated with the interprofessional team, community, providers, the patient, and their support system to ensure a successful transition in care. The ANA identifies that coordination of care is a subset of the implementation step of nursing practice. This signifies that all nursing practices should implement nursing interventions supporting managing patient care across the continuum through information sharing and person-centered care practices. Some of these nursing interventions are common practice, such as engaging in relationship- and person-centered care and using timely and effective communication (ANA, 2021). Other aspects of care coordination may be less familiar or have an unaccustomed focus to ensure coordinated continuity in care.

When coordinating care, the nurse must understand the patient outcomes identified and agreed upon by the interprofessional team, including the patient. These outcomes may determine the most appropriate next level of care and guide the nurse when advocacy or education may be needed. The nurse coordinating care comprehensively manages patient care, organizing the care delivered to meet outcomes. This is achieved by participating in person-centered care practices supporting patient autonomy and engagement in outcome development and self-management of their health, providing advocacy, guidance, and education for the patient and their support system, and assisting in navigating the complex healthcare system (ANA, 2021). The nurse care coordinator role has a significant impact on accountability in organizing, facilitating, educating, communicating, and collaborating to ensure the patient's care is managed across the continuum of care through information sharing and person-centered care practices.

Health Teaching and Health Promotion

Person-centered health teaching and promotion advance patient engagement and activation and foster self-management of health and wellness practices. Health teaching and promotion are integral to coordinated care delivery and positive patient outcomes—and this is more than reviewing discharge instructions or handing a pamphlet to a patient describing a new medication or a suggested resource. The nurse must first assess what is important to the patient, if they are willing to receive education (readiness to learn), and their health literacy needs such as reading, technology, and math (ANA, 2021). The nurse must assess these areas and prepare their health teaching to meet patient needs and priorities of care. This involves the nurse allowing the patient to discuss what is important to them, their values, preferences, and care goals. The nurse may find it helpful to focus the health education and promotion by asking permission to begin health teaching, thereby opening the conversation and allowing the patient autonomy. The nurse may also find some of the following questions/phrases helpful in engaging the patient in conversation about their health teaching and health promotion needs.

1. Can you describe what you already know about [insert health condition or situation]?
2. Is there something you would like to know more about [insert health condition or situation]?
3. Can we talk about your [insert health condition or situation]?

4. I would like to share some information with you about [insert health condition or situation]. Is this okay with you?
5. Do you have any new ideas or ways you might work with your [insert health condition or situation] when you are [discharged, return home, etc.]?
6. Have you considered doing [insert intervention] to help with your [insert health condition or situation]? (Miller & Rollnick, 2013)

Readiness to Learn

Readiness to learn refers to how a patient assimilates new knowledge and their ability to change health behaviors. Patients often must go through various stages to engage in and maintain a healthy behavior change. Health education and health promotion interventions are improved if they match the patient's state of readiness. Many things can affect a person's readiness to learn, such as physical and psychological comfort (e.g., pain or anxiety) and environmental distractors (e.g., other people in the room). The nurse will be more successful in health teaching and promotion by matching the content to the patient's readiness to learn. Often, if the nurse asks how the patient views their health and what actions they are currently taking to address their health issues, they can understand how ready the patient is to learn. (EuroMed Info, n.d.)

Agenda Mapping

Agenda mapping is a way to prepare for a health education or promotion conversation. It is a time when the patient can direct the education session by identifying what they want to focus on in the session, any barriers or successes experienced, and the purpose of the conversation. You may start by asking the patient if they would mind discussing a topic you want to provide education about or by handing the "reins" to the patient and asking what they would like to focus upon in the educational session. Or you and the patient can create a list of educational topics together, with the patient prioritizing which ones are important. Then you can begin the conversation there.

Agenda mapping is a great way to learn about what the patient is most willing to learn and what the patient is least willing to engage in. This allows for a more productive educational session, where the patient-identified priority areas can be addressed first while allowing for potential additions or changes in topic or addressing other educational areas after the relationship-building process has occurred. Remember to give the patient time to consider the question, their knowledge base, and what is important to them. Affirmation is also essential, as it supports the patient throughout the process and recognizes their strengths and efforts (Miller & Rollnick, 2013).

As the nurse provides health teaching and health promotion activities, they also provide **anticipatory guidance** (ANA, 2021). This is the practice that a nurse employs to proactively address potential health issues by educating on what to expect and how an individual can best promote their health and wellness (Edwards, 2017). Central to anticipatory guidance is the nurse assisting the patient so they are able to manage their health daily or self-management their health (McCabe, 2020). This is essential for a patient to proactively address health and wellness needs such as preventative care and screenings or managing a chronic health condition to maximize positive outcomes. Anticipatory guidance provides the education and information needed to engage and activate patients, empowering them to self-manage their health through education on "red flags," potential adverse outcomes, and coping and adaptation skills if needed (Edwards, 2017).

Evaluation

Acute care settings have been operating on a negative profit margin for the last few years. According to the American Hospital Association, hospitals in America have been operating at a –1% margin as of January 2023 (AHA, 2023). With the implementation of value-based payment reforms and the transition from the fee-for-service model, it is apparent why evaluating nursing interventions and processes is an essential part of the care coordination practice. Additionally, agencies such as the Institute of Healthcare Improvement and initiatives such as the Quintuple Aim pointedly focus on outcomes—patient outcomes, system outcomes, accessibility outcomes, staff outcomes, and cost outcomes. Nurses cannot stop the nursing process at assessment or intervention, but they must evaluate their nursing practice utilizing patient feedback, system benchmarks, and health and safety guidelines.

Evaluation is a crucial aspect of quality assurance in healthcare delivery and a critical element of the nursing process. In the evaluation step, the nurse collects and analyzes outcomes, regulatory and quality measures, and benchmark data to determine if patient outcomes have been met, what gaps are apparent, and what else could have been provided to meet outcomes. The patient and their support system must be involved in outcomes evaluation so that person-centered care is provided, which allows for patient autonomy and prioritizes patient preferences and goals of care. The nurse can collect data concerning outcomes through patient and support system interviews, discussion with the interprofessional team, review of the EHR, feedback from community stakeholders and payers, or review of organizational data provided, such as the number of return emergency room visits in the last 30 days.

Evaluation is based on monitoring the nursing process and outcomes in a structured manner. If it is determined that outcomes have not been met, the nurse must analyze the nursing practice process and identify areas of improvement, ensuring that the care coordination provided meets the seven rights and guiding principles of care coordination. Once evaluated from all perspectives (nursing, system, community stakeholders, the patient, etc.), opportunities for improvement in the care coordination process can be identified and modified to achieve outcomes and benchmarks (Porter-O'Grady & Malloch, 2018).

A key area of care coordination evaluation is that of **muda**, which is a Japanese word that means "waste" and can be seen when care coordination interventions need to be corrected or reworked, are not timely, are unnecessary, or do not contribute to identified outcome attainment (The Council for Six Sigma Certification, 2018). Suppose care coordination deficits or muda are found in the evaluation step. In that case, the nurse may need to reassess, re-diagnose, rework identified outcomes, or revise the plan of care, instituting new care coordination interventions, offering additional health teaching, or engaging in process improvement activities to ensure continuity of care and identified outcomes attainment.

Evaluation is interrelated to all aspects of the nursing process in care coordination. It is not the "end" but the overarching action informing all other aspects of care coordination and nursing practice. The plan of care is a responsive and transformative document, and the evaluative process informs revisions, additional interventions, addressing gaps in care, and determining whether identified outcomes have moved along the continuum in "state, perception, or behavior" (Moorhead, 2009, p. 869). See Figure 3.1 for a visual of the relationship of evaluation to nursing practice. As seen in the figure, evaluation encompasses and is interconnected with all aspects of nursing practice.

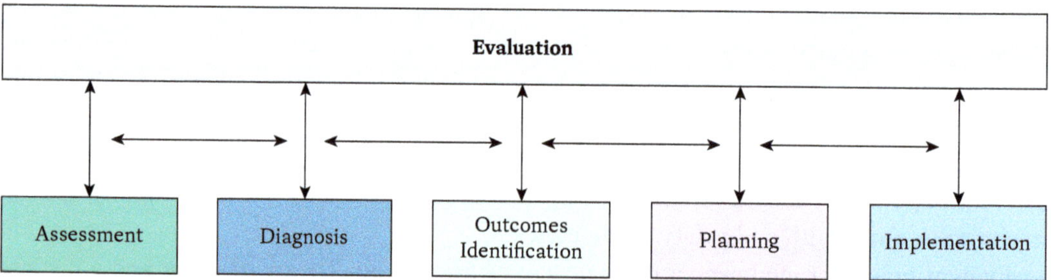

FIGURE 3.1 Relationship of Evaluation to Nursing Practice

Practice Focus: Monitoring Coordination of Care

Evaluation of the care coordination process through continuous monitoring and ensuring the care coordination process is not caught up in muda or something that is unnecessary or does not contribute to the desired identified outcome is required (The Council for Six Sigma Certification, 2018). At times, the care coordination offered may not meet identified outcomes, timelines, or goals of care. When this occurs, problem-solving concerning the process is needed. Examples of muda in care coordination may be an intervention delivered incorrectly in the care plan, causing interventions or the care plan to be redone or revised, or an unmet identified outcome. The need to make corrections to or rework the care plan, referrals, follow-up plans, or care coordination interventions also needs to be examined if this is discovered through monitoring, as this likely means there may be role overlap or diffusion in the work performed, training required, or new processes developed (The Council for Six Sigma Certification, 2018).

Eliminating Muda

Muda can be eliminated by making the care coordination process more efficient, and this is done through continuous monitoring and quality improvement. This requires determining what in the care coordination process went wrong and how this can be dealt with, consistently implementing the process change improvement, and then monitoring *again* to determine if the change made a difference (The Council for Six Sigma Certification, 2018).

The one area of muda that frequently affects care coordination efforts negatively is wait times. When the care coordinating nurse is managing a transition in care, they may be waiting for insurance authorizations, confirmation of receipt of information, acceptance of a patient by a provider, an evaluation, or an application to be completed (e.g., Medicaid application). These needed items for successful care coordination may leave the nurse waiting for periods of time only to find out a patient will not be approved for transition to a particular facility or provider. Then the referral process will need to begin again. These muda areas of incorrect timing, correction, and waiting can be dealt with through proper planning and persistent monitoring of the status of the transition plan.

The nurse can monitor the care coordination process in a variety of ways. By engaging in ongoing collaboration with the interprofessional team, the nurse can receive real-time feedback on whether there are process delays or failures. Through documentation of what has been done in the care coordination process, the nurse improves the ability of all interprofessional team members to screen for gaps in the process or identify potential barriers to coordination and continuity of care. The nurse can also frequently assess the patient and their circumstances related to the coordination of care and determine whether revisions are needed in the identified outcomes or whether there are barriers or gaps in care (New Mexico Department of Health, 2018). Through continual monitoring and surveillance of the care coordination process, the nurse can deliver safe, effective, and quality care that supports patient autonomy and provides successful transitions in care.

Practice Focus: Assessing Risk

Risk assessment is a critical aspect of care coordination and often directs the rest of the nursing process in care coordination practice. Due to life situations, literacy needs, or physical, social, or mental health needs, patients may be at risk for poor outcomes or contributing to unmet benchmarks. The care coordinator has a crucial role in assessing for these types of risks and developing a plan of care that will address them, promote outcomes attainment, and decrease risk in care delivered. The care coordinator may use various tools to assess for risk, identify potential problems, and plan and implement interventions to prevent these risks. The care coordinator may review prior patient admissions, previous plans of care, interventions offered, and also assess for safety issues.

When assessing risk in care coordination, the nurse must address potential health and wellness and social and support needs. Karam et al. (2021) developed a model of vulnerabilities in patients with high-risk social and health needs (See Figure 3.2 "Complex Health and Social Care Needs"). Although the model is based in the context of patients with complex needs, it could be argued that when assessing for risk, the nurse must holistically examine all patients, including considering vulnerabilities in physical health, social determinants of health, mental health/substance use, and individual characteristics that may affect outcomes and direct care planning and interventions. The six areas identified in this model provide a multidimensional framework nurses can follow when assessing risks in care coordination and the potential for unmet outcomes and regulatory or quality benchmark attainment.

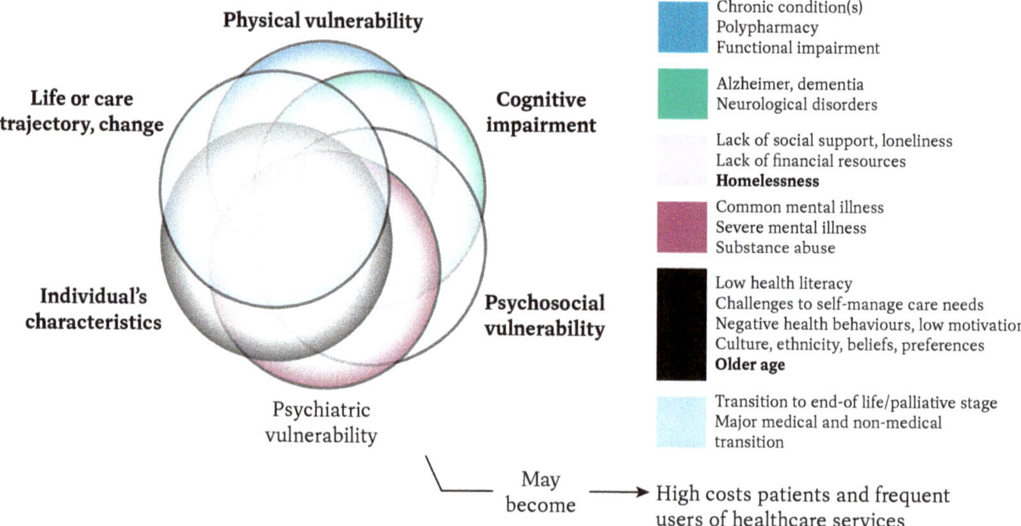

FIGURE 3.2 Complex Health and Social Care Needs

Gap Analysis

When performing the risk assessment, it may become evident to the care coordinating nurse that gaps in care need to be addressed. A gap analysis is essential to dealing with potential barriers to identified outcomes attainment and ensuring continuity and coordinated care. The gap analysis process has the following three basic steps:

1. Reviewing current and, at times, past patient records and conferring with the interprofessional team as needed to determine health issues, social determinants of health, and potential vulnerabilities.
2. Interviewing patient and support system and consulting with the interprofessional team to confirm identified potential gaps in care and to facilitate further clarification and identification of gaps in care. This is performed utilizing a strength-based approach, gathering information on prior successes, past attempts to address the potential gap, and patient priorities and preferences concerning the potential gap in care.

3. Reviewing the identified gaps in care with the patient and support system and interprofessional team, collaboratively identifying the next steps for the outcomes identification and implementation phase of the nursing process (AHRQ, 2022). See Figure 3.3—Gap Analysis Process.

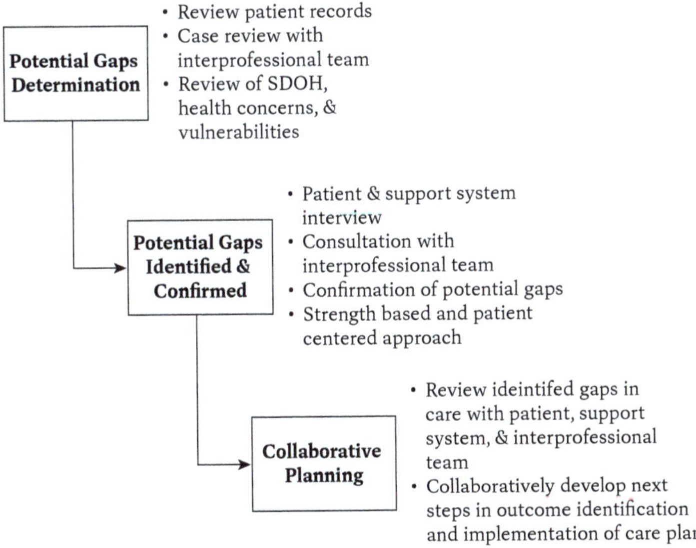

FIGURE 3.3 Gap Analysis Process

Care coordination of gaps in care often relate to communication or closing the loop of care gaps. Patients may lack understanding of what their insurance provider covers or be unaware of the services for which they are eligible. This can create a situation where the patient is not accessing care that would be helpful to their outcomes. Patients may feel that they reach out for assistance but do not receive what is needed and then ultimately either do not continue with follow-up care or return to the hospital or emergency room. There may be difficulties in transitioning a patient from one provider to another, as the provider may not be in-network or not accepting new patients. Patients may need the nurse to act as an advocate and facilitate transitions in care, ensuring all parties are aware of key issues such as insurance coverage, services to be provided, and who is accountable for follow-up. This needs to be based on relationship-centered care, which builds relationships among all involved in the care to be provided and ensures that there is an identified point person (often the care coordinator) for any difficulties or questions that arise (Tarrant et al., 2015).

Relationship Continuity

"Relationship continuity (an ongoing therapeutic relationship with one or more care providers) has been argued to be 'the antidote to an increasingly fragmented and depersonalized health care system'" (Tarrant et al., 2015, p. 85).

Practice Focus: Preparing for Transitions in Care

Transition management coordinates the patient's movement between one setting or provider and another. This requires effective communication and collaboration between providers and settings. The nurse must possess competency in person- and relationship-centered care, advocacy, assessment and critical analysis, communication, interprofessional teamwork, and quality assurance. Each of these competencies has a vital role in successful transitions of care. Critical areas of care coordination practice in transitions of care include the following:

1. Coordination of the care and interventions being received or required at the next level of care.
2. Use of empathy to understand others' perspectives on the transition and care to be provided.
3. Supporting patient autonomy in decision-making related to the transition in care, goals of care, and expression of preferences.
4. Engaging in meaningful communication and collaborative partnership with the interprofessional team, patient, and support system.
5. Ability to communicate with the interprofessional team and other stakeholders and promote active engagement and accountability in the transition of care.

(Fraser et al., 2018, p. 181)

The nurse coordinating care during transitions focuses on safeguarding the transition of the care process, ensuring high-quality and cost-effective care continues. This is done through an integrative approach in which the care coordinating nurse facilitates the transition in care through impeccable communication and collaborative practice. This ultimately promotes quality outcomes, met benchmarks, and patient and provider satisfaction.

The nurse managing the transition in care must possess care coordination competencies and a knowledge base to exercise those competencies. One key area of knowledge includes understanding the payer source and their process for pre-authorization of the level of care covered as well as which providers and agencies have a contractual relationship with the payer (Fraser et al., 2018). Often, a transition in care can be stopped before it begins if the insurance provider does not have a contract with the selected next level of care or does not believe the patient meets insurance criteria for a certain level of care. Additionally, patients often need a funding source, and the care coordinating nurse will need knowledge of state and community funding sources, the application processes, and how to assist the patient in applying for and navigating these programs.

Transitions in care involve almost continuous communication with the stakeholders and the interprofessional team to ensure the transition is successful. The nurse will need to communicate changes in the patient's condition, discharge status, funding sources, authorizations, and care plan, including medication reconciliation. These items can be fluid until the transition, and the care coordinating nurse must have their finger on the pulse of all that is going on with the patient to ensure that significant information and patient changes are communicated promptly. Some phrases often used in care coordination are "**pace the case**" or "discharge begins at admission." Both phrases indicate the need for the nurse to be ever watchful for timing issues such as length of stay or confirmation of a referral being received. It is critical to ensure that the care and interventions delivered in a transition of care are timely.

The Agency for Healthcare Quality and Research has developed the IDEAL (include, discuss, educate, assess, listen) discharge planning process to address transition timing. This process is based on patient- and relationship-centered care and engaging the patient and their support system with transition planning. The transition begins by including the patient and discussing the transition process with them, allowing them time to consider questions and articulate their preferences in care. Education is also provided throughout the transition process, assessing and listening for patient understanding of the transition plan, giving guidance for who to contact if difficulties are encountered, reviewing the follow-up plan, and addressing questions (AHRQ, n.d.a). See Table 3.4 for the application of IDEAL to the transition management process. This method can be adapted to short transitions as well as to longer ones. The key is to ensure that all aspects of the IDEAL strategy are met. Depending on the patient's situation, this could be done in one day or over several weeks.

TABLE 3.4 Pacing the Case in with IDEAL

Timing	Actions	
At Admission	1. Identify if caregivers will be needed at the next level of care and plan to identify if they will be family members or friends or paid caregivers and how they will be funded if funding is needed.	2. Determine patient goals, priorities, and preferences for the next level of care.
	3. Discuss with the patient the transition planning process and what next steps to expect.	4. Encourage questions from the patient and their support system, and provide a way for them to easily communicate their questions, such as a whiteboard or a number to call.
Daily During the Stay	1. Educate the patient and their support system (as appropriate) on health conditions, resources, or other areas needed.	2. Ensure the patient understands their medications, any changes that have or will occur, and allow time for questions.

(Continued)

TABLE 3.4 ***(Continued)***

	3. Keep the patient and their support system informed of the transition plan, any changes that have occurred, and the progress toward transition. Allow time for questions and revision of plan if needed based on patient condition, goals, and preferences.	4. Arrange for training for the patient and their caregivers if needed concerning any care needs post-transition (e.g., wound care).
Prior to the Transition in Care	1. Provide all education and training needed concerning the transition in care.	2. Ensure all equipment, transportation, or care needs are arranged for (e.g., walker, home healthcare).
	3. Meet with the patient and support system (as appropriate) to review the transition plan and timing. Allow for questions and clarification.	4. Make follow-up appointments for the patient and document them in the EHR. Communicate the follow-up plan to the patient, eliciting preferences for follow up providers, locations, and appointment timing.
Day of Transition in Care	1. Review orders, referrals, and/or discharge summary for completeness.	2. Confirm that the medication list is correct, complete, and has been reconciled.
	3. Review the transition instructions with the patient and their support system (if appropriate), assessing understanding of health conditions, medications, follow-up care, and instructions, and who to contact with questions.	4. Review follow up appointments with patient and confirm they are documented in transition instructions.
	5. Give written transition instructions to patient confirming the following are documented: follow-up appointments, who to contact with questions, what the red flags are and what to do if one occurs.	

(AHRQ, n.d.a, p. 12)

CHAPTER SUMMARY

Coordination of care utilizes a multidimensional strength-based approach to the nursing process of ADOPIE. Adding outcomes identification, care coordination, and health education and health promotion to the nursing process supports the integration of coordination and continuity of care activities into all aspects of nursing practice and settings (ANA, 2021). The combination of ADOPIE, foundational nursing theory, and the guiding principles of care coordination allows the nurse to engage with the patient, their support system, and the interprofessional team to meet challenges to the transition of care process and deliver high-quality continuity and coordination of care.

The assessment process in care coordination allows the nurse to determine resource gaps and strengths and give a global picture of the patient's situational and health needs. Assessment assists the nurse in creating strength-based diagnoses in partnership with the patient and allows the nurse to understand the patient's lifestyle, goals, and care priorities. Identified patient outcomes may be patient-oriented, system-oriented, or benchmark-oriented, based on evidence-based practices and regulatory parameters, and developed with the interprofessional team (ANA, 2021). Planning occurs with the patient as the "expert" on themselves and with a relationship-based care approach.

The care plan is dynamic and flexible, being updated and revised as needed to support identified outcomes and reflecting patient-driven and person-centered care goals. Implementation strategies for the care plan should meet evidenced-based guidelines and the patient's situational and contextual needs. All nursing practices should implement nursing actions and interventions that support coordinated care and provide anticipatory guidance to proactively address patient health and wellness needs (ANA, 2021). Evaluation of the care coordination process is all-encompassing and interconnects with each aspect of the nursing process. Quality improvement activities or plan of care revisions are warranted if deficits are found or to ensure identified outcomes are met.

Coordination and continuity of care rely upon assessing risks and performing a gap analysis of potential barriers to care or effective transitions. Risk assessment involves a comprehensive examination and analysis of the patient's vulnerabilities, including physical, social, and mental health, substance use, and individual characteristics that may affect outcome attainment (Karam et al., 2021). Through an integrative approach and utilizing interpersonal communication and collaborative practice competencies, the nurse facilitates coordinated care throughout the transition in care.

Successful care coordination also involves pacing the case and being watchful for timing issues that may be barriers to a successful transition of care. The IDEAL discharge planning process can be helpful with this and can be adapted to short-term or long-term transitions of care (AHRQ, n.d.a). As nurses must be cognizant of wasteful practice and resource use in healthcare to enhance quality, safety, and cost outcomes, they must also monitor for muda in their nursing practice, things that are unnecessary or cause the care plan to be corrected, reworked, or do not contribute to successful attainment of identified outcomes. Through continuous monitoring and surveillance of the nursing process when coordinating care, the nurse can deliver effective quality care that supports patient autonomy, meets identified patient and system outcomes and regulatory benchmarks, and create successful coordination and continuity of care across settings.

CHAPTER 3 GLOSSARY

Anticipatory Guidance: Education and information the nurse provides to proactively address health and wellness needs, empowering the patient to self-manage their health, preventing adverse outcomes, and maximizing positive outcomes.

Care Coordination Care Plan: A dynamic, flexible, and responsive plan developed with the patient and the interprofessional team that formulates and outlines person-centered goals and priorities of care, supporting meeting patient needs and identified outcomes.

Community Paramedicine: Programs that utilize paramedics and emergency medical technicians (EMTs) to assist with primary and preventative care services and improve care access for underserved or vulnerable community members.

Disease Model of Healthcare: A model of healthcare that emphasizes illness, focusing on the signs, symptoms, and diagnosis of "disease" and subsequent treatment.

Evidence-based practice (EBP): A process that reviews, analyzes, and interprets research information, with the goal of timely integration into clinical practice in combination with the nurse's clinical experience and the patient's goals and priorities of care to direct care decisions.

Fragmented Care: Care that results from poor communication and collaboration amongst providers and organizations, leading to increased costs, decreased outcome attainment, and transitions of care that do not meet patient needs or preferences.

Guiding Principles: Core standards of care coordination that provide a viewpoint or "lens" the nurse can use to guide the clinical decision-making process regarding coordination and continuity of care and address challenges to the coordination of care.

Muda: A Japanese word that means "waste" and can be seen when care coordination interventions need to be corrected, reworked, are not timely, are unnecessary, or do not contribute to identified outcome attainment.

Multidimensional Healthcare Model: A model of healthcare that is strength-based and meets the multidimensional aspects of health, including physical health—preventative, acute, and chronic health, mental health—substance use and emotional health, and social determinants of health—healthcare quality, access, and equity.

Pace the Case: A phrase used to express the need for the nurse to engage in continuous monitoring of the care coordination process, following a stepwise progression from the day of admission to the day of care transition, and to be watchful for timing, communication, and process issues that may cause delays in transitions of care.

Regulatory and Quality Measures: Standards developed by various accrediting and regulatory bodies that gauge and quantify the performance of a healthcare system, health plan, or provider in meeting coordination of care benchmarks and goals of care delivery.

Strength-Based Diagnosis: A nursing diagnosis based on the belief that all patients have strength, are resilient and capable, and recognizing the patient as the "expert" on themselves.

Unlicensed Personnel: People who are not professionally licensed but are part of the care coordination team and assist the nurse or other provider in care coordination activities. They may work directly under the supervision or direction of a registered nurse (RN). If so, the RN is accountable for delegating and supervising tasks as outlined by the American Nurses Association and the National Council of State Boards of Nursing.

DISCUSSION QUESTIONS AND ACTIVITIES

Discussion Questions

1. The current healthcare system is being transformed from the "disease" model of care. Identify and discuss at least one way you have seen this model transition affect how nurses provide care.
2. The nursing process of ADOPIE has added outcomes identification, care coordination, and health education and health promotion to the nursing process. Consider and describe how you will adapt your nursing practice to meet the outcomes identification, care coordination, health education, and health promotion steps. Identify at least one barrier to completing these steps and discuss how you plan to address it in your nursing practice.
3. Look up a care coordination guideline or standard and discuss how the guideline or standard contributes to the Quintuple Aim. You may wish to explore HEDIS, *The Care Coordination Measures Atlas*, or the HCHAPS survey to identify a guideline or standard.
4. Choose an assessment tool for care coordination practice and explore what it assesses and what interprofessional team member you would consult with concerning the tool and information gained from it. Identify how the care coordinator may use the information gained from the tool to promote positive outcomes or decrease costs or resource use. You may refer to Table 3.3 for examples of these types of tools.
5. Choose one nursing theory. It could be one of the theories presented in the chapter or another nursing theory that you believe supports care coordination practices. Apply your chosen nursing theory to care coordination. Discuss how the theory supports effective care coordination practice. Then consider and discuss how integrating the theory could promote innovative and responsive care coordination structures, processes, or interventions.

Activities

1. Strength-based nursing diagnoses are essential for patient activation, engagement, and empowerment. Consider a patient that you have worked with in one of your clinical courses or workplace, and list as many strengths as you can remember about that patient. Then, list the reasons the patient was in the clinical setting. Using your identified patient strengths, create at least two strength-based nursing diagnoses that could have been used in your nursing care. Please do not identify the patient or clinical setting. When creating your strength-based diagnoses, consider the questions the nurse could ask the patient, which are listed in the section of this chapter titled "Diagnosis."
2. In the table provided, list a guiding principle of care coordination and a nursing process (ADOPIE) step that contributes to meeting the five outcomes of the Quintuple Aim. Briefly describe how the principles and steps of the nursing process contribute to meeting the outcome.

Quintuple Aim Outcomes	**Guiding Principle**	**Description of How the Principle Contributes to Meeting the Outcome.**	**Step of the Nursing Process**	**Description of How the Step of the Nursing Process Contributes to Meeting the Outcome**
Outcome 1: Improving population health				
Outcome 2: Enhancing the care experience				
Outcome 3: Care-team well-being				
Outcome 4: Advancing health equity				
Outcome 5: Reducing costs				

3. Case Study:

   Allen is the caregiver for his wife, Betty, who is 67 years old. Betty has been diagnosed with coronary artery disease (CAD) and congestive obstructive pulmonary disease (COPD). These conditions have caused Betty to experience extreme fatigue, shortness of breath, and an inability to perform most of her activities of daily living (ADLs) and functional ADLs. Allen has converted their family room into her bedroom because she no longer can climb the stairs to their upstairs bedroom. Betty uses an electric wheelchair for mobility and has a bedside commode near her hospital-type bed in the family room. Betty needs assistance transferring to and from the wheelchair, bed, and bedside commode. Allen feels he cannot leave Betty alone, even to go to his doctor, because she often tries to transfer herself and has had numerous falls. When this happens, Allen cannot pick Betty up so he has to call emergency medical services to lift her back into bed.

   Allen has recently been diagnosed with Parkinson's disease and fears he will be unable to care for Betty much longer. He is following all the prescribed treatments, but they have not successfully managed his symptoms yet. Their only daughter Clara lives out of the country and sends some money each month to assist with expenses. Allen uses that money to cover the cost of a caregiver one day per week. Otherwise, Allen has no assistance in caring for Betty. They are not part of a church community, they have no living relatives in the area, and since his and Betty's health has declined, they have not seen any friends for over a year.

   Betty has recently been admitted to the local hospital for angina. You are meeting with Allen concerning discharge planning for Betty, and Allen expresses that he cannot care for Betty any longer but is feeling hopeless and guilty because he promised her that she would not have to leave their home. They cannot afford the cost of an assisted living or skilled nursing facility. Allen has expressed that he is constantly worried, cannot sleep, and feels there is no way out of the situation.

   1. Identify one guiding principle of care coordination that could guide your decision-making concerning Allen and Betty's situation. Describe how you would use this guiding principle in your work with Allen and Betty.
   2. Identify one or more barriers affecting Betty's health. How could this barrier to health be affecting the situation?
   3. What types of health education and health promotion would you provide Allen and Betty? Before presenting this health education and health promotion to them, what might you need to consider?

NCLEX STYLE QUESTIONS

Colton Barber is a 68-year-old male diagnosed with follicular lymphoma and recently had a bone marrow transplant. You have been assigned as his nurse care coordinator and are meeting with Colton to develop his care plan regarding his transition to home. (Questions 1 to 5 relate to this scenario)

1. Mr. Barber and you are setting person-centered goals for his care coordination plan of care. Which of the following is the best description of how you would approach creating person-centered goals of care for the transition home?
   a. Consult with the oncologist following the patient for goals of care in the home, as the oncologist is the expert on what will be needed.
   b. Ensure the patient has enough information concerning their condition before developing goals of care.
   c. Focus on reviewing the patient's electronic health record (EHR), as this has the best information on the patient's needs at home.
   d. Confirm that the interprofessional team's goals of care are in the plan of care.
2. As you discuss goals of care, Mr. Barber tells you that he is looking forward to a visit from his son with his newborn baby girl later today. Mr. Barber is excited to meet her as she is named after his late wife, Gianna. Which of the following steps in the nursing process will you need to engage in to promote health outcomes?
   a. Care coordination
   b. Health teaching
   c. Evaluation
   d. Focused assessment
3. You are considering which nursing diagnosis is most appropriate for Mr. Barber. To form your nursing diagnosis, you should ask the patient which of the following?
   a. What is already working for him?
   b. What is his vision for himself?
   c. What support does he have?
   d. All of the above.
4. You begin doing a risk assessment on Mr. Barber. You know that the purpose of the risk assessment is to do which of the following?
   a. Promote outcomes attainment
   b. Promote medically focused goals
   c. Promote identification of deficits
   d. Promote stratification of risk

5. Mr. Barber has discharge orders, and you are meeting with the patient to provide health teaching before discharge. Which of the following best describes a foundational step of health teaching?

   a. Collecting all the needed brochures and instructions before meeting with Mr. Barber

   b. Assessing if Mr. Barber is ready for and willing to receive health teaching

   c. Making sure his son is in the room while the teaching occurs in case Mr. Barber needs a reminder of what was presented

   d. Directing the health teaching session so that all outcomes are met

6. You are precepting a new nurse and describing the multidimensional health aspects of nursing practice. You know that the orienting nurse understands the multidimensional aspects of health when they say which of the following?

   a. "I must focus on understanding the signs, symptoms, and disease diagnosis to provide good nursing care."

   b. "I must focus on discovering the patient's deficits either in their home life or their characteristics as this can direct how I should provide nursing care."

   c. "I must focus on understanding the treatment options to give them information about their options."

   d. "I must focus on understanding the patient's strengths, health issues, symptom management, mental health, and socioeconomic needs."

7. When the care coordinator faces difficulty coordinating and managing a patient's care, which should be done first?

   a. Report it to the provider following the patient.

   b. Review the guiding principles of care coordination.

   c. Revisit the care plan with the interprofessional team.

   d. Both a and c.

8. You are explaining strength-based diagnosis to a fellow nurse. Which of the following is a correct description of strength-based diagnoses?

   a. Strength-based diagnoses focus on the patient's disease or diagnosis.

   b. Strength-based diagnoses are approved by the interprofessional team.

   c. Strength-based diagnoses are based on the belief that patients are capable.

   d. Strength-based diagnoses focus on what resources are needed.

9. Care coordination outcomes should be identified and based upon which of the following?

    a. Evidence-based practice
    b. Patient character
    c. Family member recommendations
    d. Intuitive practice

10. Which of the following activities does the anticipatory guidance include?

    a. Providing education on "red flags"
    b. Engaging patients in self-management of health
    c. Proactively addressing potential health issues
    d. All of the above

11. Which of the following is an example of having a gap in care?

    a. There is an identified person to contact if the patient has questions or concerns.
    b. The patient understands what their insurance provides and covers.
    c. Relationship-centered care is provided.
    d. The patient is referred to an out-of-network provider.

12. Which of the following are key areas of care coordination practice in transitions of care?

    a. Engaging in meaningful communication and collaborative partnership.
    b. Use of sympathy to see another point of view.
    c. Supporting decision-making based on medical diagnosis.
    d. Ensuring accountability in other members of the interprofessional team.

13. Which acronym identifies a strategy that can assist the care coordinator to "Pace the Case"?

    a. ADPIE
    b. IDEAL
    c. NANDA
    d. BOOST

14. Which best describes examples of muda in care coordination practice? (Select all that apply.)

    a. Surveillance

    b. Rework

    c. Timing

    d. Outcomes

15. Fragmented care is best described as:

    a. Care that leads to increased costs and decreased outcome attainment.

    b. Care that is flexible to patient needs and priorities.

    c. Care that follows a stepwise progression from the day of admission to the day of discharge.

    d. Care that does not utilize community paramedicine.

REFERENCES

Agarwal, G., Angeles, R., Pirrie, M., Marzanek, F., McLeod, B., Parascandalo, J. & Dolovic, L. (2017). Effectiveness of a community paramedic-led health assessment and education initiative in a seniors' residence building: The Community Health Assessment Program through Emergency Medical Services (CHAP-EMS). *BMC Emergency Medicine, 17*(8), 1–9. https://doi.org/10.1186/s12873-017-0119-4

Agency for Healthcare Research and Quality (AHRQ). (n.d.a) *Care transitions from hospital to home: IDEAL discharge planning implementation handbook.* https://www.ahrq.gov/sites/default/files/wysiwyg/professionals/systems/hospital/engagingfamilies/strategy4/Strat4_Implement_Hndbook_508_v2.pdf

Agency for Healthcare Research and Quality (AHRQ) (2014). *Care coordination measurement framework* (Ch.3). https://www.ahrq.gov/ncepcr/care/coordination/atlas/chapter3.html

Agency for Healthcare Research and Quality (AHRQ) (2018). *Care Coordination.* https://www.ahrq.gov/ncepcr/care/coordination.html

Agency for Healthcare Research and Quality (AHRQ) (2022). *Gap analysis facilitator's guide.* https://www.ahrq.gov/patient-safety/settings/hospital/candor/modules/facguide3.html

Agusti, A. (2018). The disease model: Implications for clinical practice. *European Respiratory Journal, 51*(1800188), pp. 1–3. https://doi.org/10.1183/13993003.00188-2018.

American Case Management Association (ACMA). (2020). *Case management standards of practice & scope of services.* http://www.acmaweb.org/forms/Standards%20of%20Care_Brochure_Case%20Management 2020.pdf

American Hospital Association (AHA). (2023). *Report: Hospitals could face new normal as financial challenges linger.* https://www.aha.org/news/headline/2023-02-28 report hospitals-could-face-new-normal-financial-challenges-linger

American Nurses Association (ANA) (2010). *ANA's principles for nursing documentation.* https://www.nursingworld.org/~4af4f2/globalassets/docs/ana/ethics/principles-of-nursing-documentation.pdf

American Nurses Association (ANA) (2021). *Nursing: Scope and standards of practice* (4th ed.). ANA.

Brydges, M., Denton, M., & Agarwal, G. (2016). The CHAP-EMS health promotion program: a qualitative study on participants' views of the role of paramedics. *BMC Health Services Research, 16*(435), 1–10. https://doi.org/10.1186/s12913-016-1687-9

Centers for Medicare and Medicaid Services (CMS), (n.d.). *Care coordination.* https://innovation.cms.gov/key-concept/care-coordination

Clinical Solutions. (2019). *Optimizing care coordination strategies to improve clinical outcomes and elevate quality performance.* https://www.elsevier.com/__data/assets/pdf_file/0004/861070/EL-CareCoordinator-WP-FINAL.pdf

Coon, R. (n.d.). *Examples of care coordination plans.* https://www.forcura.com/blog/care-coordination/examples-of-care-coordination-plans

The Council for Six Sigma Certification. (2018). *Six sigma: A complete step-by-step guide.* Author.

Dickson, K. S., Holt, T., & Arrendondo, E. (2022). Applying implementation mapping to expand a care coordination program at a Federally Qualified Health Center. *Frontiers in Public Health, 10*(844898). https://doi.org/10.3389/fpubh.2022.844898

Edwards, J. D., (2017). Anticipatory guidance on the risks of unfavorable outcomes among children with medical complexity. *The Journal of Pediatrics, 180*, 247–250. https://doi.org/10.1016/j.jpeds.2016.10.02

EuroMed Info. (n.d.). *Patient education: Learning readiness.* https://www.euromedinfo.eu/patient-education-learning-readiness.html/

Fawcett, J. (2005). *Contemporary nursing knowledge: Analysis and evaluation of nursing models and theories* (2nd ed.). F. A. Davis Company.

Finkelman, A. (2016). *Leadership and management for nurses: Core competencies for quality care* (3rd ed.). Pearson.

Finkelman, A., & Kenner, C., (2007). *Teaching IOM: Implications of the Institute of Medicine reports for nursing education.* ANA.

Fraser, K., Perez, R., & Latour, C., (2018). *CMSA's integrated case management: A manual for case managers by case managers.* Springer Publishing Company.

Fulmer, T., & Chernof, B. (Eds.). (2019). *Handbook of geriatric assessment* (5th ed.). Jones & Bartlett Learning.

Gottlieb, L.N., & Gottlieb, B. (2017). Strength-based nursing: A process for implementing a philosophy into practice. *Journal of Family Nursing, 23*(3), 319–340. https://doi.org/10.1177/1074840717717731.

Haas, S. A., Swan, B. A., & Haynes, T. S. (Eds.). (2014). *Care coordination and transition management: Core curriculum.* American Academy of Ambulatory Care Nursing.

HealthStream. (2021). *The importance of patient care coordination for outcomes.* https://www.healthstream.com/resource/blog/the-importance-of-patient-care-coordination-for-outcomes

Heath, S. (2022). *What are HCAHPS scores, why are they important to patient satisfaction?* https://patientengagementhit.com/features/patient-satisfaction-and-hcahps-what-it-means-for-providers

Johns Hopkins Medicine Alliance for Patients (2023). *Care coordination model.* https://www.hopkinsmedicine.org/population-health/alliance-patients/model-of-care.html

Karam, M., Chouinard, M. C., Poitras, M.E., Couturier Y., Vedel I., Grgurevic, N., & Hudon, C. (2021). Nursing care coordination for patients with complex needs in primary healthcare: A scoping review. *International Journal of Integrated Care, 21*(16), 1–21, https://doi.org/10.5334/ijic.5518

Lamb, G., & Newhouse, R. (2018). *Care coordination: A blueprint for action for RNs.* American Nurses Association.

McCabe, E. M. (2020). School nurses' role in self-management, anticipatory guidance, and advocacy for students with chronic illness. *NASN School Nurse, 35*(6), 338–343. https://doi.org/10.1177/1942602X209065

Medicaid.gov. (n.d.). *Preadmission Screening and Resident Review.* https://www.medicaid.gov/medicaid/long-term-services-supports/institutional-long-term-care/preadmission-screening-and-resident-review/index.html

Miller, W. R., & Rollnick, S., (2013). *Motivational interviewing: Helping people change* (3rd ed.). The Guilford Press.

Moorhead, S. A. (2009). The nursing outcomes classification. *Acta Paulista de Enfermagem, 22* (spe), 868–871. https://doi.org/10.1590/S0103-21002009000700004

NANDA International. (2023). *Glossary of terms.* https://nanda.org/publications-resources/resources/glossary-of-terms/

New Mexico Department of Health. (2018). *Instructions and guidelines for case management monitoring activities.* https://www.nmhealth.org/publication/view/guide/4738/

Porter-O'Grady, T., & Malloch, K. (2018). *Quantum leadership: Creating sustainable value in health care* (5th ed.). Jones & Bartlett Learning.

Rural Health Information Hub. (2023). *Community paramedicine.* https://www.ruralhealthinfo.org/topics/community-paramedicine

Singer, C., & Porta, C. (2022). Improving patient well-being in the United States through care coordination interventions informed by social determinants of health. *Health & Social Care in the Community, 30*(6), 2270–2281. https://doi.org/10.1111/hsc.13776

Tarrant, C., Windridge, K., Baker, R., Freeman, G., & Boulton, M. (2015). 'Falling through gaps': Primary care patients' accounts of breakdowns in experienced continuity of care. *Family Practice, 32*(1), 82–87. https://doi.org/10.1093/fampra/cmu077

Williams, M. D., Asiedu, G. B., Finnie, D., Neely, C., Egginton, J., Finney Rutten, L. J., & Jacobson, R. M. (2019). Sustainable care coordination: A qualitative study of primary care provider, administrator, and insurer perspectives. *BMC Health Services Research, 19*(92), 1–10. https://doi.org/10.1186/s12913-019-3916-5

Yale University School of Medicine Program for Recovery and Community Health (2007). *Important language considerations in developing person-centered care plans.* https://portal.ct.gov/-/media/DMHAS/Publications/PCRPLanguagepdf.pdf

Credit

Fig. 3.2: Source: M. Karam, et al, "Nursing Care Coordination for Patients with Complex Needs in Primary Healthcare: A Scoping Review," *International Journal of Integrated Care*, vol. 21, no. 16, p. 4. 2021.

CHAPTER 4

Activation, Engagement, and Health Self-Management

LEARNING OBJECTIVES

1. Examine the patient and nurse roles in activation, engagement, and health self-management.
2. Explore characteristics of activation, engagement, and health self-management.
3. Expand knowledge and skills to foster patient activation, engagement, and health self-management.
4. Apply concepts of patient engagement and activation to the promotion of health outcomes and self-management.

KEY TERMS

- activation language
- durable power of attorney
- expert trap
- health literacy
- health self-management
- motivational interviewing
- organization literacy
- patient activation
- patient engagement
- righting reflex
- self-efficacy
- shared decision-making
- social influencer of health
- universal health literacy precautions

Introduction

Self-management of health leads to helpful lifestyle changes, increases positive health outcomes, and reduces costs and resource use, meeting many care coordination goals, guiding principles, and rights. Evidence shows that providing health self-management support is associated with increased self-efficacy on the part of the patient and healthier behaviors (AHRQ, 2016). Health self-management requires knowledge, skills, attitudes, and motivation. This brings to the forefront the nurse's role in educating the patient on self-management skills and promoting patient activation and engagement. The nurse must clearly understand the relationship between patient activation, self-efficacy, engagement, and the ultimate end goal of health self-management. All are needed and work together to empower patients to take charge of their health.

This requires a nurse–patient partnership based on collaboration, respect, and valuing each patient's unique personhood. The nurse must also understand the various factors that affect activation, self-efficacy, and engagement, such as health literacy on the individual and organizational level and social influencers of health. Through assessment, critical synthesis and analysis, and evaluation, the nurse can meet patient health literacy needs and be a voice for organization health literacy, supporting initiatives such as Healthy People 2030 and the Quintuple Aim. Through appropriate health education, clarification of the nurse and patient's role in health self-management, and interpersonal strategies such as shared decision-making and motivational interviewing, the nurse can support the patient in making appropriate health choices and build the skills and self-efficacy needed for long-term success in health self-management.

Health Self-Management

The ability of patients to self-manage their health is crucial to meeting foundational coordination and continuity of care goals, such as effectively managing resources, decreasing adverse health outcomes, meeting clinical quality and benchmark measures, and increasing patient satisfaction and quality of life (Schaffler et al., 2018). **Health self-management** in care coordination practice represents the patient possessing the knowledge, skills, and attitudes that allow them to manage their health daily for positive health outcomes. Patients already manage their health in one way or another with every healthcare decision. The questions that concern nurses in coordination and continuity of care practice are how the patient manages their health and how the nurse can support patient activation, engagement, and positive health outcomes (Lorig & Holman, 2003).

Due to the link between socioeconomic status, educational level, and health, patients may need support in health self-management. Patients may be experiencing housing and food scarcity issues or access to healthcare barriers, affecting their ability to self-manage health. Furthermore, patients may have health literacy barriers that negatively impact their understanding of their health conditions and plan of care or their ability to access and utilize preventative care services (Schaffer et al., 2018). Nurses must assess for these potential barriers to health self-management and address them in the plan of care and interventions provided.

There are five core health self-management skills, including (a) problem-solving, (b) decision-making, (c) use of resources, (d) partnership development, and (e) action (Lorig & Holman, 2003). Research has shown that health self-management support interventions are more successful if they focus on problem-solving, resource use, and action, likely pointing to the fact that these skills are interconnected and dependent on each other (Schaffer et al., 2018). Patients may have difficulty taking action or developing a health action plan if they do not possess sufficient problem-solving skills or understand how to access and use resources to support their actions toward health self-management.

Core Health Self-Management Skills

1. Problem-solving: The patient must possess problem-solving skills, including problem identification and solution development.
2. Decision-making: The patient must be able to make daily decisions concerning their health. This means they must have the knowledge and information to make an informed decision.
3. Use of resources: The patient must be able to find and access resources needed for their health. In today's healthcare world, they must be able to search for resources using technology, identify contact information, send emails or text messages, send messages on a secure health portal, and use a phone.
4. Partnership development: The patient must be able to form a relationship with their healthcare providers in which a partnership for health is developed. This way, the patient and provider, in partnership, can address needed resources, information, and support.
5. Action: The patient must be able to make an action plan to meet their health goals and priorities. Usually, this is planning in the short term, identifying specific steps to meet a goal. The patient will also need readiness and confidence to implement the action plan (Lorig & Holman, 2003).

Trajectory Framework of Health Self-Management

Patient self-management of health is not a newly recognized need in healthcare, and several national organizations endorse health self-management as essential to healthcare quality and safety initiatives. Corbin and Strauss (1991) developed a trajectory framework for health self-management that focused on chronicity and chronic illness but is still relevant today as nurses work with patients to support lifelong health self-management knowledge, skills, and attitudes. The trajectory model can assist nurses in gaining a perspective on how patient health and illness experiences can affect their ability and attitudes toward self-managing their health on a day-to-day basis. This, in turn, enhances the nurse's ability to dialogue with the patient concerning treatment options, priorities of care, and preventative care and wellness actions. Central to this is the recognition that health self-management applies to all phases of the health trajectory, including times of health and illness, throughout a patient's life.

The framework recognizes that health and illness are multidimensional, including medical, behavioral, and emotional/psychological responses and actions, and that the trajectories may vary as health plateaus, declines, or improves. The trajectory framework has three components, beginning with the medical component where the patient manages their wellness or health condition, such as taking medications as prescribed or going for an annual wellness exam. The second behavioral component focuses on creating new attitudes and behaviors that support wellness and health management, such as a patient with congestive heart failure engaging in energy conservation or a person with a prediabetes diagnosis working to lose weight. The third and final component addresses a health condition's emotional or psychological impact, which may affect patient reactions and decisions (Lorig & Holman, 2003). Patients may experience frustration with not meeting a weight loss goal, or they may experience more intense emotions, such as depression and anger, when diagnosed with a untreatable form of cancer. All emotions experienced related to a patient's health or illness can affect how they view the importance of, or their ability to, engage in self-management of health. The model views health on a trajectory as it evolves and changes, and it acknowledges that patients' experiences with their health and illnesses may affect their reactions to current healthcare interventions and experiences (Corbin & Strauss, 1991).

The trajectory framework of health self-management begins with preventative care and ends with death. The pretrajectory phase is preventative and begins before illness and signs and symptoms are present. The trajectory onset phase is the diagnostic period of an illness and the related signs and symptoms. Emergency or crisis health care is required in the crisis phase due to a life-threatening situation. In the acute phase, hospitalization is necessary to manage illness or complications. The stable phase is noted when illness and symptoms are controlled. The unstable phase is when illness and symptoms are not controlled but do not require acute hospitalization. Progressive deterioration of physical and/or mental health manifested by increasing symptoms signifies the downward phase. The last phase is dying, when death is imminent in weeks, days, or hours (Corbin & Strauss, 1991, p. 163).

It is critical to understand that health follows a trajectory that all patients will eventually experience and that patients will need to self-manage their personal health needs at each phase. The patient's health needs will change over time because health is not static. However, the patient should possess the knowledge, skills, and attitudes to meet the plan of care recommendations and challenges, from preventative care and wellness recommendations to enlisting support persons or designating a **durable power of attorney (DPOA)** to advocate for them when they can no longer actively participate in their health care decisions. Nurses must adapt the care to meet the patient and their support system needs regarding health self-management as the patient travels along the health trajectory, ensuring they do not project any personal beliefs concerning the health trajectory phase on the patient and the care they deliver.

Trajectory Framework Phases

1. Pretrajectory Phase: Preventative and pre-illness.
2. Trajectory Onset Phase: Signs and symptoms of illness present.
3. Crisis Phase: Emergency or crisis care is needed.
4. Acute Phase: Acute care is needed to manage illness.
5. Stable Phase: Illness controlled.
6. Unstable Phase: Illness not controlled.
7. Downward Phase: Progressive deterioration.
8. Dying Phase: Death imminent.

(Corbin & Strauss, 1991, p. 163)

The importance of health self-management in today's environment concerns preventing chronic diseases or preventable health conditions, promoting wellness and quality of life, and meeting goals and priorities of care for patients with chronic illnesses. Self-management of health is not a one-time event. It occurs throughout the lifespan and will look slightly different depending on the trajectory of health and patient care priorities. The patient needs essential knowledge, skills, and attitudes to successfully manage their health, including problem-solving and decision-making abilities, critical healthcare information, and an understanding of how to take action regarding their health and wellness. Additionally, for successful self-management of health, the patient needs to be engaged and activated in their health.

Patient Engagement

As the healthcare system transitions to value-based care models, with coordination and continuity of care central, patients must actively manage their health. **Patient engagement** has been identified as a critical component in person-centered care, improving outcomes, decreasing resource use, and increasing patient satisfaction (Barello et al., 2017; Marzban et al., 2022). In 2007, the Joint Commission added the encouragement of the patient's active involvement in their care as a patient safety strategy (AHRQ, 2019). Patient engagement is also central to the Institute for Healthcare Improvement's Framework for Safe, Reliable, and Effective Care (Frankel et al., 2017). At the fundamental level, patient engagement means the patient takes ownership of their health (Knickman & Elbel, 2019). The end goal of patient engagement is for the patient to exercise self-management of health and to be able to make informed and appropriate healthcare decisions and actions. There are many ways of thinking about patient engagement, and it may take many forms, such as patients voicing questions and concerns, engaging in shared decision-making, and collaborative care planning.

Often, patient engagement is seen as the patient and their support system working in partnership with their healthcare providers to improve health outcomes and enhance safety. Key to patient engagement is communication and information sharing, with the goal of the patient being able to engage in self-care, collaborative goal setting, and the ability to relay concerns related to their care (Haas et al., 2014). It ensures that the care provided is right for the patient, meets their needs, goals, and priorities of care, and improves identified health outcome attainment. Patient engagement positively affects multiple aspects of health care delivery and is "correlated with better outcomes and lower long-term costs" (Marzban et al., 2022, p. 7). Patient

Patient Engagement

"Patient engagement is the involvement in their own care by individuals (and others they designate to engage on their behalf), with the goal that they make competent, well-informed decisions about their health and health care and take actions to support those decisions" (Sofaer & Schumann, 2013, p. 5).

engagement can be viewed as the foundation of a pyramid that contributes and leads to meeting several care coordination guiding principles and rights, such as promoting patient autonomy and relationship-centered care, providing evidence-based and appropriate care, ensuring the care provided is right for the patient, and using the right resources. See Figure 4.1 for a visual of the patient engagement pyramid.

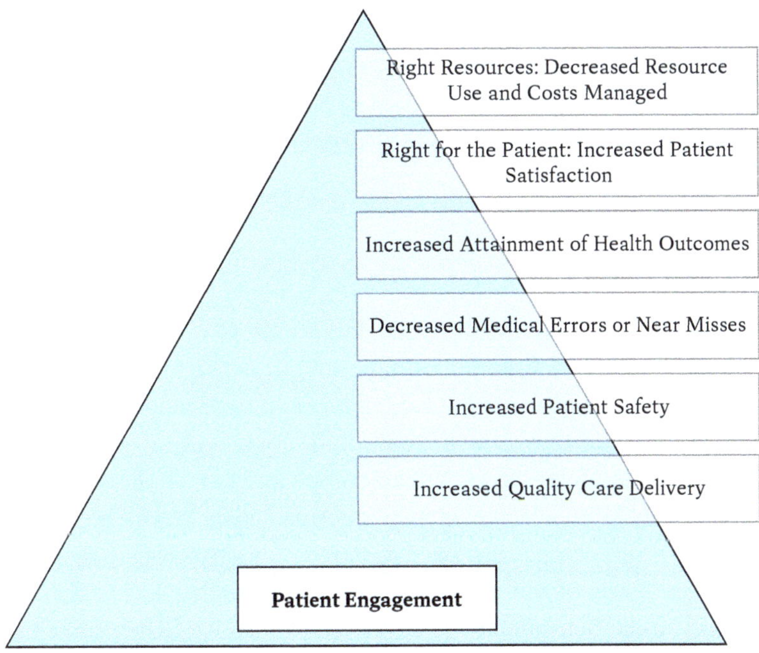

FIGURE 4.1 Patient Engagement Pyramid

Patient engagement "begins with empowering patients and healthcare providers" (WHO, 2016, p. 9). This can only be achieved through patients' understanding of their health conditions and the health system they must navigate to make informed decisions that meet their healthcare goals and priorities. This requires nurses to ensure their patients have up-to-date, evidence-based information that meets their health literacy needs. Nurses can also help patients report safety concerns and close the communication loop by providing patients with information on follow-up actions related to their concerns (WHO, 2016). Additionally, the nurse can provide information on resources in the community and for self-care assistance, such as support groups. The World Health Organization (2016) identified five factors that affect patient engagement in safety or reducing harm.

1. The patient themselves. Health literacy needs, socioeconomic factors, personal characteristics, or beliefs may support or deter patient engagement.
2. The health condition. Illness severity or symptoms may affect the patient's ability to participate in health self-management and engagement.

3. The healthcare professional. The healthcare professional's attitudes, knowledge, and skills can support or deter patient engagement.
4. The tasks required. If the behavior or task required exceeds the clinician's clinical abilities.
5. The healthcare setting. The setting itself brings its own areas of safety and harm reduction needs (p. 6).

Addressing these factors can set the patient up for success in health self-management in the long term. However, for patient engagement to flourish, it must include patient activation, where the patient has the knowledge, skills, attitudes, and motivation to self-manage their health (Abid et al., 2020).

Patient Activation

Patient activation is based on the "willingness and ability to take independent actions ..." to self-manage health (Hibbard & Greene, 2013, p. 207). It is the movement toward an action regarding health. If a patient does not have confidence in their ability to manage their health or the readiness to act, then they may have limited movement toward self-management of their health. Confidence is central to patient activation and can be thought of as **self-efficacy**, or the belief in one's capabilities to accomplish identified goals, health behaviors, or course of action (Bandura, 1997). Self-efficacy has been found to promote self-management and self-care behaviors, and higher levels of self-efficacy are related to higher levels of patient activation (Mirmazhari et al., 2022). Self-efficacy is connected to health behaviors and outcomes, as patients will choose to engage in health behaviors or not, based partly on their beliefs in their abilities to attain the health outcome.

Expectation related to outcome is another aspect of self-efficacy that can hinder health self-management (Driscoll, 2000). Will it have positive or negative effects from the patient's perspective? Albert Bandura developed the theory of self-efficacy and identified that outcome expectations fall into three categories: (a) physical effects (pain, hunger, etc.), (b) social effects (approval vs. disapproval, social group reaction to change, etc.), and (c) self-evaluation of the behavior (1997). For example, suppose a patient has decided to quit smoking, but they are part of a bowling team that meets each week for practice and all members of the team smoke. The patient may want to quit smoking but may expect to receive disapproval or pushback from their teammates (e.g., social effects outcome). This might cause the patient to rethink quitting smoking. The theory of self-efficacy has application to health behavior self-management, and the concept of self-efficacy can be applied to health outcomes. When considering health behavior change from a self-efficacy standpoint, the patient must believe (e.g., have self-efficacy) that they can perform the actions required for the health behavior change and that the outcomes will be positive or have value to them. See Figure 4.2 for the application of the theory of self-efficacy to health self-management.

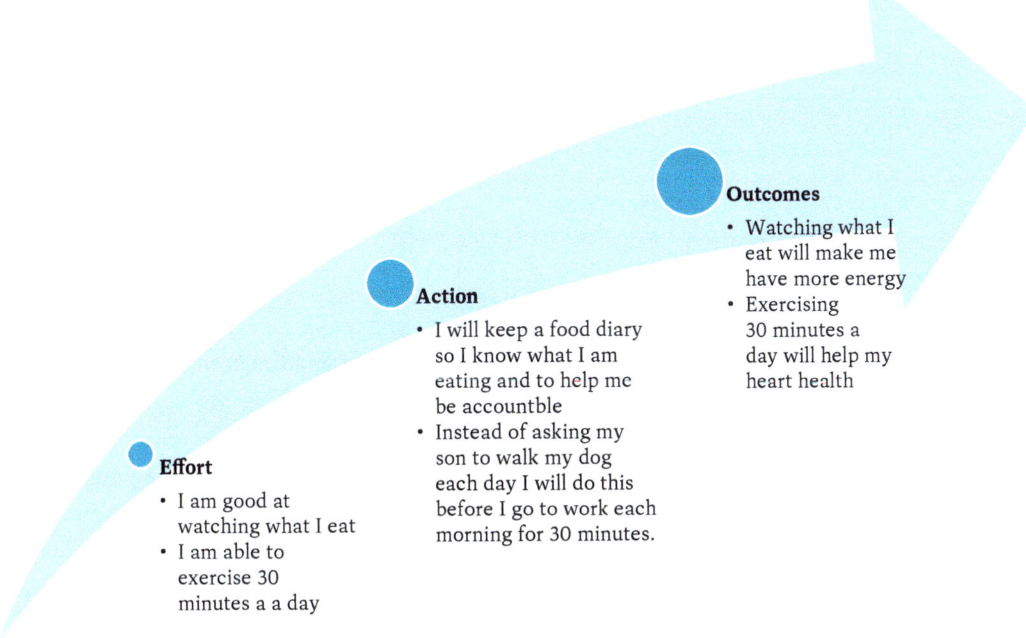

FIGURE 4.2 Theory of Self-Efficacy and Health Self-Management

Confidence

Using a confidence ruler is one way for the nurse to gauge the level of self-efficacy or how confident the patient is concerning the efforts and actions needed to meet an identified outcome. This simple exercise can be done with verbal dialogue only or visual aids (e.g., the confidence ruler). The premise is to engage the patient in conversation about how confident they are to engage in a health behavior on a scale of 0 to 10, where 0 is not at all confident and 10 is very confident. Once the patient identifies their confidence level, the nurse can delve into why a patient may be less or more confident, asking what it would take the patient to move to the next number or how they might assist the patient in getting to a higher number. These open-ended questions allow the patient to reflect upon what has worked for them in the past or what supports may be needed (Substance Abuse and Mental Health Services Administration, 2019).

The key is to find out why the patient is at a certain level and to engage the patient in dialogue about moving forward to action in health self-management. Do they need additional support? Does something in their life prevent them from being confident? Have they had unsuccessful experiences in the past? Is this what they are basing their confidence rating on? The strength-based approach to care coordination promotes patient self-efficacy in health self-management by focusing on past successes and valuing patient-generated solutions, resources, and strengths. See Figure 4.3 for an example of a confidence ruler.

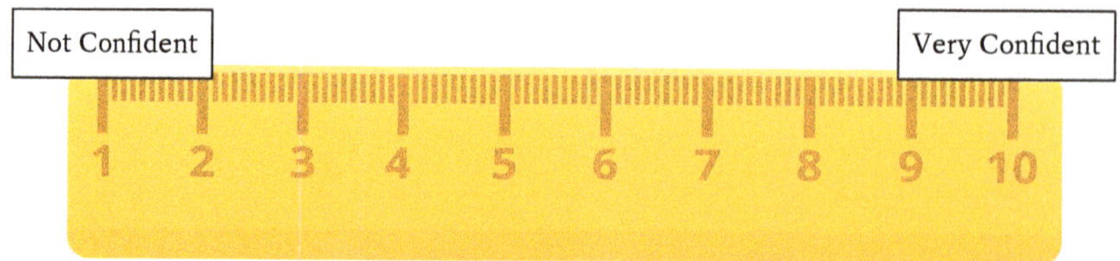

FIGURE 4.3 Example Confidence Ruler

Readiness

Not only do patients need confidence in their ability to engage in healthy behavior, but they also need to be ready to make the change or perform the action. Readiness in patient activation refers to whether the patient is ready to change health behavior. There are variations to this aspect of patient activation, focusing on how important a change is to how ready a patient is to make a health behavior change. Dialogue about how important a change is to a patient often leads to a discussion of how ready they are to change their health behaviors or self-manage their health. Importance and readiness to change are not separate from each other because, often, when something is very important to the patient, they are more ready to change their health behaviors.

The same questions in the confidence ruler example can be applied to the importance or readiness ruler. If the patient rates themselves at a lower level, what can the nurse do to support them to move to a higher level of importance or readiness? What would make something more important to them? Are there items in their life that they need to get situated to feel more ready to change their health behavior? Beginning the conversation with something's importance allows the patient not to feel pushed into being ready to change health behaviors (Miller & Rollnick, 2013). Once a patient identifies something important to them, the conversation about readiness organically enters the dialogue. These types of "ruler" assessments lend themselves well to all ages and populations and can be adapted as needed. See Figure 4.4 for example importance or readiness ruler.

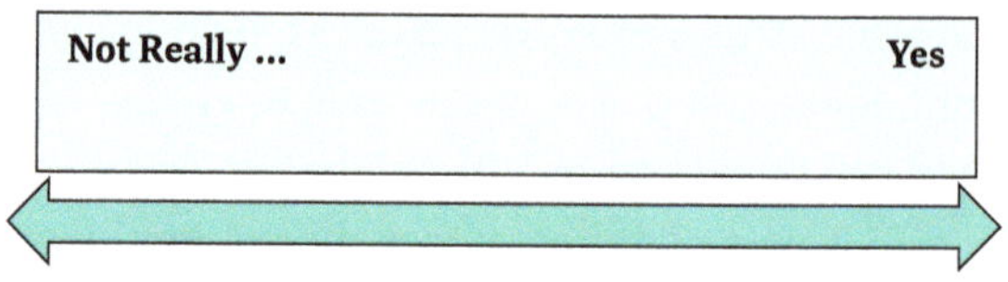

FIGURE 4.4 Example Importance or Readiness Ruler

Patient Activation Measure

The Patient Activation Measure®, or PAM®, is a common tool for quantifying patient activation levels. There is a more extended version of the PAM®, the PAM-22®, and a shorter version, the PAM-13®. The PAM-22® has 22 survey questions, and the PAM-13® has 13 questions. Questions in the survey focus on identifying beliefs concerning ownership of health, confidence in taking action and voicing questions, knowledge of treatments and health conditions, and confidence and ability to maintain lifestyle and behavior change to support health self-management (Hibbard et al., 2005, p. 1923). The survey questions identify where the patient is in relation to the four stages of activation. These stages include the following:

1. The patient holds the belief that they have an important and active role in the self-management of their health.
2. The patient possesses the confidence and knowledge needed to act.
3. The patient can act in the self-management of health.
4. The patient can continue the course even when experiencing stress (Hibbard et al., 2005, p. 1922).

The PAM® identifies four levels of patient activation that begin with not being engaged and end with the patient being fully activated and engaged in self-managing their health. "The levels are: (1) disengaged and overwhelmed; (2) becoming aware but still struggling; (3) taking action; and (4) maintaining behaviors and pushing further" (Hellström et al., 2019, p. 2). The PAM-13® has been shown to have over 90% accuracy and is a tool that some healthcare providers use to assess patient activation levels and to base their patient engagement strategies (Heath, 2017).

Activation Language

Activation occurs on a continuum, as patients may have varying levels of confidence and readiness to move toward health actions. It is essential to understand that patient activation may go back and forth along the continuum depending on the circumstances, context, and situation. Words that may signify a patient is considering action concerning their health include phrases such as "I am ready to ..." or "I am willing to ..." (Rollnick & Miller, 2013. p. 162). These types of phrases are often referred to as **activation language**, which are phrases or language that indicates the patient is considering making a health behavior action or change. Nurses must listen for activation language phrases as they provide an opening to offer support, additional information or education, and encouragement for the patient to continue movement along the activation continuum. Sometimes the activation language may take the form of a patient telling the nurse that they have taken action or made a change in their health, such as making a colonoscopy screening appointment or attending a support group.

Interventions that Increase Patient Activation

1. Skill development and peer support: Interventions that focus on developing problem-solving abilities, communication (voicing questions and concerns), and participatory decision-making with providers.
2. Social environment change: Interventions that change the environment include posters, opportunities to engage in health behaviors, and information campaigns.
3. Tailoring support to the patient's activation level: Interventions that encourage small manageable steps, matching intervention intensity to activation level, starting with small successes (Hibbard & Greene, 2013, pp. 209–210).

Ultimately, a patient needs to see the importance of the health behavior. The behavior or action must be congruent with the patient's priorities and goals of care. The patient also needs to be ready to take action toward their health. Many things can hinder action, such as lack of time, understanding, or communication. The health behavior action may also feel overwhelming to the patient or not fit well into their lifestyle or situation. Once the patient prioritizes the health action and feels ready to act, they must have confidence or self-efficacy, believing they can successfully enact the health behavior. Patient activation requires intrinsic motivation and ability, supported by self-efficacy and willingness to take action toward specific health behaviors or self-management of health. The nurse needs to understand that activation, engagement, and ultimately self-management of health build upon each other, may take time to develop, and may wax and wane as health conditions, symptoms, and life circumstances occur. See Figure 4.5 for a visual of the relationship between these conceptual building blocks and health self-management.

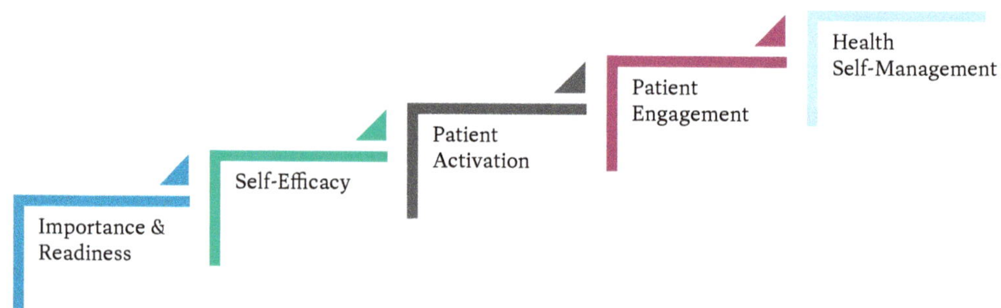

FIGURE 4.5 Health Self-Management Building Blocks

The Nurse's Role

Nurses are central to patient activation, engagement, and health self-management. The nurse builds these through giving relationship-centered care, being aware of their role in wellness and health management, educating patients about health, supporting patient autonomous decision-making, and providing connections and coordination of care (Barello et al., 2017). To do this, the nurse must participate in a joint and collaborative process with the patient, where there is a motivation for mutual partnership and accountability. The nurse's role is critical in responding to the patient or situation, assessing, recognizing patient needs, sharing information with the interprofessional team, and providing education to foster the development of health self-management (Jerofke-Owen et al., 2023).

Often in nursing—and it could be argued that in healthcare in general—providers may have an expert attitude and may fall into the "**expert trap**." They have engaged in education, sometimes for many years, and they have in-depth training in their area of expertise. So it is not uncommon for a healthcare provider or a nurse to take on the attitude that they know what is best for the patient. They may believe the patient should always do what the provider or nurse tells them to do regarding their health. They may feel that they better understand the health condition and outcomes than the patient and are giving the patient the "right" advice concerning their health. However, this brings the role of the nurse and the patient in this type of situation into question. Is the role of the nurse to tell or inform the patient what they need to do to get healthy or manage their health? Or is the role more of an interpersonal and collaborative one, where the nurse engages in dialogue, empathy, and understanding to assist in developing a plan of health self-management that works for the patient and their life circumstances and priorities, ultimately leading to the patient managing their health in the long-term? Some nurses may struggle with the expert trap if they hold the attitude or belief that they are the expert on the patient's health and situation and know what is best for the patient concerning their healthcare and which decisions or actions are most appropriate.

As a member of a profession that puts caring and helping at the center of nursing practice, many nurses may also experience the **righting reflex**, wanting to "fix" or "correct" a situation, condition, or belief. The righting reflex happens when the nurse knowingly or unknowingly shows their expertise on a subject or content area and tries to fix a situation based on their opinions, beliefs, or knowledge without first considering the situational context, circumstance, or patient's perspective (Miller & Rollnick, 2013). The righting reflex can be thought of as giving unsolicited advice that is seen as intrusive or unwelcome by the recipient. Alternatively, it could be viewed as a parent who fixes all problems for their children, sending the message to the child that they are unable to fix their own problems. The righting reflex can make the patient feel that the nurse–patient relationship is hierarchical, paternalistic, or maternalistic. It also can inhibit the patient from asking questions, sharing aspects of their lives or situations affecting their health, and decreasing patient satisfaction (Barello et al., 2017). Nurse-held attitudes and belief systems that support the expert trap or the righting reflex can decrease patient autonomy and may demotivate the patient to change or engage in health behaviors in the long term.

Nurses must promote patient engagement and activation based on caring and valuing the patient's personhood (Welch & Fournier, 2018). The relationship between the nurse and patient often acts as a barrier or a conduit for patients to learn the knowledge, skills, and attitudes necessary to manage their health effectively. Sofaer and Schumann (2013) developed a five-factor model of caring in nursing practice that supports patient engagement and activation. This model begins with the foundation of the nurse maintaining belief in the patient and their capacity and potential to achieve health self-management. Secondly, the nurse attains knowing through partnership with the patient and their support system, attaining an "informed understanding" of patient perceptions and circumstances (Welch & Fournier, 2018, p. 4). The third factor is being with the patient, being present physically, emotionally, and in a meaningful and relevant manner. This assists in relationship-building and relationship-centered care. Fourthly, the nurse must "do for" the patient. This does not mean the nurse inappropriately does tasks or activities for the patient. It means that the nurse does what is necessary to maintain the patient's dignity and sense of personhood. Lastly, the nurse engages in enabling. Again, this does not mean the nurse supports dysfunctional behaviors, as many might interpret the word "enabling." It means the nurse facilitates the patient's self-efficacy, activation, and engagement growth to improve their health (Welch & Fournier, 2018, p. 6).

Caring Practices and Patient Engagement Model

1. Maintaining belief: The nurse believes the patient has the capacity and potential to achieve health self-management.
2. Knowing: The nurse attains an understanding of the patient's perceptions and circumstances.
3. Being with: The nurse engages in relationship and person-centered care and is physically and emotionally present.
4. Doing for: The nurse does what is necessary to maintain the patient's dignity and personhood.
5. Enabling: The nurse facilitates patient self-efficacy, activation, and engagement.

(Welch & Fournier, 2018, p. 3)

The connection between the nurse and patient is critical to patient activation and engagement in self-management of health. Patients who hold positive feelings toward health and have had positive experiences are more likely to participate in self-management of health (Jiang et al., 2021). Patients and their support systems expect nurses to engage them in decision-making and respond to their questions and concerns (WHO, 2016). Nurses are in a pivotal position to provide this education and information and are vital to assisting the patient in their health self-management journey. The nurse's role coordinates care, provides transition management, advocacy, and education, communicates across settings and stakeholders, and ethically supports patient engagement, activation, self-efficacy, and health self-management.

Principles of Patient Engagement for Nurses

1. Engage with the patient in a relevant and meaningful manner, recognizing the patient's lifestyle, background, goals, and the complexity of health system navigation.
2. Engage with the patient where they are, taking time to assess their situation, barriers, strengths, and resources—NOT where you think they should be.
3. Engage with the patient early in the care planning process—NOT after you have determined the goals of care.
4. Engage with the patient regularly, providing follow-up on patient concerns or questions and giving regular updates on any changes in their care plan.
5. Engage with the patient as an equal; do not engage in paternalistic, maternalistic, or hierarchical relationships with the patient.
6. Engage with the patient beyond their "story," recognizing and respecting their unique personhood (Ennis-O'Connor, 2018).

The Patient's Role

The goal of patient engagement and activation is for the patient to effectively manage their health, make appropriate decisions, and engage in wellness or preventative care, enhancing quality of life. So the patient is central to patient engagement and activation, requiring them to act as an active agent in developing the knowledge, skills, and attitudes needed. Part of the education and teaching that nurses provide to patients should include information on the patient's role in the self-management of their health. The nurse must understand their role in promoting patient engagement and activation, and they must also understand the patients' crucial role, as part of confidence and readiness to take independent action in managing health requires an understanding of the role (Hibbard & Greene, 2013).

Patients have the right to be involved in decision-making concerning their health. This necessitates that patients use their knowledge, resources, and skills to self-manage their health. The patient is not a passive participant in healthcare; it could be argued that they should be the ones most invested and active in their health. This requires the patient to engage in a relationship with the nurse and other providers to take some control over their healthcare decisions and to be physically and emotionally involved in their health (Jiang et al., 2021).

Several factors may affect the participation of the patient in their healthcare. Patient preference is one key factor. Some patients may prefer traditionally delivered care where the patient is a passive participant and the nurse or other provider acts paternalistically, making care decisions for them. For patient engagement and activation, the patient may need support and education related to the positive aspects of having a more active and empowered role in their care. Additionally, the patient must hold the attitude that their participation will positively affect their health and that they can implement actions that will benefit them (Jiang et al., 2021). Patients' perspectives on being activated and engaged and self-managing their health may vary based on their personal characteristics, health trajectory, and healthcare experiences over time (Barello et al., 2017). This means the nurse should look and listen for cues related to patient perceptions and expectations regarding their activation, engagement, and health self-management and provide appropriate education to support the patient along their journey to active and engaged health management.

The patient brings knowledge of their experiences concerning their health and how they have dealt with any illnesses they may have. Critical to the patient's role in engagement and activation is participating in dialogue with the nurse concerning these experiences. In this way, nurses can use their training, knowledge, and skills to facilitate further patient engagement. Communication and continued dialogue are essential to enhance understanding between the patient and nurse. It should be recognized that, at times, patients may be physically unable to participate in dialogue, healthcare decision-making, or a collaborative relationship with the nurse or other providers due to the severity of illness or symptoms. In this case, the nurse must ensure the patient has a representative of their choice or a DPOA acting for them in the decision-making process or providing them the support needed to engage in their healthcare.

One central skill of the patient's role is sharing and receiving information. The patient must be able to communicate and share their needs, questions, concerns, goals, and priorities with the nurse or other providers (Jerofke-Owen et al., 2023). Recognition that they are the experts on themselves and sharing critical information concerning themselves is required for their health outcomes.

Skills in receiving information are also necessary. The patient will be the recipient of health teaching and promotion education, and for this education to be effective, the patient will need to be able to receive it, consider the information, and have the ability to apply it to their life circumstances and healthcare goals (Welch & Fournier, 2018). This will be the basis of informed decision-making concerning their health and wellness.

Jerofke-Owen et al. (2023) conceptualized patient engagement, involvement, and participation in nursing care. This conceptualization identifies attributes that the patient and nurse bring to the mutual partnership and functions each is responsible for in the process (p. 6). The nurse must bring their knowledge, training, skills, and ethical practice values to the partnership, responding to patient needs and concerns, collaborating with the patient and the interprofessional team, and recognizing when other interventions or approaches may be needed. The patient has an active role in voicing concerns, asking questions, learning from the education provided, and making decisions concerning managing their health based on their values and abilities. Investment in the process, relationship, and dialogue supports this partnership and participation model. See Figure 4.6—Conceptualization of Patient Engagement, Involvement, and Participation in Nursing.

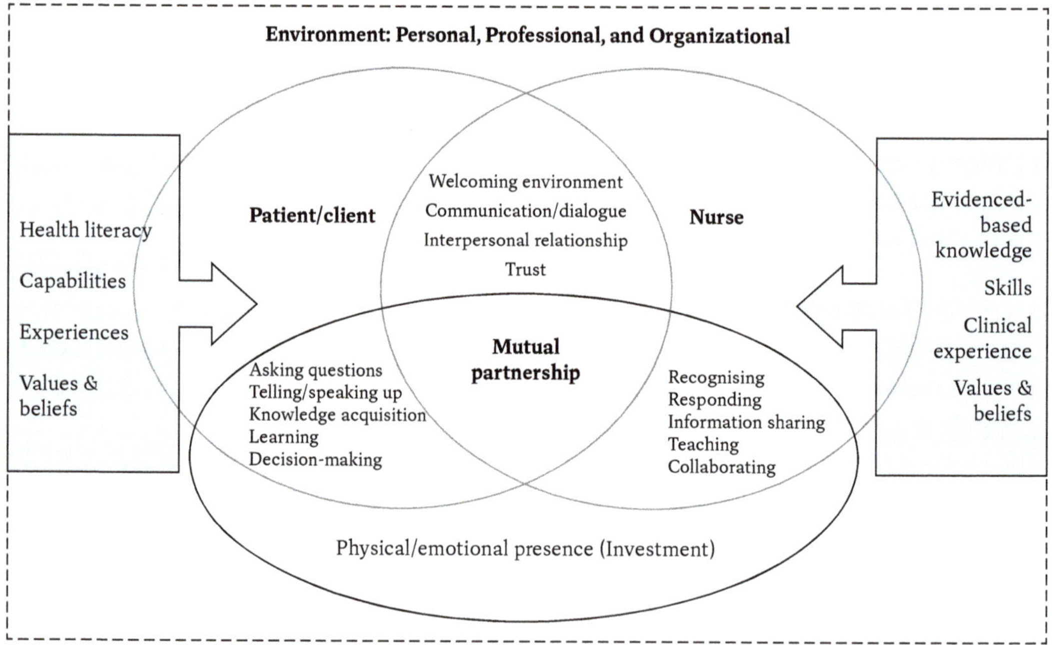

FIGURE 4.6 Conceptualization of Patient Engagement, Involvement, and Participation in Nursing

Health Literacy

Health literacy is essential for effective health teaching and education delivery, patient engagement, and activation. Over 30% of acute care hospital readmissions are linked to patients not clearly understanding discharge instructions (Amer, 2013, p. 123). Alternately, it has been shown that patients who understand their discharge instructions have a lower rate of readmission and emergency room visits. When planning health teaching, the nurse must assess for issues that could negatively affect the patient's readiness to learn. Several factors may impact the patient's ability to understand the teaching and education provided, including physical health, the severity of symptoms (e.g., pain, delirium, etc.), and emotional distress, which can affect the patient's ability to engage in and process health teaching offered (Chorrojprasert, 2020). Additionally, the teaching and education provided may not match the patient's learning style or literacy needs (Bajorek & McElroy, 2020). Assessing for and addressing readiness to learn will enhance the ability of the patient to understand the teaching or education given and to gain the knowledge, skills, and attitudes needed for positive health outcomes.

The Centers for Disease Control (CDC) defines health literacy as "the degree to which individuals have the ability to find, understand, and use information and services to inform health-related decisions and actions for themselves and others" (CDC, 2023, para. 1). This definition and focus on the use of information pulls in concepts of patient engagement and activation. Not only does the patient need to be able to understand and process the information presented, but the patient must also be able to integrate that information into making informed decisions regarding their health. The Healthy People 2030 goal of "Eliminate health disparities, achieve health equity, and attain health literacy to improve the health and well-being of all" makes the additional connection between health literacy and equity and disparities in healthcare (Healthy People 2030, n.d.a, para. 1). Inadequate health literacy impacts the patient's ability to access and navigate the healthcare system and to obtain and make decisions concerning preventive care, management of health, and illness-based care (Truglio-Londrigan & Lewenson, 2013).

Limited health literacy has also been associated with increased costs, with estimates of a patient with inadequate health literacy spending an "additional $143 to $7,798 per year" (Lopez et al., 2022, p. 6). Patients at risk of lower health literacy are likelier not to complete health forms wholly or accurately and miss follow-up appointments. They may also have difficulty reading medication labels or explaining the purpose of procedures. It is estimated that at least "88 percent of adults living in the US have health literacy inadequate to navigate the healthcare system and promote their well-being ..." (Lopez et al., 2022, p. 8).

Nutbeam (2000) identified three aspects of health literacy: (a) functional, (b) communicative, and (c) critical. Functional literacy is what nurses may often think of when considering the concept of health literacy. Functional literacy is the ability to read, write, and have numeracy or mathematical skills to make decisions concerning health. Approximately 18% of the United States population is functionally illiterate, meaning they may be able to understand simple vocabulary but struggle with basic reading skills needed, such as reading a menu (Haderline & Clark, 2017). This can cause a patient not to seek help or let the nurse know they do not understand something due to feelings of inadequacy often associated with low literacy levels. If a patient cannot read or has limited reading proficiency, handing them a brochure or a discharge packet will not support health teaching efforts. Likewise, if a person has limited numeracy skills, they may be unable to calculate sliding scale doses or adjust doses of medications based on symptoms.

Communicative literacy is connected to the self-management of health. It is the cognitive, literacy, and social skills needed to manage health daily, such as seeking health information, making meaning out of information and various forms of communication received, and applying the new knowledge to health self-management (Nutbeam, 2000). Self-management of health, engagement, and activation requires the patient to process health information through reading, writing, or speaking and have the communication skills to express concerns and questions, ensuring understanding of the information's meaning. Communicative literacy is based on person- and relationship-centered care, where there is back-and-forth dialogue and interaction about health information, education, teaching, and application to health self-management. Critical literacy requires advanced cognitive abilities and social skills (Nutbeam, 2000). These are needed for the patient to engage in critical analysis and synthesis of health information in order to engage in shared decision-making and autonomy in the self-management of health. Critical literacy enhances patient empowerment and self-efficacy.

Health literacy is the global ability of the patient to understand, seek, and use information to direct healthcare decisions and self-management. This includes reading, writing, numeracy, communication, and social and cognitive skills, allowing patients to critically analyze and apply information to their health decisions and actions. Understanding the types of health literacy enables the nurse to have a more holistic view of literacy assessment and how to deliver health teaching and education in a relevant manner for the patient. Viewing health literacy on this continuum of functional to critical points out how important it is to deliver health education in a way that is appropriate for the patient, as well as the necessity of understanding how these aspects of health literacy affect the patient's response to education provided and their activation and engagement in their health management. See Figure 4.7 for the application of Nutbeam's model on nursing actions.

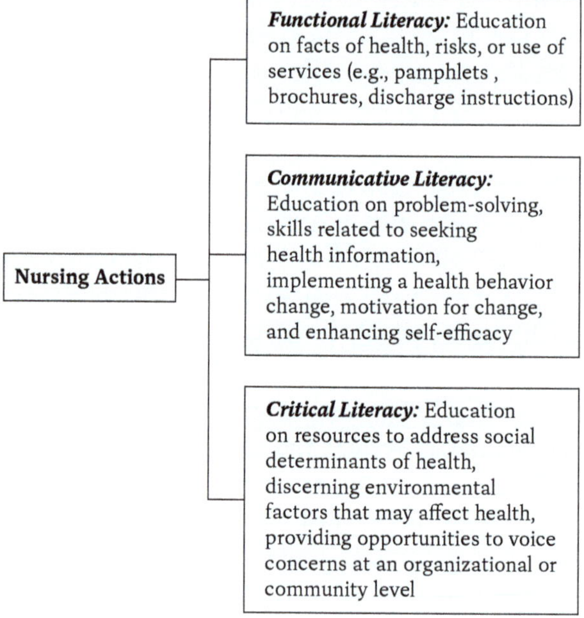

FIGURE 4.7 Types of Health Literacy and Nursing Actions

The National Action Plan to Improve Health Literacy

The National Action Plan to Improve Health Literacy is based on two core principles:

- All people have the right to health information that helps them make informed decisions.
- Health services should be delivered in ways that are easy to understand and that improve health, longevity, and quality of life.

The Action Plan contains seven goals that will improve health literacy and strategies for achieving them:

1. Develop and disseminate health and safety information that is accurate, accessible, and actionable.
2. Promote changes in the health care system to improve health information, communication, and access to healthcare, which will inform decision-making.
3. Incorporate accurate, standards-based, and developmentally appropriate health and science information and curricula in childcare and education through the university level.
4. Support and expand local efforts to provide adult education, English language instruction, and culturally and linguistically appropriate health information services in the community.
5. Build partnerships, develop guidance, and change policies.
6. Increase basic research and the development, implementation, and evaluation of practices and interventions to improve health literacy.
7. Increase the dissemination and use of evidence-based health literacy practices and interventions.

(U.S. Department of Health and Human Services, Office of Disease Prevention and Health Promotion, 2010, para. 1).

Organization Health Literacy

Organizations also need to have health literacy, supporting the role the health system has in patients' health literacy development. Healthy People 2023 defines **organization health literacy** as "the degree to which organizations equitably enable individuals to find, understand, and use information and services to inform health-related decisions and actions for themselves and others" (HRSA, 2022, para. 1). Organization health literacy is central to promoting equitable and accessible care and the ability of patients to make autonomous health decisions. Nurses can support organization health literacy by using a **universal health literacy precautions** approach, assuming all patients may have difficulty understanding the education or teaching provided. Universal health literacy precautions focus on offering simplified communication and confirming patient understanding, assisting with navigating the healthcare environment, and supporting patients in health self-management (AHRQ, 2020). When illness, symptoms, environmental

10 Elements of Competence for Using Teach-Back Effectively

1. Use a caring tone of voice and attitude.
2. Display comfortable body language and make eye contact.
3. Use plain language.
4. Ask the patient to explain back, using their own words.
5. Use non-shaming, open-ended questions.
6. Avoid asking questions that can be answered with a simple yes or no.
7. Emphasize that the responsibility to explain clearly is on you, the provider.
8. If the patient is not able to teach-back correctly, explain again and recheck.
9. Use reader-friendly print materials to support learning.
10. Document use of and patient response to teach-back.

(Always Use Teach Back, n.d., para. 1)

distractors, the complexity of the healthcare system, etc., are considered, even those with high functional, communicative, and critical literacy may have difficulty processing, understanding, and utilizing the information given in health decision-making or self-management.

The nurse should use language without jargon or acronyms and provide education in everyday language. Health education should also be supported with visual aids, pictures, or models to help understanding. Teach-back is critical to ensuring the patient understands the education received by asking them to explain the teaching in their own words. Open-ended questions should be used, encouraging patients to share information about themselves or ask questions without interruption. Offering education on what is needed, repeating the most important aspects of the education given, and supporting patients in completing forms are also part of organization health literacy (HRSA, 2022).

Social Influencers of Health

Social determinants of health (SDOH), such as economic status, educational level, community violence, etc., are often referred to when discussing factors or characteristics affecting health and quality of life. SDOH is the common phrase used to refer to these influencers of health. However, in the strength-based approach to care coordination practice, it is essential to recognize that these types of factors do not necessarily "determine" the course of a person's health. However, they can influence their health (Center for Health and Health Care in Schools, 2020).

Social influencers of health (SIOH) are those factors such as quality of education, access to healthcare, economic stability, community and social factors, and environmental factors that can influence health behaviors, health outcomes, and overall health. Words matter, and this is an essential construct around patient engagement and activation, as the nurse must believe that the patient can self-manage health and be actively engaged and motivated to improve their health outcomes. Suppose the nurse approaches the patient with the attitude that since they come from a lower socioeconomic background or education level, this determines that they cannot become health literate or activated to engage in healthy behaviors. In that case, the nurse cannot promote readiness, confidence, or self-efficacy development. This does not mean the nurse ignores traumatic experiences, unemployment, or lack of access to healthcare or other resources. It means that if the nurse identifies these as issues and potential challenges or barriers for the patient during the assessment process, these issues are addressed, in collaboration with the patient, in the care plan.

Health literacy is considered a SIOH. Research has found that those with lower health literacy levels often come from lower socioeconomic status, lower educational levels, or underserved or vulnerable populations (Lopez et al., 2022). For example, lower health literacy is associated with not having a high school diploma or living below the poverty level. Additionally, health literacy has been related to a lack of social capital, underrepresentation, or those who need accommodations (e.g., those with disabilities or non-English speaking) within society (Lopez et al., 2022). See Figure 4.8 for a visual of social determinants of health identified by Healthy People 2030.

This information directs the nurse to promote and look for organizational health literacy within their work systems, providing needed advocacy and participation in efforts to address organizational health literacy (ANA, 2015). Healthy People 2030 specifies a goal related to SDOH, "Create social, physical, and economic environments that promote attaining the full potential for health and well-being for all" (Healthy People 2030, n.d.b, para. 5). This goal calls for healthcare organizations to actively develop resources, environments, and materials that address all levels of health literacy and support the development of patient activation and

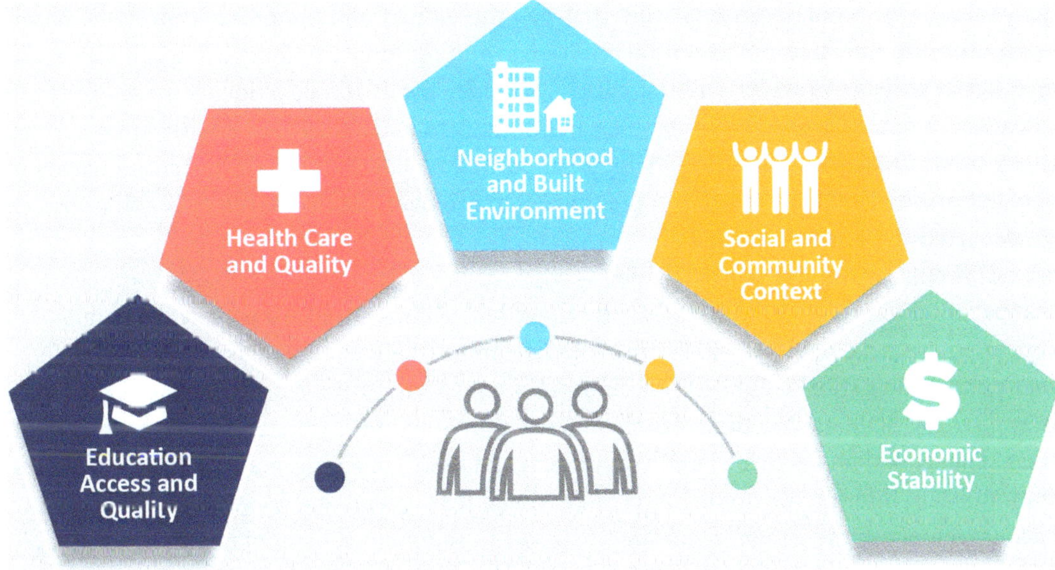

FIGURE 4.8 Healthy People 2030 Social Determinants of Health

engagement for long-term health self-management, quality of life, and wellness. Organizational actions for improving health literacy might include providing culturally and linguistically appropriate education and services, enhancing communication, and using shared and informed decision-making (Healthy People 2030, n.d.b).

Patient's life experiences, the generation into which they were born, their SIOH, the community in which they live, and their social groups influence how they will contribute to their health outcomes and engage in health self-management (Lange, 2012). Health locus of control is one way people perceive their health and events related to health as internally controllable or externally controlled by others, and this can be influenced by SIOH, life experiences, and cultural beliefs and values (Bergland et al., 2014). When working with patients to promote activation and engagement in health behaviors, the nurse must keep in mind the influence all these factors have on the patient's knowledge, skills, and attitudes toward self-management of health. For example, it is insufficient for the nurse to provide education on a new diabetic diet plan without assessing for and addressing issues such as food scarcity, ability to buy food and supplies, availability of cooking and refrigeration systems, attitudes towards a diabetes diagnosis, experience managing diabetes or with diabetes in their family or social groups, etc. These items will influence how the patient approaches the new diabetic diet plan. Without a comprehensive approach, interventions may be unsuccessful, leading to patient frustration, dissatisfaction, and lack of engagement.

Shared Decision-Making

Health literacy, organization health literacy, and patient teaching affect the ability of the patient to make appropriate informed decisions concerning their healthcare. **Shared decision-making (SDM)**, which relies upon individual and organizational health literacy, is another significant factor affecting patient engagement and health management. SDM is an informed decision-making process that occurs collaboratively between the patient and the provider or nurse based upon accurate information, potential outcomes, and options. SDM occurs when the nurse or other healthcare provider and the patient consider the available evidence-based practice information and potential care outcomes and options to make informed healthcare decisions (Kelly et al., 2018). SDM involves dialogue about the benefits, risks, and potential harms of care options, engaging the patient in the process to discover patient preferences and priorities of care (AHRQ, 2020).

SDM ensures that the care provided is right for the patient, uses the right resources, and that patient engagement and activation are supported. SDM is not only a patient right but is also supported in ethical nursing practice through developing trusting and collaborative relationships that uphold the patient's right to self-determination (ANA, 2015). Nurses have a central role in supporting SDM as they often are the ones that interact most frequently with patients and their support systems, provide health promotion and health teaching, act as patient advocates, communicate information among interprofessional team members, and provide support and encouragement to the patient regarding their role in self-management of health (Chung et al., 2021). SDM has been shown to increase patient satisfaction and adherence to the care plan and also support relationship-centered care practices (AHRQ, 2020).

The attitude and skills of the nurse can affect the quality of SDM and how engaged the patient will be in the process. Firstly, the nurse must maintain a relationship-centered focus, acknowledging that the nurse-patient relationship is essential for developing health self-management knowledge skills and attitudes. The starting point of the nurse-patient relationship is assessment, which takes time to understand the patient, their needs, and the gaps in knowledge or care. Once this is identified, the nurse can plan their health teaching and health promotion to address knowledge gaps so the patient can fully participate in SDM. In addition, the nurse can tailor the health education to meet patient learning and literacy needs and the desired level of participation in the SDM process (Truglio-Londrigan et al., 2012). Depending on patient values, preferences, cultural differences, and life experiences, the comfort level in SDM may vary among patients and their support systems. The nurse should listen to the expectations of the patient and their support system, respecting how involved the patient wants to be in the SDM process. The nurse has a crucial role as a "communication bridge," offering understandable health teaching and information for the patient and working as a conveyor and coordinator of information and expectations amongst the interprofessional team members (Chung et al., 2021, p. 5).

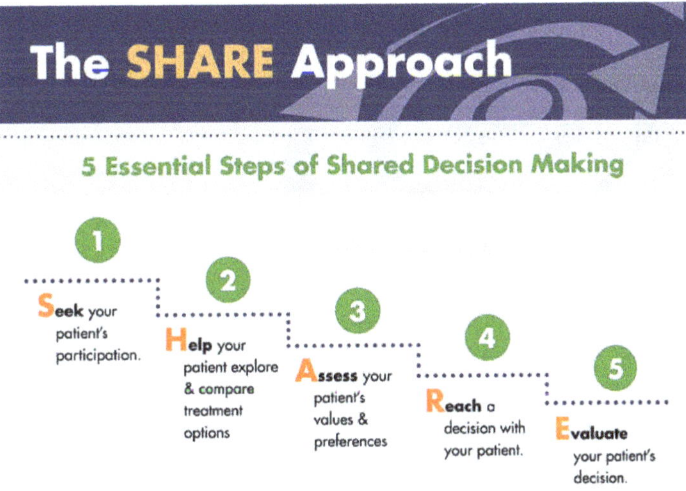

FIGURE 4.9 The SHARE Approach to Shared Decision-Making

Motivational Interviewing and Stages of Change

Motivational interviewing (MI) is a person-centered approach often used to address the common problem of ambivalence about behavior change (Miller & Rollnick, 2013). MI is conversation and dialogue that elicits intrinsic motivation to change health behavior, explores ambivalence toward health behavior change, and empowers the patient to begin health behavior change by clarifying patient care priorities and values and collaborative action planning. MI focuses on language about change, centered on patient values, preferences of care, and life situations. As part of relationship-centered care, it is an opportunity for the nurse to encourage, collaborate, and guide the patient toward activation and engagement in their health self-management based upon informed decision-making.

MI views motivation as grounded in readiness, importance, confidence, and willingness to change. These are all needed for intrinsic motivation to change health behaviors, to activate and engage in health self-management. Intrinsic motivation is based on the patient's internal desire to perform the action, not a desire built on outside reinforcement or consequences (Driscoll, 2000). The nurse may have conversations centered on MI with the patient, provide health teaching, and coordinate care, but ultimately, the patient goes home to live independently. They will not have the nurse reminding them to take medication, engage in preventative healthcare, or exercise regularly. The patient must have the intrinsic motivation to do these activities. That is why listening for activation language, or the lack thereof, is essential—it indicates the patient's level of intrinsic motivation to begin exploring activation and engagement in their health.

The phrases and language the patient uses can assist the nurse in identifying where the patient is in the health behavior change journey. Prochaska and DiClemente (1982) developed an integrative model of behavior change that identifies a continuum for stages of change beginning with precontemplation of change and ending with the maintenance of the health behavior. The nurse will need to adjust the conversation, education provided, and support offered, depending on where the patient falls in the continuum. For example, a patient who vapes may not even

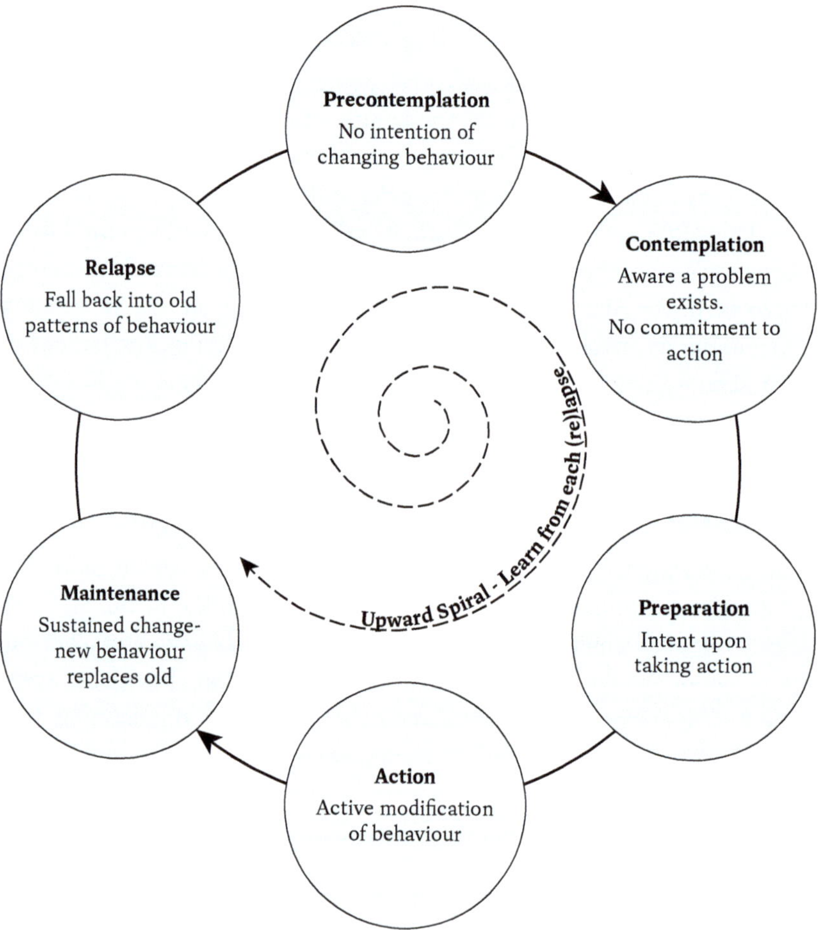

FIGURE 4.10 Stages of Change

be considering quitting due to a lack of education on the health risks or personal preferences. This is the precontemplation stage, the stage preceding a health behavior change. Next, after receiving health teaching related to the health risks of vaping, the patient may begin thinking about stopping. This is the contemplation stage. Through increased confidence and readiness, the patient may start formulating an action plan for quitting vaping and become committed to the new health behavior. This is the preparation stage. Next, the patient may attend support groups for those quitting vaping and begin cutting back on the amount of time they are vaping. This is the action stage. Lastly, the patient has quit vaping and now moves onto the maintenance stage of the health behavior.

There is also the potential for the patient to relapse and begin vaping again. This is another stage, relapse. The nurse must understand that patients may stall at one stage and not progress forward, be ambivalent about changing their health behaviors, or relapse multiple times (Prochaska & DiClemente, 1982).

MI can assist the nurse and patient to navigate the stages of change in various ways. Depending on the stage of change, the nurse may offer education and support for self-efficacy development, facilitate consideration of a health behavior change, or collaborate with the patient to create an action plan for the health behavior change, addressing barriers and challenges to the desired action (Miller & Rollnick, 2002). Utilizing a strength-based approach, the nurse may explore past experiences, support systems, and resources to boost success. No matter how MI techniques are integrated into the nurse's practice, it is based on providing the education, belief, empathy, and encouragement needed to elicit intrinsic motivation for the patient to change their health and health behaviors. Utilizing MI principles and understanding the stages of change, the nurse "evokes" intrinsic motivation already present in the patient. The role of the nurse is to enhance the patient's view of the importance of health behavior, to explore conflicting beliefs or emotions related to health behavior, and to empathize with and validate that self-management of health and health behavior change will require motivation, commitment, and engagement on the patient's part (Fraser et al., 2018).

MI is based on four principles: (a) partnership, (b) acceptance, (c) compassion, and (d) evocation (Miller & Rollnick, 2013). The principle of partnership fits well with person-centered practices, where care decisions are made with the patient rather than for the patient. This is key to guiding the patient to activate their own motivation and resources toward a health behavior change. Acceptance involves affirming the patient's worth and autonomy and empathizing with their situation (Miller & Rollnick, 2013). Viewing the patient with positive regard, respect, and trust is critical to mobilize the patient along the change continuum, believing they are capable and have a right to autonomous decision-making. The principle of compassion calls for the commitment to the patient's best interests, which is also supported by ethical nursing practice and relationship-based care. Lastly, evocation is based on the belief that the patient has what they need to meet the challenge or to self-manage their health (Miller & Rollnick, 2013). By focusing on their strengths and resources, the nurse strengthens motivations and resources already present. See Figure 4.11—The Spirit of Motivational Interviewing Application to Nursing.

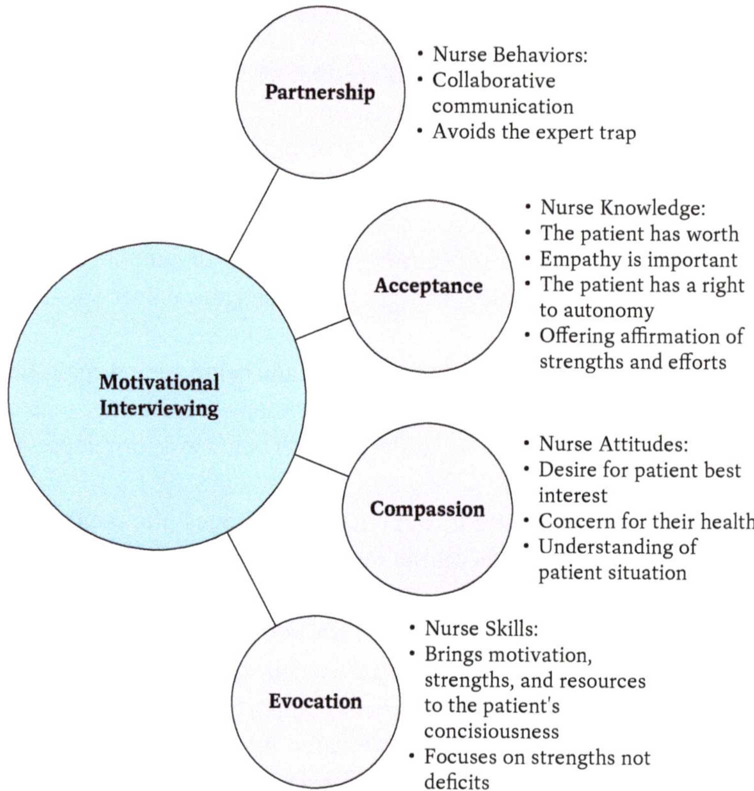

FIGURE 4.11 The Spirit of Motivational Interviewing and Application to Nursing

MI has four steps in the process: (a) engaging, (b) focusing, (c) evoking, and (d) planning (Miller & Rollnick, 2013). Engaging allows the patient to build a rapport and trust with the nurse. While engaging, the nurse assists the patient in accessing their intrinsic motivation and building self-efficacy related to health self-management. A tool to help with engaging is using OARS, open-ended questions, affirmation, reflective listening, and conversation summary. Using OARS allows the patient to explore readiness, importance, and confidence and enables the nurse to build a trusting and collaborative relationship with the patient.

The second step is focusing, which assists in clarifying and identifying patient priorities of care and values, focusing on a patient-driven agenda. This can be difficult in healthcare, as the nurse often has an agenda for health teaching and may try to direct the focus. Collaborative agenda mapping can assist with focusing, allowing the patient to identify priority topics or gaps in their knowledge.

In the third step, evoking, MI is used to bring to consciousness intrinsic motivation already present in the patient. In this step, the nurse may bring past successes to the conversation and use tools like importance and confidence rulers. Lastly, in the planning step, the nurse works with the patient collaboratively to create relevant and meaningful health goals that will assist them in managing their health, recognizing that health behavior change, activation, and engagement is a process.

A Case Manager's Experience with OARS in a Transition of Care

As I was working in an acute care setting, an elderly man who lived alone and independently was admitted inpatient. The discharge plan recommendation from the physical therapist was subacute rehabilitation (SAR) for mobility and strengthening before returning home. This was discussed with the patient; he agreed to the plan, and all moved forward. Then, the day of discharge to the SAR facility came. The patient became agitated and said he planned to leave against medical advice (AMA) and return to his home instead of the SAR facility.

I met with the patient and began using some MI principles to see if I could understand the patient's situation and how he could best be supported to receive the rehabilitation needed for good health outcomes. I began using OARS. Open-ended questions and reflective listening facilitated the dialogue, and I could see why the patient had changed his mind. As the conversation evolved, the patient expressed that he feared losing his apartment if he went to the SAR facility and was unable to pay the rent. He indicated that he needed to go to his bank because he did not have anyone else listed on his account to get the money to pay his rent. I affirmed his concern and challenge in paying his rent and told him I would work on a solution. I contacted the SAR facility to see if they could get him to the bank to pay his rent. A solution was developed to allow the patient to leave the SAR facility on a day pass to pay his rent once he was deemed safe, and they would coordinate transportation.

I met with the patient again, summarized his concerns, presented the potential solution, and allowed him to ask questions or express concerns and collaboratively adjust the plan if needed. The patient agreed to the plan and was safely discharged to the SAR facility. Using the OARS technique allowed me to understand the patient's concerns, make additional plans to meet the patient's needs, engage in relationship-centered care, and ultimately get the patient the rehabilitation he needed so he could return home and live independently. —R. W., inpatient case manager

Motivational Interviewing and Shared Decision-Making

MI and SDM share a person-centered approach, supporting patient participation and autonomy. SDM can utilize MI principles to ensure the patient is informed about their health and options for health management and assist the patient in identifying what is important to them, how ready they are to make a health decision, and how confident they are in implementing the decision or action. This increases the likelihood that the patient will adhere to the plan of care and that it will be relevant and meaningful to the patient (Fraser et al., 2018). Both MI and SDM require excellent communication skills, a trusting and respectful relationship between the nurse and the patient, and a flexible approach to promote the exploration of options and perspectives (Elwyn, 2014).

MI and SDM use similar techniques, such as exchanging information, exploring priorities and perspectives, and reflective listening. OARS (open-ended questions, affirmation, reflection, and summary) is used extensively in MI and SDM to elicit preferences and provide context to the decisions being made. Another tool used in MI and SDM is creating a pro and con list, option talk, or decisional balance exercises. These seek to draw out the patient's views concerning the positives or negatives of a decision or a health behavior change (Elwyn, 2014). This allows for a more focused examination of patient concerns and provides a springboard for further exploration of the patient's questions or evoking motivation concerning a behavior change or health decision.

Patients may move along the shared decision-making and health self-management journey at different paces and have setbacks. Sometimes the patient may experience ambivalence about their progress in the health self-management journey or appear to be at a momentary standstill in the shared decision-making process. The nurse must recognize when different approaches are needed, when to integrate methods, and when a patient may need a topic revisited, allowing them time to process and weigh the information given to further the patient along the activation, engagement, and health self-management continuum. See Figure 4.12—Application of MI to SDM.

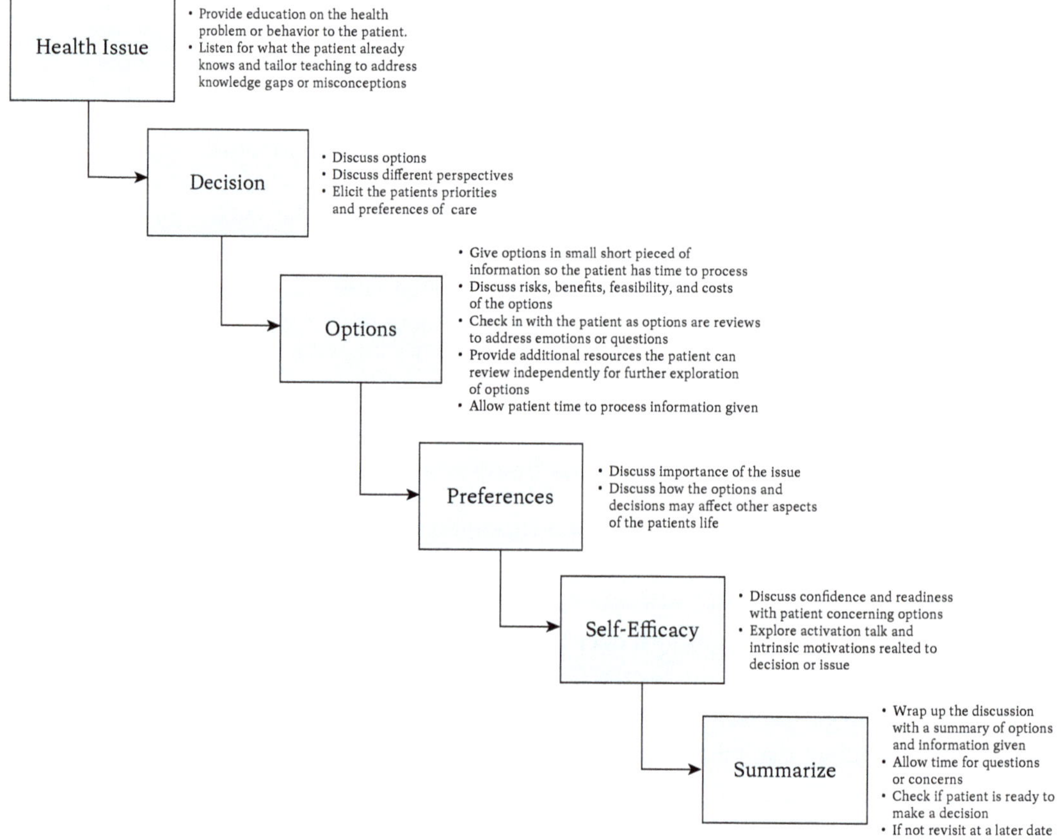

FIGURE 4.12 Application of Motivational Interviewing to Shared Decision Making

Decisional Balance, Option Talk, and Pro/Con Lists

In MI and SDM, the patient will need to engage in dialogue about the decisions or the health behavior change. Sometimes a patient may be experiencing confusion or ambivalence or feeling unable to determine what is most important to them. In these cases, using a decisional balance exercise, also known as option talk, or a pro/con list can be helpful. This can be done with a paper worksheet outlining the pros or positives of a decision or change and the cons, the negatives. Alternatively, it can be done through strategic dialogue and using visual aids if needed (e.g., whiteboard). In various forms, this exercise can assist the patient in considering the benefits and costs of a choice and may move the patient from ambivalence to action. See the example pro/con worksheet.

Pros of Not Changing Behavior*	Cons of Not Changing Behavior*
1.	1.
2.	2.
3.	3.
Short-Term Pros of Changing Behavior	**Short-Term Cons of Changing Behavior**
1.	1.
2.	2.
3.	3.
Long-Term Pros of Changing Behavior	**Long-Term Cons of Changing Behavior**
1.	1.
2.	2.
3.	3.

Source: https://opentext.wsu.edu/ldaffin/chapter/module-3-a-willingness-to-change/

CHAPTER SUMMARY

One critical goal of care coordination practice is supporting the patient in self-managing their health. This is essential in decreasing healthcare costs and resource use and increasing patient satisfaction and positive health outcomes. Empowering patients to understand their health conditions, the role of preventative and wellness care, and how to self-manage their health assists the patient in making informed, appropriate choices for their health. Understanding the critical impact of self-management of health and promoting it puts patients at the center of their care experience, sustaining collaborative and person-centered care practices.

Health self-management is not a newly recognized need and has been brought back to the forefront with the transition to value-based care and the focus on resource management and patient outcomes. Self-management of health may vary based on the patient's symptoms or health conditions but is critical to preventing chronic diseases, engaging in preventative and wellness care, and enhancing quality of life. Various skills are needed for successful self-management of health, such as problem-solving, decision-making, as well as having needed information for decision-making and understanding how to take action regarding healthy behaviors.

Self-management of health is the outcome of patient engagement and activation, is dependent upon patient self-efficacy, and is supported by the patient–nurse partnership. Patient engagement is needed to meet care coordination guiding principles and rights through promoting patient autonomy and providing evidence-based and appropriate care. Patient activation is also required for health self-management, as this is a person's internal motivation to change their health behaviors and take action. "Patient activation is a strong predictor for seeking and using health information" (CDC, 2021, para. 6). Patients have identified wanting more information about their health conditions, and research has shown that patients with higher activation levels ask more questions, seek additional health information, and better understand their treatment options for their health conditions (Greene et al., 2015; Heath, 2022). Patient activation can be determined using a confidence ruler, a readiness or importance ruler, tools such as the Patient Activation Measure®, or listening for activation language.

Understanding the nurse's role in patient engagement and activation supports independent and productive health self-management. The nurse can enhance patient engagement and activation by assessing for and meeting health literacy and social influencers of health (SIOH) needs, participating in shared decision-making (SDM), and utilizing motivational interviewing (MI) techniques. The nurse must also believe in the patient's ability to self-manage their health, support self-efficacy development, and evoke intrinsic motivation. The role of the patient also requires understanding by the nurse and the patient, acknowledging patient preferences, helping the patient share critical information, voicing questions and concerns, and engaging in continued dialogue.

Comprehending the impact of health literacy on an organizational and individual level is a critical component to the growth of health self-management knowledge, skills, and attitudes. Recognizing the essential need for health literacy assessment and viewing health literacy more expansively, including functional, communication, and critical literacy, will assist the nurse in proactively meeting patient educational needs. Using organization-literate practices such as teach-back, the nurse can utilize a strength-based approach to engage the patient in health self-management. Knowledge of the SIOH on patient engagement, activation, and health literacy is central to providing exemplary patient education, teaching, and supporting SDM and patient autonomy. Nurses are ethically bound to ensure that organizationally literate practices are offered that uphold the patient's right to self-determination and SDM. This may require the nurse to participate in self-reflective practice to ensure that person- and relationship-based care is provided or to advocate proactively for organizational health literacy policies and processes.

MI techniques can encourage collaboration and guide the patient toward self-efficacy, activation, and engagement in their health. Using the principles of partnership, acceptance, compassion, and evocation, the nurse can assist the patient in accessing their internal motivation and confidence in health self-management. In the end, through a clear understanding of roles, the relationship between self-efficacy, activation, and engagement, the influence of health literacy and SIOH, and the use of collaborative techniques such as MI and SDM, the nurse can empower the patient toward long-term growth and success in health self-management.

CHAPTER 4 GLOSSARY

Activation Language: Phrases or language that indicate the patient is considering making a health behavior action or change, such as "I am thinking about ..." or "It is important that I ..."

Durable Power of Attorney: A person identified to act on the person's behalf and make healthcare or other decisions for that person when they are incapacitated and unable to make decisions for themselves.

Expert Trap: An attitude on the part of the nurse where they believe that they are the "expert" on the patient's health and situation and know what is best for the patient concerning health self-management and healthcare decisions.

Health Literacy: The global ability of the patient to understand, seek, and use information to direct healthcare decisions and self-management. This includes reading, writing, numeracy, communication, social, and cognitive skills, allowing patients to critically analyze and apply information to their health decisions and actions.

Health Self-Management: The possession of knowledge, skills, and attitudes that allows patients to manage their health daily for positive health outcomes.

Motivational Interviewing: Engaging in dialogue that elicits intrinsic motivation to change health behavior, explores ambivalence toward health behavior change, and empowers the patient to begin health behavior change by clarifying care priorities and values and collaborative action planning.

Organization Literacy: The degree to which organizations facilitate the patient's ability to seek, find, understand, and apply health information and navigate healthcare services to inform healthcare decisions and actions, promoting equitability and accessibility in healthcare.

Patient Activation: Intrinsic motivation and ability, supported by self-efficacy and willingness to take action toward specific health behaviors or self-management.

Patient Engagement: Taking ownership of one's health to make informed and appropriate healthcare decisions and actions; exercising self-management of health.

Righting Reflex: The nurse trying to correct or "fix" a situation based on their opinions, beliefs, or knowledge without considering the audience, situation, patient preferences, or circumstances.

Self-Efficacy: The belief that one is capable and can accomplish identified goals or health actions.

Shared Decision-Making: Informed decision-making that occurs collaboratively between the patient and the provider or nurse and is based upon accurate information concerning potential outcomes and options.

Social Influencer of Health: Factors such as quality of education, access to healthcare, economic stability, community and social factors, and environmental factors that can influence health behaviors, health outcomes, and overall health.

Universal Health Literacy Precautions: Assuming all patients may have difficulty understanding health teaching, utilizing simplified communication, confirming patient understanding, assisting with navigating the healthcare system, and supporting health self-management.

DISCUSSION QUESTIONS AND ACTIVITIES

Discussion Questions

1. Discuss why it is vital for nurses to understand patient activation, engagement, and health self-management.
2. Consider the issue of health literacy. Identify one complication of health illiteracy or functional literacy regarding the cost of healthcare, patient outcomes, or patient quality of life. Discuss how you will address this potential complication and the issue of health illiteracy in your nursing practice.
3. Social determinants and influencers of health can affect health outcomes as well as the ability of a person to engage in health self-management. Choose one of the social determinants of health outlined by Healthy People 2030: (a) education access and quality, (b) health care access and quality, (c) neighborhood and built environment, (d) social and community context, or (e) economic stability. Then discuss
   - the definition of the selected social determinant of health and how it could affect patient health outcomes.
   - how it could create a challenge in or affect the ability of a person to engage in health self-management.
4. The World Health Organization recognizes that a healthcare professional's attitudes, knowledge, and skills can support or deter patient engagement.
   - Identify one attitude, area of knowledge, or skill a nurse could possess to support patient engagement and explain how it promotes patient engagement.
   - Identify one attitude a nurse could possess or an area of knowledge or skill a nurse could lack that might deter patient engagement and explain how it might prevent patient engagement.

5. Some nurses may fall into the "expert trap" or engage in the "righting reflex." Think of a time you saw this in your clinical experiences or your personal healthcare experiences. Identify what attitude or belief system the nurse seemed to hold that led to them participating in the "expert trap" or "righting reflex." Then discuss the following:
   - Do you hold this attitude or belief system?
   - If not, do you hold another attitude that could encourage you to participate in the "expert trap" or "righting reflex" in your nursing practice?
   - How will you address the "expert trap" or "righting reflex" if you see them exhibited by another nurse?

Activities

1. Create a mind map of health self-management.
   a. Put the concept of health self-management in a circle in the middle.
   b. Select three to five main concepts or ideas affecting health self-management and circle them around your main circle.
   c. Draw a line from the outside circle concepts or ideas to the main concept of health self-management.
   d. Brainstorm ideas, skills, tasks, attitudes, and questions for each main concept or idea.
   e. Draw lines connecting each main concept or idea to the supporting brainstormed ideas, skills, tasks, attitudes, and questions.
2. Using the following scenario, role-play with fellow students using OARS.
   a. You are a transition coordinator meeting with a palliative care patient and his wife concerning potentially transitioning to hospice care. The patient receives blood transfusions three times a week to address extreme fatigue related to his lymphoma diagnosis, which is without benefit as the fatigue continues to increase. When you mention that the blood transfusions may not be continued on hospice care, the wife becomes upset and states, "I am not just going to let him die."
   b. Utilize the OARS (open ended questions, affirmation, reflective listening, and summary) technique to explore the issue and potential transition with the patient and his wife.
   c. Switch roles and repeat the process.
   d. Reflect on the experience and identify what you have learned about the OARS strategy related to health decision-making and whether there is anything that you want to know more about concerning the use of OARS in your nursing practice.

3. Work in groups to create a social environment change to increase patient activation. Complete the following steps:

    a. Identify a health behavior issue.

    b. Provide a background on why this is an issue and why a change in this health behavior is needed for positive health outcomes.

    c. Design a poster, an interactive session, or an information campaign to address the issue and promote health education and patient activation via social media delivery.

    d. Ensure that health literacy is addressed in the design and that the intervention focuses on one specific, manageable ability related to patient activation.

NCLEX STYLE QUESTIONS

1. Which answer reflects patient engagement in health self-management?

    a. The patient understands that their pharmacy monitors their medication adherence and relays any concerns they may have to the patient's primary care provider.

    b. The patient writes down questions for their primary care provider before their annual wellness exam and brings the list to the appointment.

    c. The patient utilizes the emergency room to get their immunizations.

    d. The patient knows there is a "sick day" dose for their insulin and uses it whenever someone around them is sick.

Questions 2–4 relate to the scenario below.

Ms. Dawson is visiting her primary care provider for her annual wellness exam. The results of her examination showed that Ms. Dawson has hypothyroidism and osteoporosis. You are the nurse giving the health teaching and education related to her new medications. She has been prescribed levothyroxine sodium 137mcg daily, one hour before breakfast, and alendronate 70 mg, weekly on Friday, taken 30 minutes before the Levothyroxine Sodium.

2. What is the BEST way to assess Ms. Dawson's health literacy as you prepare to begin health teaching?

    a. Ask Ms. Dawson about her education level and how well she can read.

    b. Ask Ms. Dawson if she will read the instructions herself at home.

    c. Ask Ms. Dawson what she knows about hypothyroidism and osteoporosis.

    d. Ask Ms. Dawson how she learns best when learning something new.

3. Ms. Dawson tells you that it will be difficult for her to remember that on Fridays she must take one medication 30 minutes before the other and which is which. Which is the BEST way to assist Ms. Dawson and encourage patient engagement?

   a. Ask her primary care provider to meet with her and explain the need for the dosage times.

   b. Encourage the patient to use the Internet to learn the importance of taking the medications at the times prescribed so she will understand the why.

   c. Explain to Ms. Dawson that she needs to take her medication at the times prescribed and refer her to a medication reminder system application for cellular phone use.

   d. Acknowledge the potential difficulty and engage Ms. Dawson in dialogue about what things she might be able to do at home to help her remember when and how to take her medications.

4. You have provided Ms. Dawson with health teaching concerning her new medications and want to validate that she understands how to take the medications. Which of the following is the BEST question to evaluate Ms. Dawson's understanding?

   a. Ask Ms. Dawson to explain the purpose, dosage, order of administration, and timing of the medications to you in her own words.

   b. Ask Ms. Dawson if she understood the health teaching provided and allow time for questions and answers.

   c. Ask Ms. Dawson if she has any concerns about taking her new medications.

   d. Ask Ms. Dawson if she has someone at home to remind her of the medication administration order and timing on Fridays.

5. The nurse knows that health self-management is needed to do which of the following? (Select all that apply.)

   a. Health self-management ensures patient adherence to the plan of care.

   b. Health self-management assists in managing resources.

   c. Health self-management increases patient quality of life.

   d. Health self-management decreases poor health outcomes.

6. The five core health self-management skills include which of the following?

    a. Problem identification, decision-making, motivational interviewing, self-efficacy, and action.

    b. Problem-solving, shared decision-making, use of resources, partnership development, and self-efficacy.

    c. Problem-solving, decision-making, use of resources, partnership development, and action.

    d. Problem-identification, shared decision-making, use of resources, action, and self-efficacy.

7. The trajectory framework of health self-management has three components. Which of the following is a component of the trajectory framework?

    a. Mental

    b. Behavioral

    c. Engagement

    d. Activation

8. Which of the following has been identified as critical to patient engagement? (Select all that apply.)

    a. Increasing patient satisfaction

    b. Increasing resource use

    c. Increasing positive outcomes

    d. All of the above

9. You are precepting a new nurse and have just finished reviewing the concept of activation language related to patient activation. You know the new nurse understands the concept when they say to you which of the following?

    a. My role as the nurse is to teach the patient how to use activation language and phrases.

    b. My role as the nurse is to discover why the patient is not using activation language and phrases.

c. My role as the nurse is to offer support and encouragement when I hear activation language and phrases.

d. My role as the nurse is to educate the patient's support system and the interprofessional team on listening for activation language and phrases.

10. In which of the following ways does the nurse assist in building patient activation, engagement, and self-management of health? (Select all that apply.)

 a. Awareness of the nurse's role in the process

 b. Supporting patient autonomous decision-making

 c. Ensuring the patient knows expert recommendations

 d. Engaging in the "righting reflex"

11. You are meeting with a patient and discussing their role in patient activation, engagement, and self-management of health. Which of the following should you NOT include in the discussion?

 a. The patient's role includes engaging in dialogue and conversation.

 b. The patient's role includes sharing information and asking questions.

 c. The patient's role recognizes that the healthcare provider is the health expert.

 d. The patient's role is to believe their participation will positively affect their health.

12. You are assessing the health literacy needs of a patient and want to assess for communicative literacy. Which of the following knowledge, skills, or attitudes would you assess for?

 a. The patient shows interest in the health topic.

 b. The patient can listen without interrupting.

 c. The patient recognizes the importance of paying attention to the teaching.

 d. The patient can receive and process new information and apply it to their situation.

13. Your organization has just started a task force on organization health literacy. You have been assigned as the task force chair and must outline the definition of organization health literacy. Which phrase BEST defines organization health literacy?

a. Organizations have a role in developing health literacy policies and processes and assisting patients in navigating the healthcare system.

b. Organizations have a role in facilitating the ability of patients to seek, find, understand, and apply health information to inform healthcare decisions, promoting equitability and accessibility in healthcare.

c. Organizations have a role in using universal health literacy precautions and supporting accessible and equitable care.

d. Organizations have a role in supporting patient health literacy development and their ability to make autonomous health decisions, assisting with navigating the healthcare system and creating processes that address equity and accessibility.

14. You are interviewing for a job as a nurse care coordinator, and the interviewer asks you to identify two ways you can enhance patient activation and engagement. Which of the following is the most appropriate answer?

a. I would assess for medical needs and utilize motivational interviewing techniques.

b. I would hold the belief that the patient can self-manage their health and work to build their self-efficacy.

c. I would help the patient voice concerns and document their preferences.

d. I would assess for social determinants of health and functional illiteracy as this determines health outcomes.

15. You are a school nurse meeting with a 15-year-old student who was diagnosed with Type 1 diabetes 5 years earlier and manages the disease well. As part of your role, you are to provide continued health education to promote long-term self-management of health. You have just attended a motivational interviewing (MI) training and want to use MI principles in your health teaching practice. Which MI tools would be the MOST appropriate to use with this student?

a. OARS (open-ended questions, affirmation, reflection, summarize)

b. Collaborative agenda mapping

c. Evoking (bringing to consciousness intrinsic motivation)

d. Importance and confidence rulers

REFERENCES

Abid, M. H., Abid, M. M., Surani, S., & Ratnani, I. (2020). Patient engagement and patient safety: Are we missing the patient in the center? *Cureus, 12*(2), e7048. https://doi.org/10.7759/cureus.7048

Agency for Healthcare Research and Quality (AHRQ). (2016). *Why is self-management support important?* https://www.ahrq.gov/ncepcr/tools/self-mgmt/why.html

Agency for Healthcare Research and Quality (AHRQ). (2019). *Patient engagement and safety.* https://psnet.ahrq.gov/primer/patient-engagement-and-safety?.com

Agency for Healthcare Research and Quality (AHRQ). (2020). *AHRQ health literacy universal precautions toolkit.* https://www.ahrq.gov/health-literacy/improve/precautions/index.html

Always Use Teach Back. (n.d.). *10 elements of competence for using teach-back effectively.* Iowa Health System. http://higherlogicdownload.s3.amazonaws.com/HEALTHLITERACYSOLUTIONS/b33097fb-8e0f-4f8c-b23c-543f80c39ff3/UploadedImages/docs/Teach_Back_-_10_Elements_of_Competence.pdf

Amer, K. S. (2013). *Quality and safety for transformational nursing: Core competencies.* Pearson.

American Nurses Association (ANA). (2015). *Code of ethics for nurses with interpretive statements.* American Nurses Association.

Bajorek, S. A., & McElroy, V. (2020). Discharge planning and transitions of care. *Patient Safety Network.* https://psnet.ahrq.gov/primer/discharge-planning-and-transitions-care

Bandura, A. (1997). *Self-efficacy: The exercise of control.* W.H. Freeman.

Barello, S., Graffigna, G., Pitacco, G., Mislej, M., Cortale, M., & Provenzi, L. (2017). An educational intervention to train professional nurses in promoting patient engagement: A pilot feasibility study. *Frontiers in Psychology, 7,* 2020. https://doi.org/10.3389/fpsyg.2016.02020

Berglund, E., Lytsy, P., & Westerling, R. (2014). The influence of locus of control on self-rated health in context of chronic disease: A structural equation modeling approach in a cross-sectional study. *BMC Public Health,14*(492). http://doi.org/10.1186/1471-2458-14-492

Center for Health and Health Care in Schools, School-Based Health Alliance, National Center for School Mental Health (2020). Understanding social influencers of health and education: A role for school-based health centers and comprehensive school mental health systems. *School Health Services National Quality Initiative.* https://www.schoolmentalhealth.org/media/SOM/Microsites/NCSMH/Documents/Resources/Understanding-Social-Influencers-of-Health-and-Education.pdf

Centers for Disease Control and Prevention (CDC). (2021). *Patient engagement.* https://www.cdc.gov/healthliteracy/researchevaluate/patient-engage.html

Centers for Disease Control and Prevention (CDC). (2023). *What is health literacy?* https://www.cdc.gov/healthliteracy/learn/index.html

Chorrojprasert, L. (2020). Learner readiness: Why and how should they be ready? *Language Education and Acquisition Research Network Journal, 13*(1), 268–274. https://files.eric.ed.gov/fulltext/EJ1242968.pdf

Chung, F. F., Wang, P. Y., Lin, S. C., Lee, Y. H., Wu, H. Y., & Lin, M. H. (2021). Shared clinical decision-making experiences in nursing: A qualitative study. *BMC Nursing, 20*(1), 85. https://doi.org/10.1186/s12912-021-00597-0

Corbin, J. M., & Strauss, A. (1991). A nursing model for chronic illness management based upon the Trajectory Framework. *Scholarly Inquiry for Nursing Practice, 5*(3), 155–174. https://pubmed.ncbi.nlm.nih.gov/1763239/

Driscoll, M. P. (2000). *Psychology of learning for instruction* (2nd. Ed). Allyn and Bacon.

Elwyn, G., Dehlendorf, C., Epstein, R. M., Marrin, K., White, J., & Frosch, D. L. (2014). Shared decision making and motivational interviewing: Achieving patient-centered care across the spectrum of health care problems. *Annals of Family Medicine, 12*(3), 270–275. https://doi.org/10.1370/afm.1615

Ennis-O'Connor, M. (2018). *A patient engagement manifesto—6 principles of partnership.* Patient Empowerment Network. https://powerfulpatients.org/2018/09/19/a-patient-engagement-manifesto-6-principles-of-partnership/

Frankel A., Haraden C., Federico F., & Lenoci-Edwards J. (2017). *A framework for safe, reliable, and effective care.* [White paper]. Institute for Healthcare Improvement and Safe & Reliable Healthcare. https://www.ihi.org/resources/Pages/IHIWhitePapers/Framework-Safe-Reliable-Effective-Care.aspx

Fraser, K., Perez, R., & Latour, C. (2018). *CMSA's integrated case management: A manual for case managers by case managers.* Springer.

Greene, J., Hibbard, J. H., Sacks, R., Overton, V., & Parrotta, C. D. (2015). When patient activation levels change, health outcomes and costs change, too. *Health Affairs (Project Hope), 34*(3), 431–437. https://doi.org/10.1377/hlthaff.2014.0452

Haas, S. A., Swan, B. A., & Haynes, T. S. (2014). *Care coordination and transition management core curriculum.* American Academy of Ambulatory Care Nursing.

Haderline, C., & Clark, A. (2017). Illiteracy among adults in the US. *Ballard Brief, 2017*(3). 1–29. https://scholarsarchive.byu.edu/ballardbrief/vol2017/iss3/2

Health Resources and Services Administration (HRSA). (2022). *Health literacy.* https://www.hrsa.gov/about/organization/bureaus/ohe/health-literacy

Healthy People 2030. (n.d.a). *Health literacy in Healthy People 2030.* Office of Disease Prevention and Health Promotion, U.S. Department of Health and Human Services. https://health.gov/healthypeople/priority-areas/social-determinants-health/literature-summaries/health-literacy

Healthy People 2030. (n.d.b). *Social determinants of health.* Office of Disease Prevention and Health Promotion, U.S. Department of Health and Human Services. https://health.gov/healthypeople/priority-areas/social-determinants-health

Heath, S. (2017). *What is the patient activation measure in patient-centered care?* https://patientengagementhit.com/news/what-is-the-patient-activation-measure-in-patient-centered-care

Heath, S. (2022). *96% of nurses lack tools needed for patient engagement, education.* https://patientengagementhit.com/news/96-of-nurses-lack-tools-needed-for-patient-engagement-education

Hellström, A., Kassaye Tessma, M., Flink, M. Dahlgren, A., Schildmeijer, K., & Ekstedt, M. (2019). Validation of the patient activation measure in patients at discharge from hospitals and at distance from hospital care in Sweden. *BMC Public Health, 19*(1701). https://doi.org/10.1186/s12889-019-8025-1

Hibbard, J. H., & Greene, J. (2013). What the evidence shows about patient activation: Better health outcomes and care experiences; fewer data on costs. *Health Affairs (Project Hope), 32*(2), 207–214. https://doi.org/10.1377/hlthaff.2012.1061

Hibbard, J. H., Mahoney, E. R., Stockard, J., & Tusler, M. (2005). Development and testing of a short form of the patient activation measure. *Health Services Research, 40*(6 Pt 1), 1918–1930. https://doi.org/10.1111/j.1475-6773.2005.00438.x

Jerofke-Owen, T. A., Tobiano, G., & Eldh, A. C. (2023). Patient engagement, involvement, or participation—entrapping concepts in nurse–patient interactions: A critical discussion. *Nursing inquiry, 30*(1), e12513. https://doi.org/10.1111/nin.12513

Jiang, N., Sun, M. M., Zhou, Y. Y., & Feng, X. X. (2021). Significance of patient participation in nursing care. *Alternative Therapies in Health and Medicine, 27*(5), 115–119.

Kelly, P., Vottero, B. A., & Christie-McAuliffe, C. A. (2018). *Introduction to quality and safety education for nurses: Core competencies for nursing leadership and management* (2nd ed.). Springer Publishing Company.

Knickman, J. R., & Elbel, B. (Eds.). (2019). *Jonas & Kovner's health care delivery in the United States* (12th ed.). Springer Publishing Company.

Lange, J. W. (2012). *The nurse's role in promoting optimal health of older adults: Thriving in the wisdom years.* F.A. Davis.

Lopez, C., Bumyang, K., & Sacks, K. (2022). *Health literacy in the United States: Enhancing assessments and reducing disparities.* Milken Institute. https://milkeninstitute.org/report/health-literacy-us-assessments-disparities

Lorig, K. R., & Holman, H. (2003). Self-management education: History, definition, outcomes, and mechanisms. *Annals of Behavioral Medicine: A Publication of the Society of Behavioral Medicine, 26*(1), 1–7. https://doi.org/10.1207/S15324796ABM2601_01

Marzban, S., Najafi, M., Agolli, A., & Ashrafi, E. (2022). Impact of patient engagement on healthcare quality: A scoping review. *Journal of Patient Experience, 9*, 23743735221125439. https://doi.org/10.1177/23743735221125439

Miller, W. R., & Rollnick. S. (2002). *Motivational interviewing: Preparing people for change* (2nd ed.). The Guilford Press.

Miller, W. R., & Rollnick, S. (2013). *Motivational interviewing: Helping people change* (3rd ed.). The Guilford Press.

Mirmazhari, R., Ghafourifard, M., & Sheikhalipour, Z. (2022). Relationship between patient activation and self-efficacy among patients undergoing hemodialysis: A cross-sectional study. *Renal Replacement Therapy, 8*(40), 1–11. https://doi.org/10.1186/s41100-022-00431-6

Nutbeam, D. (2000). Health literacy as a public health goal: A challenge for contemporary health education and communication strategies into the 21st century. *Health Promotion International, 15*(3), 259–267. https://doi.org/10.1093/heapro/15.3.259

Prochaska, J. O., & DiClemente, C. C. (1982). Transtheoretical therapy: Toward a more integrative model of change. *Psychotherapy: Theory, Research & Practice, 19*(3), 276–288. https://doi.org/10.1037/h0088437

Schaffler, J., Leung, K., Tremblay, S., Merdsoy, L., Belzile, E., Lambrou, A., & Lambert, S. D. (2018). The effectiveness of self-management interventions for individuals with low health literacy and/or low income: A descriptive systematic review. *Journal of General Internal Medicine, 33*(4), 510–523. https://doi.org/10.1007/s11606-017-4265-x

Sofaer, S., & Schumann, M. J. (2013). *Fostering successful patient and family engagement: Nursing's critical role.* [White paper]. https://www.nursingworld.org/~4aa949/globalassets/naqc/naqc_patientengagementwhitepaper.pdf

Substance Abuse and Mental Health Services Administration (US). (2019). *Enhancing motivation for change in substance use disorder treatment* (Treatment Improvement Protocol (TIP) Series, No. 35.). https://www.ncbi.nlm.nih.gov/books/NBK571071/

Truglio-Londrigan, M., & Lewenson, S. B. (2013). *Public health nursing: Practicing population-based care* (2nd Ed.). Jones & Bartlett Learning.

Truglio-Londrigan, M., Slyer, J. T., Singleton, J. K., & Worral, P. (2012). A qualitative systematic review of internal and external influences on shared decision-making in all health care settings. *JBI Library of Systematic Reviews, 10*(58), 4633–4646. https://doi.org/10.11124/jbisrir-2012-432

U.S. Department of Health and Human Services, Office of Disease Prevention and Health Promotion. (2010). *National Action Plan to Improve Health Literacy.* Author. https://health.gov/our-work/national-health-initiatives/health-literacy/national-action-plan-improve-health-literacy

Welch, J., & Fournier, A. (2018). Patient engagement through informed nurse caring. *International Journal for Human Caring, 22*(1), 1–10. DOI:10.1891/1091-5710.22.1

World Health Organization (WHO). (2016). *Patient engagement: Technical series on safer primary care.* Author. https://apps.who.int/iris/bitstream/handle/10665/252269/9789241511629-eng.pdf

Credits

Fig. 4.2: A. Bandura, "Bandura's Theory of Self-Efficacy and Health Self-Management," *Self Efficacy: The Exercise of Control.* Copyright © 1997 by Macmillan Publishing Company.

Fig. 4.3a: Copyright © 2020 Depositphotos/Nsit0108.

Fig. 4.6: Source: T. A. Jerofke-Owen, G. Tobiano, & A. C. Eldh, "Patient Engagement, Involvement, or Participation — Entrapping Concepts in Nurse-patient Interactions: A Critical Discussion," *Nursing Inquiry*, vol. 30, no. 11, p. 6, John Wiley & Sons, Inc., 2023.

Fig. 4.7: Source: D. Nutbeam, "Health Literacy as a Public Health Goal: A Challenge for Contemporary Health Education and Communication Strategies into the 21st Century," *Health Promotion International*, vol. 15, no. 3, p. 266, Oxford University Press, 2000.

Fig. 4.8: U.S. Department of Health and Human Services, Office of Disease Prevention and Health Promotion, https://www.cdc.gov/public-health-gateway/php/about/social-determinants-of-health.html.

Fig. 4.9: AHRQ, https://www.ahrq.gov/health-literacy/professional-training/shared-decision/index.html, 2023.

Fig. 4.10: Source: https://hinsd.blogspot.com/2018/02/the-stages-of-change.html.

CHAPTER 5

The Continuum of Care

LEARNING OBJECTIVES

1. Classify the various levels of care available throughout the continuum of care.
2. Conceptualize how the levels of care meet differing needs across the continuum of care.
3. Examine requirements for various levels of care.
4. Reflect upon how the level of care, continuum of care, and patient needs affect care coordination practice.

KEY TERMS

- acute rehabilitation
- continuum of care
- grave disability
- involuntary admission
- level of care
- long-term acute care hospital (LTACH)
- personal care services
- preventative and maintenance level of care
- primary level of care
- quaternary level of care
- rehabilitative level of care
- restorative level of care
- secondary level of care
- spheres of care
- subacute rehabilitation (SAR)
- swing beds
- tertiary level of care
- voluntary admission

Introduction

A central goal of care coordination in all settings is effective patient-care transitions. The nurse must understand the overarching healthcare system and how healthcare needs are met throughout the patient's lifespan. Patients and their families/caregivers will need education related to healthcare choices, expectations of care, and what is required to transition between care settings. Additionally, once a transition in care is determined to be appropriate and the patient has been educated on what to expect, timelines, etc., they or their family/caregivers will likely have further questions concerning what happens after discharge or transfer, who is responsible for scheduling appointments or managing medications at the next level of care, and depending on the circumstances, they may need continued emotional support throughout the transition (Callister et al., 2020).

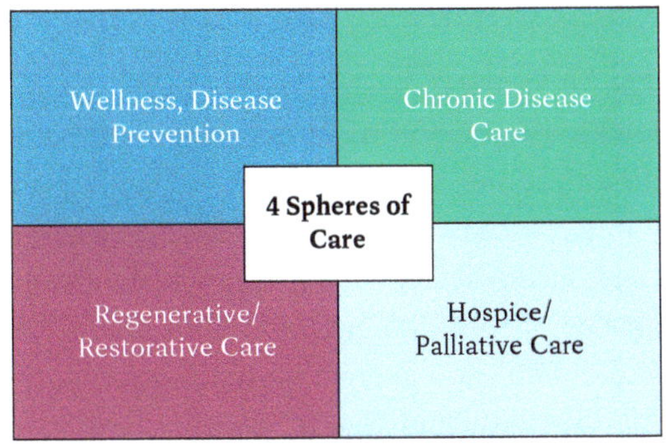

FIGURE 5.1 The Four Spheres of Care

Several terms are used to refer to the various types and settings of healthcare offered to meet patient needs throughout their lifespan. The American Association of Colleges of Nursing (AACN, 2021) has identified the need for nurses to be educated in four **spheres of care** that meet patient health needs across the lifespan, including (a) wellness and disease prevention, (b) restorative and regenerative care, (c) chronic disease care, and (d) hospice and palliative care (p. 19). See Figure 5.1—The Four Spheres of Care. Other times, this may be referred to as the continuum or continuity of care that signifies a system of care services providing integrated and comprehensive healthcare over time, settings, and intensity of care needs, with the goal of high-quality and cost-effective care delivered (Evashwick, 1989). The **level of care** may also be referred to, which identifies the acuity of care required, the amount of expertise needed, and the intensity of care and service required to meet healthcare needs and goals of care.

The nurse must have a foundational knowledge of how these concepts of care spheres, continuum, and levels encompass the patient's lifespan to encourage patient autonomy and engagement and participate in collaborative care planning. Care transitions must be connected and uninterrupted and provide informational and relational continuity amongst settings, providers, and services (Khatri et al., 2023). Knowledge concerning how to link and interconnect care settings and services to meet patient needs over the trajectory of health from conception to end-of-life care is essential for the care coordinating nurse.

The nurse must exercise their skills in interprofessional facilitation, cross-setting communication, and follow-up processes, ensuring the next steps in the care plan and current or newly prescribed medications are clear to the patient and their family/caregiver as well as the receiving next level of care (Swan et al., 2019). Awareness of community resources and the care settings and services available in the community is critical, as well as knowledge of common policies or guidelines that may affect facility acceptance of the patient when transitioning to a new level of care or setting. For a smooth transition between settings and services and to continue integrated care, the nurse must exercise the nursing process, first assessing patient choice and understanding, ensuring the next level of care meets patient health needs and priorities of care, identifying barriers or challenges in meeting outcomes, planning the transition, and implementing it seamlessly, and this requires the nurse to understand the key features and benefits of each sphere, setting, and level of care on the continuum.

The Continuum of Care

The United States healthcare system has many complex and moving parts that at times can lead to fragmentation of care. Elements of the healthcare system include public and private organizations, state and federally-funded components, and some community-supported segments. National and local legislation and government funding requirements affect many of these health system organizations. Yet, the United States does not have a central governmental agency of control regarding the healthcare system. This leads to an increasingly complicated and difficult-to-navigate system, affecting the continuum of care (Knickman & Elbel, 2019).

One may think that the **continuum of care** is linear and solely focuses on care delivered over the trajectory of health or the lifespan—conception to death. Still, the nurse must be cognizant of considerations with the care delivered to provide appropriate advocacy and education for their patients. The continuum of care is a system of healthcare that matches patient healthcare needs with the appropriate level of care and services across all stages of the lifespan and settings, delivering person-centered, integrated, and continuity of care to achieve optimal outcomes and use of resources. Understanding the continuum of care from a systems viewpoint can promote prevention of adverse outcomes and proactively identify the care services and settings most appropriate for the patient (Lane et al., 2009).

A general definition of the continuum of care is "how providers follow a patient from preventative care through medical incidents, rehabilitation, and maintenance" (Primary Care Development Corporation, 2023, para. 1). This definition points to how continuity of care is provided across healthcare settings and organizations. However, we must consider whether it is only the primary care provider (PCP) or other provider who needs to "follow" the patient and be concerned and accountable for their continuity of care across the continuum. Coordination and continuity of care depend on an interprofessional team approach and collaborative practice so that all involved in the patient's care should be invested in seeing the patient through any healthcare transitions. The continuum of care focuses on "maintaining continuity of the medical care delivered to the patient at all touchpoints ..." (SYNZI, 2018, para. 1). This may include multisectoral touchpoints, including healthcare services and supportive services such as financial, legal, psychosocial, or community resources across various settings (Case Management Study Guide, 2023; Khatri et al., 2023).

The continuum of care is a global concept that requires a holistic view of the patient experience and needs. It integrates and supports continuity of care and services to promote quality and cost-effective care as the patient navigates a variety of services and healthcare settings. A person may need many types of care over their lifespan, such as outreach services like emergency medical services (EMS), health screenings, and general health information and referrals. These types of services assist with the person's ability to engage in healthy living. Prevention of health issues and health maintenance are supported by services such as support groups, respite programs for caregivers, and educational or exercise programs. Ambulatory or routine care addresses the treatment of minor illnesses, specialist referrals, and health promotion through outpatient clinics, urgent care clinics, PCP care, counseling, and substance use disorder services. Acute illness and injury care include emergency room services, psychiatric hospitalization, or medical/surgical hospitalization. Recovery and rehabilitation services are often provided through home health or extended care services such as skilled nursing care, subacute rehabilitation, or **swing beds**, which are rooms in rural or critical access hospitals that can be "switched" from an acute care status to a skilled care or rehabilitative status (Evashwick, 1989, p. 38). Patients with chronic illness or health decline may receive care from home health, case management, or personal care services. Once palliative and end-of-life care is needed, it can be provided in the patient's residence, such as hospice care, an outpatient palliative care clinic, or acute care or long-term care setting.

The continuum of care relates to health, which slowly changes over time but includes many parts. Patients are not only well or ill, but on a continuum from illness to wellness. The continuum may be experienced by the patient in various ways and intensities, at times enjoying maximum wellness and other times requiring interventions to address physical or emotional health issues to continue their wellness journey in a manner that is meaningful to them (The Wellspring, 2018). Health is not a static and siloed experience but involves all aspects of the person's being and lived experience (e.g., physical health, mental/emotional health, substance use, SDOH). The range of healthcare services needed varies depending on the life circumstances and issues the patient is experiencing. It does not just work linearly, beginning with wellness and preventative care and moving to end-of-life care. There are many parts in the continuum of care, and a patient may move back and forth, depending on their health needs and priorities of care, as long as they are alive. It is care that is delivered in an integrated manner, utilizing interprofessional teams to tailor services to the patient's needs, resources, strengths, and care priorities (Khatri et al., 2023). See Figure 5.2 for a visual of the care and services offered across the continuum.

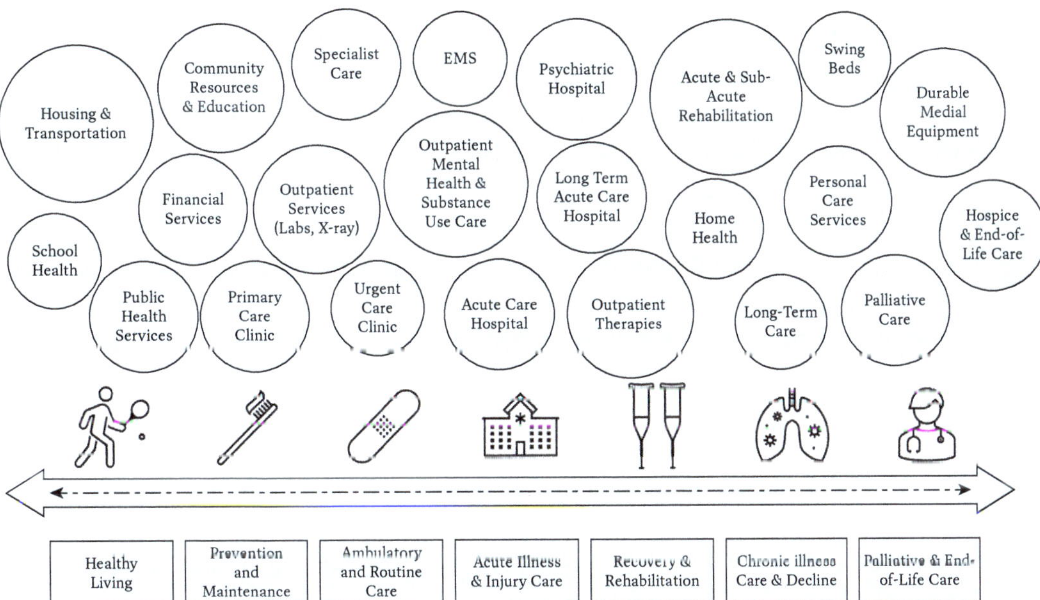

FIGURE 5.2 Types of Care and Services Across the Continuum

Levels of Care

The level of care is defined by the amount of expertise and intensity of effort required to meet a patient's healthcare needs and preserve or maintain their health (Case Management Study Guide, 2023). When considering the levels of healthcare, one may think of the concepts of primary, secondary, and tertiary care. However, with the advent of value-based healthcare systems and the integration of care coordination and continuity of care into healthcare practices, nurses must also consider preventative and maintenance care, rehabilitation and restorative care, and quaternary care, as these are needed to promote effective resource use and outcomes such as patient quality of life and satisfaction.

The preventative and maintenance level of care provides services that prevent or screen for healthcare issues early to avoid severe or negative outcomes, therefore maintaining health and preventing illness (Department of Managed Healthcare, 2023). **Prevention and maintenance level of care** involves health and wellness promotion, patient self-management of health, and other activities to sustain health and prevent injury and illness. Examples of this could be well-child exams, immunizations, mammogram screenings, dental cleanings, bicycle helmet use education, or clinics offering smoking cessation classes to the community. Preventative and maintenance care can be delivered by various entities, including community organizations, school nurses, public health clinics, or a PCP.

The **primary level of care** is healthcare that provides treatment for a wide range of health issues, including wellness, prevention, and common illnesses and injuries, usually provided by a PCP (Healthcare.gov, n.d.a). In primary care, the PCP may also act as the gatekeeper for referrals to specialists or different levels of care and be the point person for maintaining continuity of care throughout the continuum. For example, suppose a patient had been recently diagnosed with diabetes and the PCP felt that a home health nurse was needed for a short period to provide teaching regarding the new diagnosis and medication management. In that case, the PCP may order and coordinate these home health services. Other times, a patient may need a referral to a specialist provider. This is the **secondary level of care**, where the PCP has transferred the patient's care to a specialist who is an expert in the disease process or illness. For example, suppose a patient had a mammogram screening that pointed to possible breast cancer. In that case, the PCP might refer and transfer the patient's care concerning this health issue to an oncologist who could address any further testing or treatments the potential breast cancer diagnosis might require.

The **tertiary level of care** addresses healthcare needs in an acute care hospital setting that provides specialized care requiring specific expertise and equipment (Torrey, 2022). A PCP or a specialist provider may directly admit a patient to the hospital, or a patient may arrive via ambulance or personal vehicle and then be admitted for care. For example, a patient with a pancreatic cancer diagnosis may be directly admitted to the hospital by the secondary level of care specialist oncologist for acute pain management or a surgical procedure, such as a Whipple procedure to remove a cancerous part of the pancreas (American Cancer Society, 2019). Alternatively, a patient may arrive at the emergency room of an acute care hospital via police escort related to active suicidal thoughts and actions. The emergency room provider then would transfer the patient to a specialty tertiary-level psychiatric hospital for treatment and stabilization.

The **quaternary level of care** is more specialized than tertiary-level services, focusing on uncommon conditions, very specialized or rare surgeries, clinical trials, or innovative healthcare technologies and treatments (Mallender, 2022). Usually, the patient is referred to and transferred from the tertiary care setting to a quaternary level of care setting. For example, suppose a patient was admitted to the tertiary acute care hospital following a severe chemical burn, and the tertiary hospital did not have a burn unit or the equipment or expertise to meet the patient's needs. The tertiary hospital would then transfer the patient to the closest facility with a burn unit. Quaternary care facilities are usually connected to large teaching hospitals or care facilities affiliated with a hospital system (Mallender, 2022). Specialist secondary-level care could also refer a patient to a quaternary care facility for specific health conditions that need very specialized care, such as a pediatric patient with leukemia being referred to a children's cancer care center to participate in a clinical trial.

Rehabilitation and restorative levels of care are related but offered for different purposes. The **rehabilitative level of care** aims to improve lost or impaired functioning due to an illness or injury (Healthcare.gov, n.d.b.). Often, rehabilitative care involves multiple therapies, such as occupational, physical, and speech-language therapy. Rehabilitative care can be delivered in an inpatient setting, such as an acute rehabilitation center, where the patient stays until their rehabilitation is complete. It can also be provided in the home or outpatient settings through home health therapies or a community therapy provider, such as a concussion clinic. For example, suppose a patient is admitted to tertiary care through the emergency room after a motor vehicle accident and is found to have a concussion. The tertiary facility may refer them to outpatient concussion rehabilitation care and therapies at discharge.

The **restorative level of care** is an integrated care approach that focuses on assisting patients to optimize and maintain functional abilities and prevent a decline in function and independence (Talley et al., 2015). A therapist, nurse, or family member could perform this. Actions might include range of motion (ROM) exercises, cognitive retraining, or the use of splints and other devices to promote safety and independence in the home and community. An example of restorative care would be a home health physical therapist providing training to a family member on ROM exercises for their parent to maintain mobility or doing an environmental assessment to determine if additional durable medical equipment, such as a shower chair, is needed in the home to prevent injury and promote independence in activities of daily living.

Levels of care are dynamic, moving back and forth along the continuum of care depending on the patient's needs and priorities of care. Health is not linear; patients may experience acute illness, receive treatment, and arrive back at the prevention and maintenance level of care. Wherever the patient is in the care continuum, care coordination practice promotes optimum outcomes and resource utilization through active preventative care, healthy living, and health maintenance interventions. Once a patient experiences an acute illness or injury, restoring health and functional abilities is prioritized. Suppose a patient has a chronic disease or is declining in health. In that case, the goal is to provide education and support for

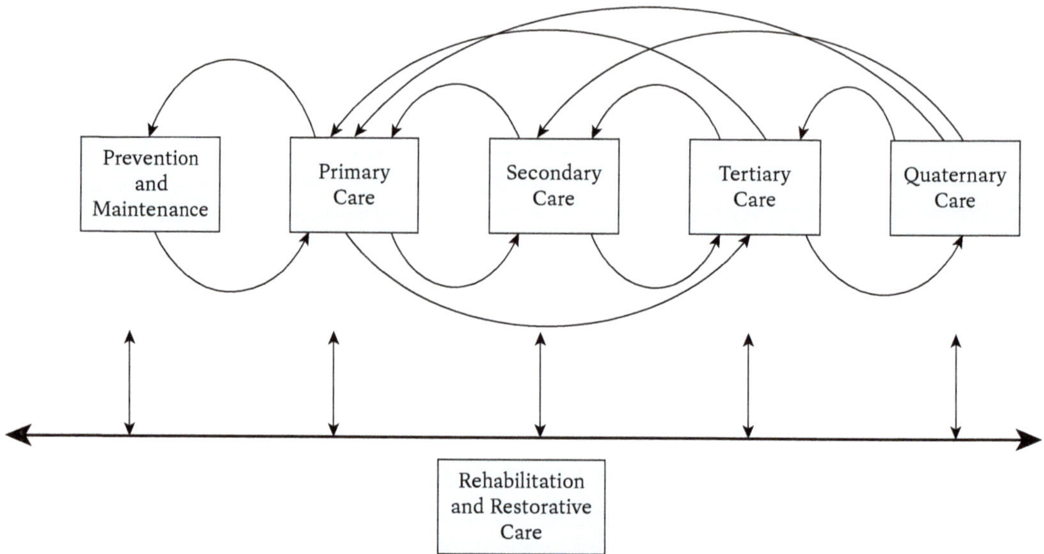

FIGURE 5.3 Interconnecting Levels of Care

patient self-management of the condition for optimal outcomes and to offer restorative care to prevent further decline in function or independence. If the patient has moved along the trajectory of health and palliative or end-of-life care services are appropriate, effort is spent in collaborative care planning and goals of care clarification to meet patient and family/support system needs and preferences. See Figure 5.3 for a visual of the levels of care and how they are interconnected.

The essential concept related to spheres of care, levels of care, or a view of the continuum of care is that healthcare is delivered in a system of services, each having a unique purpose in providing high-quality and cost-effective care. Each aspect of the healthcare system is designed and organized to meet the needs of specific patient populations and community requirements. Care coordination efforts emphasize delivering quality and cost-effective care through integrating and linking healthcare services and resources across all spheres, levels, and the continuum of care (Khatri et al., 2023). This model supports person-centered care, allows the patient to have an optimal choice of services, and ensures that care transition decisions are based on patient needs and preferences (CMS, 2006). This requires the nurse care coordinator to make sure that the patient and their family/support system have adequate information concerning the situation, interprofessional recommendations, and any relevant guidelines to make informed choices of care setting and delivery in the continuum of care. The nurse care coordinator must understand how each part of the healthcare system works together to meet the patient's health needs across the lifespan, leverage additional resources and services (e.g., housing, support groups, transportation, financial, etc.), and make sure that the patient is receiving care at the most appropriate level for their healthcare needs. Through a health systems framework and perspective, the nurse care coordinator will promote good outcomes, limit unnecessary resource use, and further successful continuity of care practices.

Common Transitions in Care Coordination Practice

The interprofessional care coordination plan of care will identify services and resources the patient may need and the most appropriate level of care and setting in the care continuum for patient transitions. There are always those more complex and infrequent transitions to a very specialized level of care, such as transferring a patient via helicopter to a transplant center or a quaternary level of care. However, most times, patients transition to common care settings such as rehabilitation, home health, or hospice care. The care coordinator must understand the services offered and defining factors of these commonly used levels of care on the continuum to provide the education and support needed for the patient to make an appropriate and informed choice concerning the transition, as well as ensure they are pacing the case and addressing any unique features or needs for the next care setting, supporting a successful transition of care. This will include all seven care coordination rights, guiding principles, and foundational care coordination competencies.

Acute Care Hospitals

The defining characteristics of a hospital include maintaining a facility whose primary function is to provide diagnostic and therapeutic services, has an organized staff of physicians, and offers continuous nursing care under the supervision of a registered nurse. The hospital must also maintain patient records and provide pharmacy, nutrition, and therapy services to meet the patient's healthcare needs (Shi & Singh, 2019). There are various types of hospitals: teaching, public, community, specialty, critical access/rural, or general hospitals. The hospital can be private for-profit, private not-for-profit, or locally, state or federally owned. Acute care hospitals provide intensive and expert care for a brief period of time related to acute illness, injury, trauma, surgery, recovery, or exacerbation of chronic disease processes. Often the provider caring for patients is a hospitalist or specialist who has not seen the patient previously unless they had a previous hospital admission (Knickman & Elbel, 2019).

Acute care hospitals receive payment/reimbursement for care provided by private insurance companies, Medicare and Medicaid, and sometimes via private pay from the patient. Various organizations are involved in developing and maintaining standards for operation and accreditation for hospitals, such as The Joint Commission (JCAHO), the National Committee for Quality Assurance (NCQA), the American Medical Accreditation Program (AMAP), the American Accreditation Health Care Commission/Utilization Review Accreditation Commission (AAHC/URAC), and the Accreditation Association for Ambulatory Health Care (AAAHC) (Viswanathan & Salmon, 2000)

Unique Considerations of the Acute Care Hospital

Most acute care hospitals accept Medicare and Medicaid payments and must follow the Centers for Medicare and Medicaid (CMS) guidelines. The care coordinating nurse must be aware of several specific guidelines related to these payment models. One regulatory guideline that can create a potential barrier to the level of care transfers is that of inpatient versus outpatient admission status. Inpatient admission status means the patient is expected to be in the acute care setting for two midnights or more. When admitted, the provider attests to this in the admission documentation.

The critical point to this admission status determination is that the provider attests that the patient's health or safety would be negatively impacted if they were treated at a less intensive level of care, such as outpatient care (Medicare Program Integrity Manual, 2020). At admission, the level of care must be evaluated for appropriateness through utilization review, and there must be documentation in the patient record supporting the admission status. This is not only an important issue related to reimbursement for care provided, but it can also be used to determine whether the patient will be eligible for certain post-discharge services, such as rehabilitation.

For example, Medicare requires a 3-consecutive-day inpatient stay for a patient to qualify for admission to rehabilitation post-acute care. The rule requires that Medicare recipient patients be admitted inpatient status for 3 days. The day of admission counts toward the 3 days but not the day of discharge. Any time the patient spends in the emergency room, in observation, or outpatient status does not count toward the 3 days. The days are calculated using a 24-hour time period from midnight to midnight, and any part of the day counts as a full day (American Hospital Association, 2023, p. 3). So suppose a patient was admitted to observation status and not inpatient status and stayed 3 days. In that case, Medicare may not approve a discharge to a rehabilitation facility due to the patient not meeting inpatient status.

Furthermore, if the patient was admitted inpatient, let's say on September 22, spent two days and was discharged on September 24, they likely would also be denied coverage for rehabilitation placement at discharge because they did not stay three days. In this case, the patient may only be eligible for insurance coverage for outpatient therapy services post-discharge. Of course, there are waivers and exceptions to this rule. Still, it is vital for the care coordinating nurse in the acute care hospital setting to understand the patient's admission status and insurance requirements for placement options post-discharge.

Another critical aspect to consider in care coordination activities is the CMS conditions of participation (CoP), which directs acute care discharge planning processes. Several requirements need to be documented to meet the CoP. If coordinating care in an acute care hospital, the nurse must screen all patients to determine those most in need of discharge planning and identify discharge needs, including the ability to self-care or return to the previous setting and any potential post-discharge services needed. A registered nurse, social worker, or another qualified person must also develop and evaluate a discharge plan for effectiveness. The hospital must also provide the initial implementation of the post-acute care discharge plan, such as arranging for durable medical equipment, follow-up appointments, transportation to the next level of care, etc. (Department of Health and Human Services, 2013).

When creating the discharge plan for another level of care, the care coordinating nurse must provide the patient with a "choice." This means that the nurse cannot decide for the patient or recommend to the patient which facility or agency they prefer or believe is the best. They must provide the patient with a list of choices or options that accept the patient's insurance, are in the geographic area or area the patient requests, and meet the level of care needs of the patient. Furthermore, they must disclose if the hospital has any financial relationship with the agencies listed (McAlister, 2023). Lastly, the discharge plan needs frequent reassessment to pace the case and adjust the plan if required, producing a smooth transition of care that promotes patient satisfaction, outcomes, benchmark attainment, and resource management.

Long-Term Acute Care Hospitals (LTACH)

Long-Term Acute Care Hospitals (LTACH) are another type of tertiary level of care that offers specialized care for those with serious health conditions requiring longer-term specialized and expert care. LTACHs are acute care hospitals that provide care for patients who need more than 25 days of intensive care, with an average length of stay of 30 days. Most patients transferred to LTACHs are transferred from a critical or intensive care unit and have serious health conditions that require continued specialized and expert care but have the potential to improve over time and allow return to their place of residence or discharge to a lower level of care such as a skilled nursing facility (SNF) for rehabilitation (Department of Health and Human Services, 2019). LTACHs provide care such as ventilator weaning or prolonged ventilator use, intensive respiratory care, or complex wound or burn care. LTACHs may also provide up to a few hours a day of rehabilitation to assist in recovery (Compton, 2020).

As an acute care hospital, the LTACH must meet CMS conditions of participation (CoP) for Medicare patients. CMS suggests specific criteria for LTACH transfers/placements. These include the need for daily provider intervention, intensive treatment, and the presence of complex conditions with too high of acuity for an SNF to meet, use of an interprofessional team, including physical, occupational, speech, and respiratory therapy, and continuous registered nursing staffing, 24 hours a day (Healthcare Roadmap, n.d.). LTACHs receive payment/reimbursement for care provided by private insurance companies, Medicare and Medicaid, and sometimes via private pay from the patient. Various organizations are involved in developing and maintaining standards for operation and accreditation for LTACHs, such as The Joint Commission (JCAHO), the American Accreditation Healthcare Commission (AAHC), and the Center for Improvement in Healthcare Quality (CIHQ).

Unique Considerations of the Long-Term Acute Care Hospital (LTACH)

Because there are several criteria for a patient to be eligible for placement or transfer to an LTACH the care coordinator must ensure that the eligibility criteria are well documented. This may mean that before the insurance provider approves an LTACH, they will want assurance that the patient's needs cannot be met at a lower level of care, such as an SNF. LTACHs have clinical liaisons who will meet with the patient and their family/support system, review their medical records and condition, discuss potential treatment options, and determine if the patient meets eligibility criteria (Compton, 2020). Therefore, the care coordinator must meet with the patient and their family/support system concerning what the LTACH provides, give the patient a choice of the facility if there is more than one LTACH in the area, discuss how transportation and other coordination of care activities might look, address any insurance coverage questions, and explain to them in advance the need for the clinical liaison meeting.

Once a patient is accepted for transfer to the LTACH, prior authorization from the insurance provider on the LTACH side will occur, and the providers and interprofessional team will work to determine a timeline for transition to the facility and continue to assess for ongoing needs during the transition of care. Coordinating activities like arranging transportation and a provider-to-provider report will need to occur. This is not a nurse-to-nurse

The Value of the Long-Term Acute Care Hospital (LTACH)

"LTAC hospitals definitely have a role [in value-based care]. A lot of times it is the most appropriate site of care for a patient, and this can prevent readmissions ... if [LTAC hospital utilization] is appropriate, it is necessary" (ATI advisory, 2022, p. 15).

report, although that will happen as well as a standard of practice. The provider-to-provider report is one where the provider following the patient in the hospital connects with and gives a detailed report of the patient's condition and needs to the "accepting" provider at the LTACH as part of transferring care. Once the patient arrives at the facility, the LTACH provider will follow the patient concerning their healthcare needs until discharge from the LTACH. There are many steps and areas to coordinate for a smooth transfer to an LTACH as the patient has serious health conditions, and continuity of information and care is critical for positive outcomes.

Psychiatric Hospitals

A psychiatric hospital is a specialty hospital at the tertiary level that provides care and services for a specific patient population with mental health and illness needs. Psychiatric hospitals are required to provide psychiatric, psychological, and social work services and support for their patients (CMS, 2023a). Psychiatric hospitals may have specific units for those with substance use disorders (SUD), offering medical management of withdrawal or voluntary SUD treatment. The hospital may also provide specific services and designated units for certain age groups, such as geriatric populations or children and adolescent populations. The psychiatric hospital generally is required to have an agreement or memorandum of understanding with a local general acute care hospital for the transfer of patients who may exceed the level of care they can provide or have specific needs, such as pregnancy, withdrawal or medication management concerns, or other acute health conditions (Shi & Singh, 2019).

Psychiatric hospitals must maintain patient records, meet all general hospital requirements, and provide sufficient staffing to provide active treatment for patients receiving services from the hospital. They must also meet the conditions of participation (CoPs) to receive reimbursement from Medicare and Medicaid, including meeting restraint and seclusion rules (CMS, 2023a). An Inpatient Psychiatric Facility Quality Reporting Program (IPFQR) sponsored by CMS provides healthcare consumers with data about the quality of care and measures that the psychiatric facility meets (CMS, 2023b). Psychiatric hospitals receive payment/reimbursement for care provided by private insurance companies, Medicare, Medicaid, and sometimes via private pay from the patient. Various organizations are involved in developing and maintaining standards for operation and accreditation for psychiatric hospitals, such as The Joint Commission (JCAHO), the National Integrated Accreditation for Healthcare Organizations (NIAHO) program, and The Center for Improvement in Healthcare Quality (CIHQ).

Unique Considerations of the Psychiatric Hospital

One critical aspect of coordinating a transfer or admission to a psychiatric hospital is whether the admission is voluntary or involuntary. **Voluntary admission** is when a patient has given consent, by their own choice, to be placed in a psychiatric hospital for treatment. Voluntary admission to treatment at the psychiatric hospital should be offered unless the patient's mental health or condition makes the offer inappropriate.

If a person has been determined to need psychiatric hospitalization by a mental health examiner or provider and refuses voluntary admission, then involuntary admission should be pursued. **Involuntary admission** is when the patient is placed in a psychiatric hospital setting due to meeting specific criteria but does not agree to the hospitalization. The specific criteria for involuntary admission include the person suffering from a mental health disorder, defined by the *Diagnostic and Statistical Manual of the American Psychiatric Association*, and that it is believed that inpatient psychiatric treatment will improve or prevent deterioration of the psychiatric symptoms, that hospitalization is the least restrictive appropriate level of care, that the person is unwilling or unable to consent to voluntary admission, and that the person is likely to harm themselves or others, or be unable to care for their activities of daily living, medical conditions, or provide self-protection due to psychiatric symptoms, or the person will suffer significant deterioration involving impairment of judgment or behaviors that will interfere with their ability to function (APA, 2020, pp. 1–2).

All states in the United States have emergency psychiatric hold laws and regulations to protect individuals deemed a danger to themselves or others, but these vary by state. Some states also add the condition of grave disability to their laws and regulations. **Grave disability** is when the patient cannot provide self-care, self-protection, or basic personal needs due to a mental health condition. Ideally, these laws allow time for a qualified mental health examiner to evaluate and determine if the patient meets the criteria for involuntary admission, if they want to be voluntarily admitted, or if there is no identifiable mental health concern. Some states may only mandate a 24-hour hold, others up to 72 hours, and there are differences in oversight processes and patient rights during this emergency psychiatric hold time (Hedman et al., 2016). This delineation of voluntary versus involuntary admission and emergency psychiatric holds is important for the care coordinating nurse to understand, as it is essential that the patient is evaluated and assessed by a qualified mental health professional to determine symptoms and diagnoses and provide recommendations for services and care settings while having patient rights respected.

Another factor to consider as the care coordinator is the actual transition of the care process. Usually, healthcare agencies and providers will have procedures and policies outlining the steps of transition to a psychiatric hospital and how continuity of information will be addressed. It is essential to be aware of these identified processes as several common areas are challenging in transitioning care to a psychiatric hospital. One key challenge is transferring medication and prescription information to ensure quality care and medication safety. Timely sharing of patient information and treatment provided is critical so that the multiple providers who may be involved in the patient's psychiatric care can access critical information during their assessment and care planning process (SAMHSA, 2023). This is necessary to avoid a lag

Factors Affecting the Decision to Admit to Psychiatric Hospitalization

Nathan et al. (2021) conducted focus groups with providers involved in decision-making regarding admission to inpatient psychiatric hospitalization. Four themes emerged regarding the factors considered during the decision-making process: (a) clinical and risk factors, (b) fear/threat factors, (c) interpersonal dynamics, and (d) contextual factors. Clinical and risk factors referred to the presentation of symptoms and issues and whether the risk of harm and safety issues were considered in decision-making. Threat/fear factors pointed to the provider seeking to avoid an adverse event or outcome, such as a death by suicide. Interpersonal dynamics focused upon when providers felt the patient might be attempting to manipulate them into an inpatient admission decision or whether they thought the patient was not being truthful concerning symptoms or plans. The following focus group member quotation expresses an aspect of the interpersonal dynamics factor: "The patient can push you in a corner and say, well if you send me home, I'm going to kill myself" (p. 5). Contextual factors concerned barriers to the provider having the time and support to thoroughly assess and evaluate or the lack of resource availability for inpatient care or outpatient follow-up. The following quotations from a focus group member outline contextual factors affecting the decision-making process: "Our community teams are really struggling with their capacity as well" or "People feel a lot of pressure because there's less inpatient beds" (p. 5).

between the transfer to the psychiatric facility and assessment and treatment. Furthermore, if appropriate or permission is given, family and support system members should be updated regarding the transfer of care timeline, plan, and setting. Transportation may also need to be arranged if the patient is an involuntary admission, and each work setting likely will have a policy related to how this is organized and if specific vendors or companies are used to provide involuntary admission transportation, such as a non-emergent ambulance service.

Rehabilitation Across the Continuum of Care

Rehabilitation services are designed to optimize and restore functional abilities, returning patients to as close to baseline functioning as possible post-illness or injury, enhancing quality of life and independence. This can be offered in various settings, through outpatient therapy and rehabilitative services, home health therapy services, or inpatient settings such as acute and subacute rehabilitation. Rehabilitative services selected depends upon interprofessional recommendations, the patient's ability to participate in rehabilitation, the extent of rehabilitation needed, and insurance considerations (e.g., inpatient vs. outpatient status, preauthorization of rehabilitation, etc.). In whichever setting rehabilitative services are provided, they are very person-centered with interventions and therapies designed individually to meet identified goals and preferences. Rehabilitative services vary based on patient needs. For example, the rehabilitation could target therapies to enhance functioning or the physical environment for risk reduction purposes, or the rehabilitation may focus on reducing complications and improving patient self-management and adaptation to prosthetics or assistive devices. Rehabilitation is a central part of the health care system, decreasing complications, improving quality of life, and reducing readmissions and hospital length of stays (WHO, 2023).

Rehabilitative services receive payment/reimbursement for care provided by private insurance companies, Medicare, Medicaid, and sometimes via private pay from the patient. Organizations that maintain standards for operation and accreditation for rehabilitative services vary with the setting. If the rehabilitation facility is connected to a hospital, it may be accredited through The Joint Commission (JCAHO). Many rehabilitation facilities are accredited by the Commission on Accreditation of Rehabilitation Facilities (CARF). They may be facilities certified as a Medicare and/or Medicaid Inpatient Rehabilitation Facility (IRF) or accredited through the National Outpatient Rehabilitation Facility Accreditation (NORFA). Whatever setting is providing the rehabilitative services, and however they are accredited, their goal is to "achieve the highest level of functional independence and to improve the quality of life ..." (Tombak et al., 2023, p. 101).

Unique Considerations of Inpatient Rehabilitation

When considering inpatient rehabilitation, it is essential to understand the differences between acute and subacute rehabilitation services. **Acute rehabilitation** is an inpatient rehabilitative service often connected to or associated with a hospital, which requires the patient to participate a minimum of 3 hours a day for at least 5 days a week in an intensive, interprofessional, and coordinated rehabilitation program. Several specific criteria exist for a patient's eligibility to be transitioned to an inpatient acute rehabilitation facility. The patient must have a "new" acute injury or illness or an acute exacerbation of a chronic condition, causing a marked decrease in functional abilities. The patient must have medical and rehabilitation needs that cannot be met in alternative lower-level care settings, such as with outpatient therapies. There should also be the expectation that patient improvement will be seen within 7 to 14 days from admission. Lastly, the patient must be medically stable enough to no longer need medical services in the hospital setting. The acute rehabilitation facility provides services prescribed by a provider, close medical supervision, and skilled nursing care with 24-hour availability of a physician and nurse skilled in rehabilitative medicine. Typical conditions that receive acute rehabilitation are brain and spinal cord injuries, stroke, or significant traumatic injuries (The Patient Choice, 2020).

A skilled nursing facility (SNF) often offers **subacute rehabilitation (SAR)**, a rehabilitative service requiring a lower level of patient participation in the rehabilitation program, with only about 2 hours of therapy daily. The SNF may be solely a subacute rehabilitation facility or have a unit designated for subacute rehabilitation and other units for long-term care, hospice care, or respite care. The main difference between acute and subacute rehabilitation is the required number of daily therapy hours. Subacute rehabilitation is a good choice for those patients who still need collaborative, interprofessional rehabilitative care but require a decreased intensity of service due to health or other issues that prevent them from more intense active participation in the rehabilitative process. They may also need rehabilitative care for a more extended period, with an average length of stay 27 days. Typical conditions requiring subacute rehabilitation are joint replacements, hip fractures, sepsis, or heart failure (Stefanacci, 2015).

The 60% Rule

Inpatient rehabilitation facilities (IRF) must follow a 60% rule for Medicare reimbursement. This means that 60% of the IRF's patient population must have one of the 13 following primary conditions or comorbidities: stroke, spinal cord injury, congenital deformity, amputation, major multiple traumas, hip fracture, brain injury, certain neurological conditions (e.g., Parkinson's disease), burns, arthritis conditions in which aggressive outpatient therapy has failed, or bilateral hip or knee replacement and the patient's BMI is greater than 50, or the patient is 85 or older (Medpac, 2021, p. 3). This rule is used to differentiate the IRF from an acute care hospital. Still, some argue that this is an outdated rule and does not promote person-centered care based on patient rehabilitative needs and how those are best met (Federation of American Hospitals, 2023).

Both acute and SAR facilities often have a clinical liaison who will meet with the patient and family or support system to determine eligibility for admission, discuss services provided, and explain the insurance preauthorization process and benefits. This is an important conversation and one the care coordinator should prepare the patient for, as well as follow up with the patient and clinical liaison after the meeting to answer any concerns and questions. Inpatient rehabilitative services usually must be preauthorized by the insurance provider and may have some copayment or cost. The patient should receive an explanation of benefits that discusses how much will be billed, what the insurance provider covers, and any copayments or deductibles (Busch, 2018).

Once the transfer to the rehabilitation facility is authorized and the patient is medically cleared, the care coordinator will ensure continuity of information and care, verifying the receiving facility has the essential information to begin rehabilitative care. Additionally, the care coordinator will regularly communicate with the patient, their family or support system if involved, the receiving facility, the discharging provider, and the interprofessional team, ensuring a smooth transition of care.

Home Health Services

Home health services and care are delivered in the patient's residence. This could be a private home, assisted living facility, or shelter. Home health services are short-term and intermittent and usually include skilled services such as nursing care for medication management or disease process education and rehabilitative care such as physical, occupational, or speech therapy. Some home health agencies may also offer as-needed social work, dietician, specialized wound care, or other ancillary or specialty services. In addition, some home health agencies may offer a home health aide that can assist with bathing or other activities of daily living while the patient is receiving service (Shi & Singh, 2019).

If your patient is a Medicare beneficiary, there are criteria for eligibility for home health care services. In addition, many insurance policies follow Medicare guidelines concerning eligibility and authorization of home health care services. The most critical and often misunderstood requirement is that of being homebound. This means the patient has extreme difficulty in leaving their home and likely needs help to leave their home. If this is the case, then the patient cannot

Homebound Criteria Documentation Example

Medicare considers a patient homebound if they meet one of the following criteria:

Criterion One: The patient must need the aid of supportive devices such as crutches, canes, wheelchairs, and walkers; the use of special transportation; or the assistance of another person to leave their place of residence. Or the patient must have a condition that leaving their home is medically contraindicated.

If the patient only meets one of the criteria one requirements, they must also meet the following in criterion two.

Criterion Two: There must be a normal inability to leave home, which requires a considerable and taxing effort (Medicare Benefit Policy Manual, 2022, pp. 23–24).

Example Documentation: *"The patient is temporarily homebound secondary to status post total knee replacement and currently walker dependent with painful ambulation. PT is needed to restore the ability to walk without support. Short-term skilled nursing is needed to monitor for signs of decomposition or adverse events from the new COPD medical regimen"* (Health Care Compliance Association, 2014, slide 16).

make it to appointments for outpatient therapies or nursing care, and therefore, home health care is the appropriate level of care to meet the patient's healthcare needs. Home health care is also an intermittent and skilled service, meaning the patient occasionally needs skilled care from a licensed therapist or nurse on a short-term basis. Home health care cannot be provided for only a home health aide or ancillary services; skilled nursing or therapies must always be ordered. When home health is ordered, the provider must have a face-to-face encounter with the patient to determine they meet homebound status and need intermittent skilled services and care (Medicare Interactive, 2023a).

Home health services receive payment/reimbursement for care provided by private insurance companies, Medicare, Medicaid, and sometimes via private pay from the patient. Organizations that maintain standards for operation and accreditation for home health care services include The Joint Commission (JCAHO), the Community Health Accreditation Partner (CHAP) program, and the Accreditation Commission for Health Care (ACHC). Many home health care agencies are certified as Medicare and/or Medicaid home health providers. Home health services are a critical component of the continuum of healthcare delivery and can provide a quality and safe alternative to inpatient care (Young & Kroth, 2018).

Unique Considerations of Home Health Services

Just as there are several specific eligibility requirements for home health services, there are also several stipulations and limitations to home health services. One such stipulation is that although home health services offer occupational therapy, patients are not eligible for Medicare coverage for home health services if this is the only skilled service needed. This means a Medicare beneficiary patient must have either skilled nursing or physical therapy ordered on the initial home health order and occupational therapy if needed. Once the patient has met their skilled nursing or physical therapy needs, they can continue with occupational therapy only, but this cannot be their only initial skilled need (Medicare Interactive, 2023a). This is an essential stipulation for the care coordinating nurse to be aware of because if the clinic, rehabilitation, or hospital provider orders only occupational therapy on the initial home health order, the patient will not be approved to home health services, and there will be a delay in the start of care.

Another critical aspect of home healthcare services requires that a provider follow the patient. For example, a patient may come to the emergency room and be admitted for an injury after a fall in the home. The patient may receive physical therapy in the hospital, but at discharge, the therapist recommends continued therapies via home health. The hospitalist provider may order the home health at discharge and provide the face-to-face documentation. The home health agency will still need to send orders related to the plan of care developed after assessment and evaluation by the home health nurse or therapist to be signed by the following provider, which will not be the hospitalist or emergency room provider. The care coordinating nurse must ensure the patient has a PCP they see regularly. If the patient does not have a PCP to sign the plan of care orders and follow the patient for home health services, they will be unable to provide those services. This can lead to a significant delay in the start of care.

Suppose the patient does not have a PCP. In that case, the care coordinator will need to set up an appointment with one to establish care as soon as possible and communicate to the patient the appointment time, place, etc., and the importance of attending the appointment. Sometimes, the care coordinator may set up an appointment to establish care with the PCP, but then the clinic may contact the patient to reschedule, delaying the appointment several weeks. This also likely delays the start of home healthcare as well. The patient must understand the purpose and importance of the follow-up PCP appointment and communicate that understanding to the care coordinating nurse.

When the ordering provider certifies that the patient is homebound in the face-to-face documentation, frequently there can be confusion on the part of the patient or their family as to what this means. The care coordinator must clearly understand "homebound" status to provide education regarding the requirements and limitations and evaluate whether the patient meets homebound status. A home health agency will also evaluate this on the initial visit, and if the patient does not meet homebound status, they will not open the patient to services. Again, this can delay needed therapies and skilled nursing care needs, potentially leading to poor patient outcomes, readmissions, and increased resource use.

Being homebound does not mean the patient can never leave their home. But it does mean that they can only leave home for short and intermittent periods, such as for a medical appointment, religious services, a haircut appointment, or special nonmedically related events such as a wedding or funeral (Medicare Interactive, 2023b). If the patient communicates to the care coordinator that they are going on a long weekend trip, this will likely disqualify them from being considered homebound. Additionally, suppose the patient or provider is requesting home health services due to the patient not having a vehicle to drive to outpatient appointments. This also does not necessarily qualify them as homebound. If the patient does not meet homebound status requirements, the care coordinator will need to look at alternatives, such as outpatient therapies, and work to address any transportation or other issues the patient may have in making it to their outpatient appointments.

A Clinical Resource Manager's Discharge Plan Gone Awry

I was working on the discharge of a patient with a cancer diagnosis who was admitted to the hospital with an opportunistic infection. The following oncologist cleared the patient for discharge and wrote discharge orders for home health nursing to administer daily antibiotic infusions over the next few weeks. The nurse clinical resource manager who had previously been working with the patient had already sent the referral to the home health agency but had yet to hear back if they had accepted the patient to service. I called the home health agency to confirm they would be out to see the patient the next day for their antibiotic infusion. I was told they did not receive authorization from the patient's insurance company for home health services, as they would not authorize daily visits for an infusion and they could not open the patient to service.

At that point, I had to talk to the patient and the oncologist about the issue and the fact that insurance would not authorize a home health nurse for daily visits. The only alternative was for the patient to go to the infusion clinic each day for their antibiotic infusion. When discussing this with the patient, I discovered they had no transportation and would not have an easy way to get to the infusion clinic. It was also late in the day by this time, and the infusion clinic near their home did not have any appointments open for the next day, so the patient would have to drive to a clinic about 30 miles from their house the next day for their antibiotic infusion. After much discussion, a friend of the patient agreed to change their work schedule and take them to the appointment the next day. Once the daily appointments were closer to home, the patient felt they could work with neighbors to assist with transportation for the duration of the antibiotic infusion needs.

All that was left was to get the order for the antibiotics over to the infusion clinic … but there was no order. I contacted the oncologist, who said the infectious disease specialist was writing the order. Then, I contacted the infectious disease specialist, who said the order was in their notes and to contact their clinical assistant. I then contacted the clinical assistant who worked the next hour to get the needed order to the infusion clinic and miraculously got the next day's appointment switched to the closer infusion clinic.

In the end, all was organized. The patient had transportation for the next day and a plan for transportation for the rest of the infusion days; orders were where they needed to be, and the patient was going to get the daily antibiotic infusion required. But there were care coordination issues. Only with ongoing communication and teamwork did the patient get their needs taken care of so they could be discharged on time. —E. L., inpatient clinical resource manager

Personal Care Services

Often, older people, those with chronic conditions, or those recovering from a significant injury or illness may need assistance with their activities of daily living (ADLs). This has led to a growing need for personal care services because many people want to stay in their homes as they age and recover (Office of the Assistant Secretary for Planning and Evaluation, 2019). **Personal care services (PCS)** provide nonmedical assistance or caregiving for ADLs, such as help with bathing and dressing, light housekeeping, meal preparation, transportation to medical appointments or grocery stores, and companionship. PCS can be provided up to 24 hours a day, 365 days a year. Most times, PCS is provided by a personal care aide. This is an unlicensed person with varying experience and education levels. Personal care aide required training or certification varies by state regulation and law, with some states having no training or certification requirements. Sometimes, PCS are provided by certified nursing assistants or home health aides, who can provide more medically based interventions, such as assisting with wound care or medications. These types of PCS aides must possess and follow state regulations and laws regarding the number of hours of training required, type of certification needed, and scope of practice limitations or stipulations (Sadick, 2021).

Patients, nurses, and providers often use the term "home health" interchangeably with PCS. This can be problematic in coordinating care, ensuring the patient has the correct services, and providing appropriate health education and promotion services. Home health services have specific eligibility requirements and focus on providing skilled services, occasionally with a home health aide's support for specific interventions, depending on the patient's needs, the home health agency services offered, etc. Home health services are also designed to be intermittent and short-term. The patient and their family/caregiver must understand that PCS are not the home health services covered under most insurance programs. This is because PCS are primarily privately funded, meaning the patient pays for the personal care aide services out of pocket (Paying for Senior Care, 2022). Most insurance policies do not cover the cost of these services. This is critical information for the patient and their family or support system to understand, as PCS is costly, although not as expensive as living in a long-term care facility. See Table 5.1 for a comparison of the costs. Many states have licensing requirements for PCS agencies and guidelines for the delivery of PCS. Still, unless they are also associated with a home health service agency, they likely will not be accredited through a national organization.

TABLE 5.1 PCS, HHA, ALF, & LTC Cost Comparisons in the United States

Service Provided	Median Daily Cost 2021	Median Monthly Cost 2021	Median Annual Cost 2021	Projected Annual Cost in 2031
Personal Care Services (PCS)	$163	$4,957	$59,488	$79,947
Home Health Aide (HHA) Services (Certified Aide)	$169	$5,148	$61,776	$83,022
Assisted Living Facility (ALF)	$148	$4,500	$54,000	$72,571
Long-Term Care Facility (LTC) (Semi-private room)	$260	$7,908	$94,900	$127,538

(Genworth, 2022, interactive cost calculator)

Unique Considerations of Personal Care Services

Although PCS are often privately paid for, some insurances may cover this service as a benefit, with Medicaid being one of them. Depending on the state Medicaid benefit, PCS may be authorized as a benefit for those with chronic or temporary conditions requiring assistance with their daily living activities to remain in their home and avoid an institutional setting, such as long-term care (CMS, 2017). However, it can be a longer-term process to have PCS authorized. Often, the patient must be evaluated by a provider or nurse who works for the state Medicaid program, and the evaluation must show that PCS services are needed. Suppose a patient may need PCS and they are a Medicaid beneficiary. In that case, the care coordinating nurse will need to coordinate referrals for the evaluation process and provide the Medicaid agency with any required information to determine eligibility for the PCS. This can take some time, and in the meantime, the care coordinating nurse may need to assist in arranging alternate PCS if they are essential for patient needs, outcomes, and safety.

Other ways to fund the payment for PCS is through long-term care insurance, or if the patient is a veteran, they may be eligible for covered services. Long-term care insurance is private insurance, with the patient paying the premium. However, usually a patient cannot elect to carry long-term care insurance after PCS is needed. It may not be affordable for the patient, and the policies vary on how much will be covered, when the patient is eligible to receive services, and what types of services are required to be eligible for benefit use. If the patient is a veteran or surviving spouse of a veteran, they may be eligible for the Aid and Attendance or Housebound benefits through the Veterans Administration. This benefit provides a monthly payment to the veteran or surviving spouse to assist with the cost of PCS (U.S. Department of Veterans Affairs, 2022). If the patient or the survivor still needs to apply for this benefit, the application may take some time to be processed. In the meantime, the care coordinator may need to assist in organizing PCS until the veterans benefit is authorized. There are a variety of other avenues for funding PCS, such as blended life insurance and long-term care insurance policies, annuities, and reverse mortgages. Still, all of these are personal financial decisions the patient will make with their financial advisor or family/caregiver (Cress, 2017).

If assessment and evaluation shows need of a PCS, or the patient requests them, the care coordinator will need to investigate all avenues of funding and work with the patient on any applications required. Or the care coordinator may need to work with the patient and the family/support system on designing a plan for PCS that family members, friends, or others provide, or ensure the patient understands how much the PCS services will cost and discuss whether this is affordable for the patient.

Palliative and Hospice Care

Palliative and hospice care are often considered the same or equated with end-of-life care. However, there are essential distinctions between palliative and hospice care that the care coordinator must understand as they discuss goals of care, preferences, and options with patients. Both palliative and hospice care are based on a holistic view of care for the patient, integrating care and support for the family and caregiver. However, the care types are delivered at different stages of the continuum of care. Hospice care is a type of palliative care, but palliative care is not hospice care (Hopkins, 2021). Palliative care is for any patient with a serious illness and can be offered anytime during a disease process. Patients receiving palliative care can receive treatment for their symptoms and pursue curative measures. Still, the focus is on the quality of life for the patient and their family/caregiver (National Institute of Aging, 2021). Many serious illnesses may last years, and patients and their families/caregivers can benefit from the holistic and quality-of-life approach of palliative care. Palliative care is usually provided in a healthcare setting, such as a clinic or hospital, by specialist providers.

Hospice care is for those patients who are approaching their end-of-life and either no longer want to pursue curative treatment or the disease process is no longer responding to treatments offered. There are criteria for hospice care eligibility for Medicare beneficiaries, and many private insurance companies follow Medicare guidelines concerning eligibility for hospice care. Hospice care is designed for patients who have 6 months or less to live as documented in a face-to-face encounter by the provider who states that the patient's prognosis is that their life expectancy is 6 months or less if the illness runs its normal course (Medicare Benefit Policy Manual, 2021b). Medicare also requires that all curative treatment be discontinued for eligibility. A patient may live longer than 6 months and still be eligible for hospice, but they must show evidence of continued decline in health and advancement in the end-of-life process. If a patient who elects hospice care does not decline in health, then the hospice agency will be required to discharge them from hospice care, and the patient can then transition back to palliative care or other types of healthcare. Hospice care is provided wherever the patient resides (e.g., a private residence, an assisted living facility (ALF), or a long-term care (LTC) facility). See Table 5.2 for a comparison of palliative and hospice care.

TABLE 5.2 Comparison of Palliative vs. Hospice Care

	Palliative Care (PC)	Hospice Care (HC)
Focus	PC is adjunctive to curative treatment, focuses on pain and symptom management.	HC focuses on pain and symptom management at the end of life.
Time	Is not time limited	HC is for those who are expected to have a 6-month or less lifespan if the disease runs its natural course.
Service eligibility	Anyone with a serious illness regardless of prognosis	Those with a terminal prognosis
Curative treatments	PC allows curative treatments.	HC does not allow curative treatments as it is deemed no longer beneficial, or the patient no longer chooses to pursue curative treatment.

Services provided	Pain and symptom management, patient navigation services, advanced care planning, and referrals to community resources	Pain and symptom management, 24-hour on-call service, in-person visits, durable medical equipment, related medications, volunteer services, respite care and bereavement services
Service Provider	A specialist provider with consultative support from an interprofessional team. The specialist may comanage care with the patient's primary provider.	An interdisciplinary team including nurses, social workers, chaplains, volunteers, and hospice aides, with medical director oversight in collaboration with the patient's primary provider
Medicare Coverage	PC is covered through Medicare part B and is subject to copays and deductibles.	HC is covered through the hospice benefit, which is a per diem benefit that is inclusive of all hospice costs related to terminal care, without copays or deductibles. Some medications or equipment may not be included under the hospice benefit.

(National Hospice and Palliative Care Organization, 2019)

Both palliative and hospice care provide holistic, interprofessional care, with physicians, nurses, social workers, chaplains, and other ancillary service members as needed, to meet the patient and their families/caregivers' needs throughout the illness trajectory and during the bereavement process after the patient's death. See Figure 5.4—The Palliative Care Continuum. Holism is integrated all through palliative and hospice care philosophy, from the point of person-centered assessment and evaluation of symptoms and suffering, which could be based on physical, psychological, social, emotional, spiritual, or even existential pain and discomfort (Rosser & Walsh, 2014). Patients and their families/caregivers who receive palliative and hospice care identify more satisfaction with the care they receive, have their symptoms better controlled, and avoid unnecessary tests or treatments, assisting with decreasing resource use and increasing quality and person-centered care delivery (National Institute of Aging, 2021). Palliative and hospice care are critical but often underutilized services due to providers, nurses, and patients misunderstanding the care benefits and when to refer to or request a referral to these types of care.

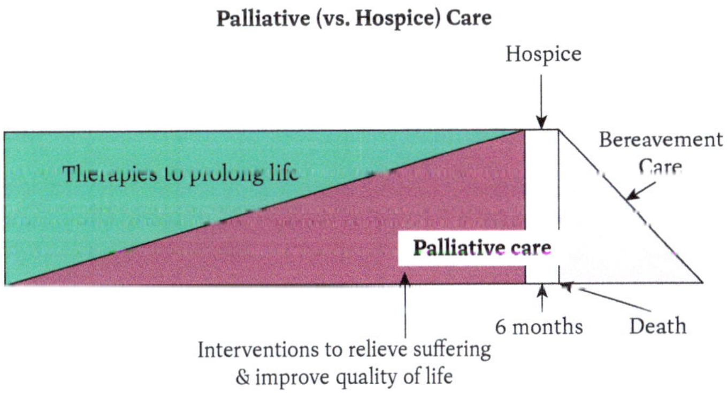

FIGURE 5.4 The Palliative Care Continuum

Palliative and hospice care services receive payment/reimbursement for care provided by private insurance companies, Medicare, Medicaid, and sometimes via private pay from the patient. Organizations that maintain standards for operation and accreditation for palliative and hospice care services include The Joint Commission (JCAHO), the Community Health Accreditation Partner (CHAP) program, and the Accreditation Commission for Health Care (ACHC). Many hospice agencies are also certified as Medicare and Medicaid hospice providers.

Unique Considerations of Palliative and Hospice Care

Palliative and hospice services will meet with the patient and their family/support system before enrolling them in the service. These information sessions go over the patient's goals of care, the diagnosis and prognosis, a description of services and the philosophy of care, and a discussion of insurance benefits, if any. This is a critical conversation that the care coordinating nurse should prepare the patient for because potentially difficult subject areas will be raised, such as if curative treatment is to be continued, how symptoms will be managed, and how the care will be delivered. If the patient has a family or caregiver involved, it is prudent to ensure they are also in attendance at this meeting with the palliative or hospice care provider, if the patient is agreeable, so they can ask questions, share concerns, and receive education and information on the services to be provided.

Palliative and hospice care goals of care and informational conversations can be emotionally charged, with differing opinions among the patient and different family or support system members on the best course of treatment or care to be sought. Often, patients may want to discontinue curative treatments, focus on quality of life, and transition to palliative or hospice care. Still, their family or support system members may not agree. Working to get the provider, patient, family, and support system on the same page can proactively address challenges to care delivery. The care coordinating nurse must possess essential communication competencies to assist in navigating these crucial conversations concerning goals of care and may also need to provide advocacy to ensure the patient's voice is heard.

When a patient is considering transitioning to hospice care, the care coordinator needs to understand the patient's insurance coverage to provide appropriate education and referrals to community resources if needed. Unlike Medicare and Medicaid, many private insurance companies offer a hospice benefit, but it is often a set dollar amount over the lifetime, such as a $10,000 lifetime hospice benefit. The patient will likely also have copays and need to meet deductible requirements. If the patient outlives their lifetime hospice benefit, they will have to discontinue hospice services or pay out of pocket for hospice care with their own funds. This is a critical conversation to have with a patient and their family/caregiver so that they can best determine, with their provider and the interprofessional team, when a transition to hospice care is best for them.

If the patient does not have private insurance and is not eligible for Medicare or Medicaid, they can privately pay for hospice care services. Often, hospice agencies have a price list of what a nursing visit costs, a hospice aide visit, etc., that can be reviewed with and given to the patient. The patient will then need to sign a form agreeing to pay the rates for each visit they receive. In this case, the hospice agency may only visit the patient at their request (due to the cost of the visit) or create a service plan outlining services and costs for a period of time, providing transparency of costs and putting the patient in control of the costs of their care. Awareness of the patient's funding sources, limitations, or requirements is crucial for successful transition to palliative or hospice care so that if additional connections to community or state resources need to be pursued, the care coordinator can do this in a proactive and timely manner, ensuring the patient receives the most appropriate level of care possible that meets their medical needs and personal goals of care.

CHAPTER SUMMARY

The healthcare system in the United States is complex and provides for a variety of health needs across the health trajectory and lifespan. It is a "system ... of interacting, interrelated, or interdependent components that form a complex and unified whole" (Johnson et al., 2020, p. 3). Whether the care being delivered is viewed as a sphere or level of care, all healthcare falls on the care continuum, and the nurse care coordinator's role is to maintain continuity and coordination of patient care throughout the healthcare system. This requires the nurse to have a keen understanding of the myriad of parts, components, and services offered across the continuum of care and to ensure the care being provided is at the most appropriate level to meet patient needs and goals. To provide information and care continuity across the continuum, the nurse must engage in person- and relationship-centered care, interprofessional collaboration, cross-setting communication, while interconnecting care and services to meet patient needs over the trajectory of health.

The care continuum includes care and services across the lifespan, including healthy living, routine care, acute care, rehabilitation, and end-of-life care. Health is not linear; patients move back and forth across the continuum of care as their health needs and goals of care change. Levels of care signify the intensity of service and expertise needed to meet the patient's healthcare needs, including prevention and maintenance, primary care, secondary care, tertiary care, quaternary care, and rehabilitative and restorative care. Each level is interconnected but requires differing expertise and equipment, each focusing on specific populations of patients to meet healthcare needs across the lifespan. Each part of the continuum of care and level of care contributes to a unified whole of healthcare services.

There are common transitions to different levels of care and settings in care coordination practice. These include acute care hospitals, long-term acute care hospitals, psychiatric hospitals, rehabilitation services, home health care, personal care services, and palliative and hospice care. Each care setting and service has unique considerations for care coordination practice. The nurse has an ethical role in promoting, advocating for, and protecting patients' rights, health, and safety (ANA, 2015, p. v). The nurse care coordinator must have foundational knowledge concerning insurance coverage requirements, eligibility criteria, legal guidelines, and organizational considerations and policies for all settings in which they transition patients' care across the continuum of care to meet this ethical role. Insurance criteria, such as inpatient versus outpatient admission status or length of stay, can affect the ability of patients to receive needed care, and legal status, such as involuntary admission, can affect the patient's rights.

Nurses must use the nursing process to ensure that patients receive the most appropriate level of care to meet their needs and goals of care and ensure quality and cost-effective care delivery. Through assessment and diagnosis of potential issues or barriers to care and transitions, the nurse can create a transition plan that meets patient healthcare needs across the continuum of care and will also meet identified patient outcomes and organizational benchmarking criteria. Providing effective health teaching and education supports the patient's right to choose, and autonomous decision-making and critical analysis of the plan of care implementation are also necessary. Using foundational knowledge concerning spheres, levels, and the continuum of care with skills in interprofessional collaborative practice, communication, and informational continuity, the nurse can successfully coordinate care across the continuum.

CHAPTER 5 GLOSSARY

Acute Rehabilitation: Inpatient rehabilitative healthcare services, usually associated with a hospital, which requires the patient to participate a minimum of 3 hours a day for at least 5 days a week in an intensive, interprofessional, and coordinated rehabilitation program.

Continuum of Care: A system of healthcare that matches patient healthcare needs with the appropriate level of care and services across all stages of the lifespan and settings, delivering person-centered, integrated, and continuity of care to achieve optimal outcomes and use of resources.

Grave Disability: Due to a mental health condition, the patient cannot provide self-care, self-protection, or their own basic personal needs.

Involuntary Admission: An admission status where the patient is placed in a psychiatric hospital setting due to meeting specific criteria but does not agree to the hospitalization.

Level of Care: This identifies the acuity of care required, the amount of expertise needed, and the intensity of care and service needed to meet healthcare needs and goals of care.

Long-Term Acute Care Hospital (LTACH): A type of tertiary level of care that offers specialized care for those with serious health conditions requiring longer-term specialized and expert care, such as prolonged ventilator use or complex wound care.

Personal Care Services (PCS): Nonmedical assistance that provides support for those with chronic conditions or recovering from illness or injury through assistance with activities of daily living, such as bathing, dressing, or meal preparation. Unlicensed caregivers provide PCS and are mostly privately funded, with the patient paying out of pocket for the PCS.

Preventative and Maintenance Level of Care: Healthcare services that promote wellness, patient self-management of health, and other activities that sustain health and prevent injury and illness.

Primary Level of Care: Healthcare services that can treat a wide range of health issues, including wellness, prevention, and common illnesses or injuries. It may include "gatekeeping" services for referrals to specialists or other levels of care as needed.

Quaternary Level of Care: Healthcare services focused on uncommon conditions, very specialized or rare surgeries, clinical trials, or innovative care and treatments. Quaternary facilities are usually associated with teaching hospitals or other hospital systems.

Rehabilitative Level of Care: Healthcare services that focus on improving lost or impaired functioning due to illness or injury, involving multiple therapies, such as physical, occupational, and speech-language therapies.

Restorative Level of Care: Healthcare services that offer an integrated approach to maintain and prevent the decline of functional abilities, promoting safety and independence.

Secondary Level of Care: Healthcare services provided by a provider who is an "expert" or specializes in a specific disease process or illness.

Spheres of Care: The spheres of care include wellness and disease prevention, restorative and regenerative care, chronic disease care, and hospice and palliative care. These spheres of care meet healthcare needs across the lifespan.

Subacute Rehabilitation (SAR): Inpatient rehabilitative healthcare services, usually associated with a skilled nursing facility (SNF), which requires a lower level of patient participation in the rehabilitation program, with only about 2 hours of daily therapy.

Swing Bed: A room in a rural or critical access acute care hospital that can be "switched" from an acute care status to a skilled care or rehabilitative status as needed and often used for patients from rural areas who need skilled nursing facility (SNF) level rehabilitation care post-acute-care discharge so that they can receive rehabilitation closer to their homes or while they wait for an SNF bed opening in their community of residence.

Tertiary Level of Care: Healthcare services provided in an acute care hospital that provides specialized care requiring specific expertise and equipment. It may be a general acute care hospital or a specialty hospital such as a psychiatric hospital.

Voluntary Admission: An admission status where the patient has given consent, by their own choice, to be placed in a psychiatric hospital setting.

DISCUSSION QUESTIONS AND ACTIVITIES

Discussion Questions

1. Discuss how each part of the continuum of care and level of care contributes to a "unified whole" of healthcare services.
2. Discuss how your understanding of the role of care coordination and the concept of person-centered care have changed when considering care coordination practice in the continuum of care.

3. Select one of the following common settings that patients are transitioned to:

   Acute care hospital
   LTACH
   Psychiatric hospital
   Home health
   Palliative care
   Hospice

   Review the unique considerations for care coordination practice presented in the chapter concerning this setting. Then discuss the implications of how these unique considerations may affect patient health and safety.

4. Discuss the similarities and differences between the four spheres of care, the continuum of care, and levels of care.

5. Choose one of the following environmental factors:

   Resource availability
   Time constraints
   Access to medical information/records
   Complexity of the transition

   Then discuss how these may affect the ability of the nurse to coordinate a smooth transition of care with continuity of information and care ensured.

Activities

1. Divide into four groups. Each group selects one of the following "hat" colors as their group's identity. Then consider the following scenario. You are a nurse care coordinator discussing the option to transition to palliative care with a patient with HIV/AIDS. Using your group's "hat" color designation, outline what you would present to the patient and their family/support system concerning transitioning to palliative care.

   Hat Color Descriptions:

   a. White hat: It is objective and focuses on facts and logic about transitioning to palliative care.

   b. Red hat: It is in tune with the emotional aspects of the palliative care transition and discusses the emotional reasons or feelings that may come with the transition.

   c. Black hat: It is cautious, considering any negative aspects of the transition to palliative care.

   d. Yellow hat: It is optimistic and discusses the positive aspects and outcomes of the transition to palliative care.

Present your findings to the class after your group has outlined what information or education you would present to the patient and their family/support system. As a class, discuss what this type of information might mean to a patient and their family/support system when making decisions about healthcare choices.

2. Consider the story "A Clinical Resource Manager's Discharge Plan Gone Awry." Then review the foundational care coordination competencies of person-centered and relationship-centered care, advocacy, assessment and critical analysis, communication, interprofessional practice, and quality assurance. Identify one positive or negative action the clinical resource manager made regarding each care coordination competency. Discuss what the clinical resource manager could have done differently for each negative action identified to ensure a smooth transition and informational and care continuity across the continuum of care.

3. Case Study:

   You are the care coordinator in the local emergency room department. A 75-year-old woman arrives via ambulance with a left humeral fracture. She lived at a local assisted living facility and was hit by another resident in their electric scooter, causing her to fall and, break her humerus. She reports a previous left shoulder replacement about 10 years earlier. The orthopedic surgeon provides consultation and recommends surgical repair. The patient has been prescribed oral medications to control pain and is stable. The patient is a Medicare beneficiary.

   After discussing with her family, the woman decides not to pursue surgical intervention and wants to receive rehabilitation services. The patient has been assessed and evaluated by the physical and occupational therapists, and they are recommending home health therapy services be provided at discharge. However, the assisted living facility refuses to accept the patient back to their service as she exceeds their level of care. No one in the patient's family can provide for her care in their homes, and you have exhausted any potential friends or other relatives who may be able to house her while she recovers from her injury and receives rehabilitative therapies. The emergency room doctor admits her in observation status until you can arrange for the patient to be transitioned to an inpatient rehabilitation facility.

   a. What is the priority for this patient's health?
   b. What considerations do you need to bear in mind regarding the emergency room doctor's admission plan?
   c. What information or education would you provide to the patient and their family/support system regarding the situation and interprofessional recommendations so they can make an informed choice of care setting and delivery?
   d. What would you do as the care coordinator in this scenario to support the delivery of quality and cost-effective care delivery?

NCLEX STYLE QUESTIONS

1. A patient has been hospitalized for pneumonia and will be discharged today. The physical therapist recommended home health physical therapy to regain strength and mobility post-illness. The care coordinator has sent the referral to the home health agency, and they have accepted the patient. As the nurse care coordinator reviews the discharge notes, they notice the patient has a history of Type 2 diabetes and congestive heart failure. Which of the following is the best answer concerning how the nurse care coordinator should communicate this finding to the next level of care?

   a. Since the patient is not at significant risk of readmission for pneumonia, the nurse care coordinator should send only the discharge orders to the home health agency.

   b. The nurse care coordinator should collect all pertinent information and ensure the family has this to share with the home health agency at the first visit.

   c. The nurse care coordinator knows that lack of information continuity can lead to fragmented care and should address any gaps in information with the home health agency before discharge.

   d. Since the home health agency will see the patient, the care coordinator knows they will discover this information on their initial assessment.

2. An outpatient nurse care coordinator receives a call from a patient with congestive heart failure who reports they have gained 4 pounds overnight and are having shortness of breath. They have taken additional doses of their diuretic medication without effect. The nurse care coordinator recommends that the patient go to the emergency room for treatment and admission. How should the nurse care coordinator facilitate the transfer of care to the emergency room?

   a. Notify the patient's primary care provider in the outpatient clinic of the patient's condition.

   b. Ask the patient about their choice of home health agency, as they likely will need this once they receive treatment in the emergency room.

   c. Ask the patient to call them once they are in the emergency room so the outpatient nurse care coordinator can give a report to the assigned emergency room nurse.

   d. Ensure that the shared electronic health record for the patient has the most up-to-date medication list.

3. The nurse care coordinator is working with a student nurse and is explaining the concept of the continuum of care and how it relates to care coordination practice. The nurse care coordinator knows the student understands the continuum of care concept when they say which of the following?

   a. The following provider is responsible for ensuring patients' continuity of care through illness, injury, rehabilitation, and health maintenance.

   b. The continuum of care involves all aspects of healthcare services but not support services.

   c. The continuum of care is a linear concept, and patients progress along it throughout their lifespan.

   d. The continuum of care is the system of healthcare matching patient needs with the appropriate level of care across the lifespan.

Questions 4 through 7 apply to the following scenario.

Mr. Gomez has been life-flighted to the regional trauma center after an all-terrain vehicle (ATV) accident. He had several surgeries to repair internal organ damage and an open reduction internal fixation (ORIF) surgery to repair a broken ankle. He is now ready to be discharged and will need subacute rehabilitation services. He lives in a remote state area with only one skilled nursing facility within a 100-mile radius.

4. Mr. Gomez was admitted on October 12th at 11:50 p.m. and was discharged on October 15th at 12:10 p.m. Does Mr. Gomez meet the 3-day rule according to the Medicare conditions of participation?

   a. Yes

   b. No

5. The local critical access hospital has agreed to accept Mr. Gomez until there is an opening in the closest skilled nursing facility. What type of bed will Mr. Raymond be admitted to at the critical access hospital?

   a. Inpatient bed

   b. Observation bed

   c. Swing bed

   d. Outpatient bed

6. As Mr. Gomez will need subacute rehabilitation, this indicates that he can participate in how many hours of therapies per day?

   a. 2 hours

   b. 1 hour

   c. 3 hours

   d. 5 hours

7. After discharge from subacute rehabilitation, Mr. Gomez must be followed by an orthopedic surgeon in his local area. Which level of care is this referred to?

   a. Quaternary level of care

   b. Secondary level of care

   c. Restorative level of care

   d. Primary level of care

Questions 8 through 10 apply to the following scenario.

Cody Freeman, a 36-year-old male Medicaid beneficiary, has experienced an aneurysm and has been admitted to the intensive care unit (ICU). Cody was put on a ventilator due to his failing respiratory status. The ICU has attempted to wean Cody off the ventilator several times unsuccessfully. The ICU hospitalist believes Cody will require longer-term ventilator support than the current ICU can offer.

8. Which care setting is the most appropriate for the ICU hospitalist to recommend Cody to be discharged to?

   a. Acute rehabilitation, as they can provide therapies to enhance the respiratory musculature

   b. Palliative care, as this may be a long-term condition and they can focus on quality-of-life goals

   c. Home health, as they can provide continuous nursing support in Cody's home

   d. Long-term acute care hospital, as they can provide for ventilator weaning

9. Cody Freeman has been weaned off the ventilator and is being discharged home with home health and personal care services recommended. Which of the following best describes personal care services (PCS)?

a. Most private insurance companies cover PCS after co-pays and deductibles are met.

b. Once a Medicaid nurse/provider determines a need for PCS, this may be a Medicaid benefit.

c. PCS services are usually provided by personal care aides who are certified or licensed.

d. The Joint Commission accredits all PCS organizations.

10. The nurse care coordinator explains home health services and the need for homebound status to Cody Freeman. Which of the following descriptions of homebound status requirements indicate that Cody understands the education given?

a. Cody states, "Being homebound means that I can leave my home for short, infrequent periods, for things like medical appointments or to attend church."

b. Cody states, "Being homebound means that I cannot leave my home at any time while receiving home health services, unless it is an emergency."

c. Cody states, "Being homebound means I can go to my upcoming weekend-long family reunion, as long as I have someone there to help me and I return home as soon as it is over."

d. Cody states, "Being homebound means that I can receive home health services as long as I do not have transportation to my medical appointments."

Questions 11 through 13 apply to the following scenario:

Gwen Grant was found by her partner attempting to cut her wrists in the kitchen. Her partner called the police for help, and she was brought to the emergency room. Gwen Grant is a 24-year-old female who is 5 months pregnant and has a history of heroin use.

11. As the nurse care coordinator, you know that Gwen may meet the criteria for an involuntary psychiatric admission if she meets which of the following? (Select all that apply.)

a. Gwen has a defined mental health disorder.

b. Gwen can care for her activities of daily living.

c. Gwen will improve if she is sent to outpatient treatment.

d. Gwen is likely to harm herself.

12. Gwen is being evaluated by a mental health examiner, Dr. Doran, to determine the most appropriate level of care and make treatment recommendations. Dr. Doran has already been working 12 hours this shift and has three more evaluations to conduct before being done for the day. Which of the following factors describe Dr. Doran's situation and may affect the doctor's decision to admit a patient to psychiatric hospitalization?

    a. Clinical and risk factors
    b. Threat/fear factors
    c. Interpersonal dynamic factors
    d. Contextual factors

13. Gwen will be transferred to the local psychiatric hospital for treatment, and her partner is concerned about her pregnancy and if she begins to have heroin withdrawals. Which is the best response by the nurse care coordinator?

    a. "That is a valid concern. I will talk with the attending provider and see if we can keep her in the hospital until we know she will not have withdrawal symptoms."
    b. "The psychiatric hospital will send Gwen back to this hospital if she begins having withdrawal symptoms that they cannot address or if there is an issue with the pregnancy."
    c. "Pregnant women should not be in a psychiatric hospital. It would be better to have her treated by an outpatient therapist."
    d. "There is no need to be concerned. Don't you want her to get better?"

Questions 14 through 15 apply to the following scenario:

Thomas Yeoh, an 81-year-old male with stage 4 prostate cancer, has indicated to the nurse care coordinator that he would like to consider transitioning to hospice care. He tells the nurse care coordinator that his family disagrees with him transitioning to hospice care, and he is concerned about how they will deal with his death.

14. The nurse care coordinator knows families who receive hospice care report which of the following outcomes. (Select all that apply.)

    a. Increased person-centered care
    b. Increased satisfaction with care
    c. Increased treatments or tests.
    d. Increased resource use and costs

15. Mr. Yeoh and his family have scheduled a hospice information session with the hospice agency. The nurse care coordinator knows that this information session will review which of the following. (Select all that apply.)

    a. The services provided by the hospice agency

    b. Types of curative treatments that can be offered

    c. The philosophy of hospice care

    d. Request family questions be addressed once the patient is signed onto hospice service

REFERENCES

American Association of Colleges of Nursing (AACN). (2021). *The Essentials: Core competencies for professional nursing education.* https://www.aacnnursing.org/Portals/0/PDFs/Publications/Essentials-2021.pdf

American Cancer Society. (2019). *Surgery for pancreatic cancer.* https://www.cancer.org/cancer/types/pancreatic-cancer/treating/surgery.html

American Hospital Association. (2023). *Skilled nursing facility 3-day rule billing.* https://www.cms.gov/files/document/skilled-nursing-facility-3-day-rule-billing.pdf

American Nurses Association. (2015). *Code of ethics for nurses with interpretive statements.* American Nurses Association.

American Psychiatric Association (APA). (2020). *Position statement on voluntary and involuntary hospitalization of adults with mental illness.* https://www.psychiatry.org/getattachment/46011d52-de5d-4738-a132-f5aaa249efb5/Position-Voluntary-Involuntary-Hospitalization-Adults.pdf

ATI Advisory. (2022). *Long-term acute care (LTAC) hospitals as part of the value-based solution: A case study of Kindred LTAC hospitals in Las Vegas.* https://atiadvisory.com/resources/long-term-acute-care-ltac-hospitals-as-part-of-the-value-based-solution-a-case-study-of-ltac-hospitals-in-las-vegas/

Busch, R. M. (2018). Critical elements of healthcare costing. *Journal of Life Care Planning, 16*(2), 37–42. https://rehabpro.org/page/JLCP_16_summary/Journal-of-Life-Care-Planning-Volume-16.htm

Callister, C., Jones, J., Schroeder, S., Breathett, K., Dollar, B., Sanghvi, U. J., Harnke, B., Lum, H. D., & Jones, C. D. (2020). Caregiver experiences of care coordination for recently discharged patients: A qualitative metasynthesis. *Western Journal of Nursing Research, 42*(8), 649–659. https://doi.org/10.1177/0193945919880183

Case Management Study Guide. (2023). *Levels of care: CCMC glossary of terms related to levels of care.* https://casemanagementstudyguide.com/ccm-knowledge-domains/healthcare-management-delivery/levels-of-care/

Centers for Medicare and Medicaid Services (CMS). (2006). *Post-acute care reform plan.* https://www.cms.gov/Medicare/Medicare-Fee-for-Service-Payment/SNFPPS/downloads/pac_reform_plan_2006.pdf

Centers for Medicare and Medicaid Services (CMS). (2017). *Preventing Medicaid improper payments for personal care services.* https://www.cms.gov/Medicare-Medicaid-Coordination/Fraud-Prevention/Medicaid-Integrity-Education/Downloads/pcs-prevent-improper-payment-factsheet.pdf

Centers for Medicare and Medicaid Services (CMS). (2023a). *Psychiatric hospitals.* https://www.cms.gov/medicare/health-safety-standards/certification-compliance/psychiatric-hospitals

Centers for Medicare and Medicaid Services (CMS). (2023b). *Inpatient psychiatric facility quality reporting (IPFQR) program.* https://www.cms.gov/medicare/quality/initiatives/hospital-quality-initiative/inpatient-psychiatric-facility-quality-reporting-ipfqr-program

Compton. P. (2020). *Understanding care: Long-term acute care hospitals 101.* https://harmony.solutions/understanding-care-long-term-acute-care-hospitals-101/

Cress, C. J. (2017). *Handbook of geriatric care management* (4th ed.). Jones & Bartlett Learning.

Department of Health & Human Services. (2013). *Revision to state operations manual (SOM), hospital appendix a—interpretive guidelines for 42 cfr 482.43, discharge planning.* https://www.hhs.gov/guidance/sites/default/files/hhs-guidance-documents/SC13-32.combinedHospital%20DP%20memo.pdf

Department of Health & Human Services. (2019). *What are long-term care hospitals?* https://www.medicare.gov/Pubs/pdf/11347-Long-Term-Care-Hospitals.pdf

Department of Managed Healthcare. (2023). *Preventative care.* https://www.dmhc.ca.gov/healthcareincalifornia/getthebestcare/preventivecare.aspx

Evashwick, C. J. (1989). Creating the continuum of care. *Health matrix, 7(1), 30–9.*

Federation of American Hospitals. (2023). *Inpatient rehabilitation hospitals.* https://www.fah.org/issues-advocacy/medicare/inpatient-rehabilitation-hospitals/

Genworth. (2022). *Cost of care survey.* https://www.genworth.com/aging-and-you/finances/cost-of-care.html/

Health Care Compliance Association. (2014). *Home care and hospice: Compliance update: 2014* [PowerPoint]. https://assets.hcca-info.org/Portals/0/PDFs/Resources/Conference_Handouts/Compliance_Institute/2014/mon/303print2.pdf

Healthcare.gov. (n.d.a). *Primary care.* https://www.healthcare.gov/glossary/primary-care/

Healthcare.gov. (n.d.b). *Rehabilitative/rehabilitation services.* https://www.healthcare.gov/glossary/rehabilitative-rehabilitation-services/

Healthcare Roadmap. (n.d.). *Long-term acute care (LTAC) criteria checklist.* https://myhealthcareroadmap.com/wp-content/uploads/2019/04/Criteria-Checklist-Long-Term-Acute-Care-LTAC.pdf

Hedman, L. C., Petrila, J., Fisher, W. H., Swanson, J. W., Dingman, D. A., & Burris, S. (2016). State laws on emergency holds for mental health stabilization. *Psychiatric Services, 67*(5), 529–535. https://doi.org/10.1176/appi.ps.201500205

Hopkins, L. (2021). *Hospice: A critical end-of-life service (part 1).* https://endoflifeoptionsnm.org/hospice-a-critical-end-of-life-service-part-1/

Johnson, J. A., Anderson, D. E., & Rossow, C. C. (2020). *Health systems thinking: A primer.* Jones & Bartlett Learning.

Khatri, R., Endalamaw, A., Erku, D., Wolka, E., Nigatu, F., Zewdie, A., & Assefa, Y. (2023). Continuity and care coordination of primary health care: A scoping review. *BMC Health Services Research, 23*(1), 750. https://doi.org/10.1186/s12913-023-09718-8

Knickman, J. R., & Elbel, B. (Eds.). (2019). *Jonas & Kovner's health care delivery in the United States* (12th ed.). Springer Publishing Company.

Lane, K. L., Kalberg, J. R., & Menzies, H. M. (2009). *Developing schoolwide programs to prevent and manage problem behaviors: A step-by-step approach.* Guilford Press.

Mallender, J. (2022). *What are levels of care? A simple guide.* https://www.economicsbydesign.com/levels-of-care/

McAlister, L. (2023). *Understanding patient choice and your rights.* https://blog.encompasshealth.com/2021/09/21/what-does-patient-choice-mean/

Medicare Benefit Policy Manual. (2021a). *Inpatient hospital services covered under part A* (ch. 1). https://www.cms.gov/Regulations-and-Guidance/Guidance/Manuals/Downloads/bp102c01.pdf

Medicare Benefit Policy Manual. (2021b). *Coverage of hospice services under hospital insurance* (ch. 9). https://www.cms.gov/regulations-and-guidance/guidance/manuals/downloads/bp102c09.pdf

Medicare Benefit Policy Manual. (2022). *Home health services* (ch. 7). https://www.cms.gov/Regulations-and-Guidance/Guidance/Manuals/downloads/bp102c07.pdf

Medicare Interactive. (2023a). *Home health basics.* https://www.medicareinteractive.org/get-answers/medicare-covered-services/home-health-services/home-health-basics

Medicare Interactive. (2023b). *The homebound requirement.* https://www.medicareinteractive.org/get-answers/medicare-covered-services/home-health-services/the-homebound-requirement

Medicare Program Integrity Manual. (2020). *Medicare contractor medical review guidelines for specific services* (ch. 6). https://www.cms.gov/Regulations-and-Guidance/Guidance/Manuals/Downloads/pim83c06.pdf

Medpac. (2021). *Inpatient rehabilitation facilities payment system.* https://www.medpac.gov/wp-content/uploads/2021/11/medpac_payment_basics_21_irf_final_sec.pdf

Nathan, R., Gabbay, M., Boyle, S., Elliott, P., Giebel, C., O'Loughlin, C., Wilson, P., & Saini, P. (2021). Use of acute psychiatric hospitalization: A study of the factors influencing decisions to arrange acute admission to inpatient mental health facilities. *Frontiers in Psychiatry, 12*, 696478. https://doi.org/10.3389/fpsyt.2021.696478

National Hospice and Palliative Care Organization. (2019). *Palliative care or hospice? The right service at the right time for seriously ill individuals.* https://www.nhpco.org/wp-content/uploads/2019/04/PalliativeCare_VS_Hospice.pdf

National Institute of Aging. (2021). *What are palliative care and hospice care?* https://www.nia.nih.gov/health/what-are-palliative-care-and-hospice-care

Office of the Assistant Secretary for Planning and Evaluation. (2019). *How many older adults can afford to purchase home care?* https://aspe.hhs.gov/reports/how-many-older-adults-can-afford-purchase-home-care-0#main-content

The Patient Choice. (2020). *What are acute care rehab facilities?* https://www.thepatientchoice.com/elderly-care-facilities/what-are-acute-care-rehab-facilities/

Paying for Senior Care. (2022). *What is home care and how much does it cost?* https://www.payingforseniorcare.com/homecare

Primary Care Development Corporation. (2023). *Primary care: The health care continuum every community needs.* https://www.pcdc.org/primary-care-the-health-care-continuum-every-community-needs/

Rosser, M., & Walsh, H. C. (2014). *Fundamentals of palliative care for student nurses* (1st ed.). Wiley Blackwell.

Sadick, B. (2021). *Home health aides: When your loved one needs help with personal care: What family caregivers need to know about hiring.* https://www.aarp.org/caregiving/home-care/info-2019/home-health-aides.html

SAMHSA. (2023). *Care coordination agreements and care transitions.* https://www.samhsa.gov/certified-community-behavioral-health-clinics/section-223/care-coordination/agreements-transitions#

Shi, L., & Singh, D. (2019). *Essentials of the U.S. health care system* (5th ed.). Jones & Bartlett Learning.

Stefanacci, R. G. (2015). Admission criteria for facility-based post-acute services. *Annals of Long-Term Care.* https://www.hmpgloballearningnetwork.com/site/altc/articles/admission-criteria facility-based-post-acute-services

Swan, B. A., Haas, S., & Jessie, A. T. (2019). Care coordination: Roles of registered nurses across the care continuum. *Nursing Economic$, 37*(6), 317–323.

SYNZI. (2018). *6 ways to optimize the continuum of care.* https://synzi.com/wp-content/uploads/2018/11/6-Ways-to-Optimize-the-Continuum-of-Care.pdf

Talley, K. M., Wyman, J. F., Savik, K., Kane, R. L., Mueller, C., & Zhao, H. (2015). Restorative care's effect on activities of daily living dependency in long-stay nursing home residents. *The Gerontologist, 55 Suppl 1*(Suppl 1), S88–S98. https://doi.org/10.1093/geront/gnv011

Tombak, Y., Karaahmet, O. Z., Umay, E., Tombak, A., & Gurcay, E. (2023). Factors influencing the willingness to participate in rehabilitation in patients with subacute stroke. *Journal of Clinical Neuroscience: Official Journal of the Neurosurgical Society of Australasia, 116*, 99–103. https://doi.org/10.1016/j.jocn.2023.09.001

Torrey, T. (2022). *Differences between primary, secondary, tertiary, and quaternary care levels of care.* https://www.verywellhealth.com/primary-secondary-tertiary-and-quaternary-care-2615354

U.S. Department of Veterans Affairs. (2022). *VA aid and attendance benefits and housebound allowance.* https://www.va.gov/pension/aid-attendance-housebound/

Viswanathan, H. N., & Salmon, J. W. (2000). Accrediting organizations and quality improvement. *The American Journal of Managed Care, 6*(10), 1117–1130.

The Wellspring. (2018). *Key concept #1: The illness-wellness continuum.* http://www.thewellspring.com/wellspring/introduction-to-wellness/357/key-concept-1-the-illnesswellness-continuum.cfm.html

World Health Organization (WHO). (2023). *Rehabilitation.* https://www.who.int/news-room/fact-sheets/detail/rehabilitation

Young, K. M., & Kroth, P. J. (2018). *Sultz & Young's health care USA: Understanding its organization and delivery* (9th ed.). Jones & Bartlett Learning.

Credits

Fig. 5.1: Source: https://www.aacnnursing.org/Portals/0/PDFs/Publications/Essentials-2021.pdf.

Fig. 5.2a: Copyright © by Microsoft.

Fig. 5.4: Source: https://endoflifeoptionsnm.org/hospice-a-critical-end-of-life-service-part-1/.

CHAPTER 6

Quality, Quality Measures, and Value in Care Coordination

LEARNING OBJECTIVES

1. Explain how care coordination practice is affected by quality measures.
2. Differentiate needed aspects of documentation in relation to quality measures.
3. Examine continuous quality improvement (CQI) strategies and apply them to care coordination practice.
4. Recognize the benefits of meeting care coordination quality measures.

KEY TERMS

- care coordination measurement framework
- continuous quality improvement (CQI)
- data-driven decision-making
- FACT (Factual, Accurate, Complete, Timely)
- Kaizen
- Lean
- meaningful measures
- measurement gaps
- quality measure
- quality measure sets
- report card
- workaround

Introduction

Care coordination practice is based on the desire and need to provide and receive quality healthcare across the continuum of care. Various governmental agencies, healthcare payers, national nursing certification organizations, and the American Nurses Association (ANA) have all identified that quality care coordination is central to nursing practice. The Institute of Medicine (IOM) has recognized care coordination as one of the top priorities in healthcare transformation (IOM, 2011). The ANA goes on to identify person-centered care coordination as a professional standard for all nurses and state that nurses should be involved in informing and designing care coordination quality measures (ANA, 2021).

Specific components of the care coordination process are essential to quality healthcare, such as cross-setting communication, risk screening, comprehensive assessment, and person- and relationship-centered care delivery. Additionally, the care coordinating nurse must utilize data to inform practice and assess risks and potential for adverse outcomes or inappropriate resource use (Singer & Porta, 2022). We know that quality care coordination supports patient outcomes and mitigates risks. However, sometimes this is lacking, with approximately 30% of patients needing clarification about follow-up directions and required care after an acute care discharge (Singer & Porta, 2022, para. 1), which contributes to medical errors, readmissions, and adverse health outcomes. The reverse has also been found to be true, with patients receiving quality care coordination reporting that they have enough information to manage their health, improved access to care, and better outcomes (Elliott et al., 2021; Wells et al., 2020, p. 62).

The care coordinating nurse must understand quality measures, the data the measures provide, and their application to quality healthcare to inform practice and identify opportunities for quality improvement. A **quality measure** is a standard designed to measure a specific performance area or indicator to monitor, evaluate, and improve healthcare quality. Implementing quality care coordination in nursing practice is integral to achieving quality care and meeting identified outcomes and quality benchmarks for reimbursement, certification, and organizational ratings. Quality care coordination provides for better care, and the nurse needs to understand that quality measures may affect how their nursing care is delivered and evaluated and how nursing interventions support patient and organizational outcomes.

Quality Healthcare and Care Coordination

Quality healthcare can be viewed from an organizational viewpoint in the perspective of **continuous quality improvement (CQI)** methods, like **Lean** or other quality frameworks, from the actual outcomes of the care delivered or a combination of these perspectives. When considering the quality of care from a care coordination practice perspective, it encompasses preventing disease or complications, increasing patient safety, minimizing risks and poor outcomes, and increasing quality of life, all of which contribute to cost and resource management and patient satisfaction (Shi & Singh, 2019). Whichever perspective or approach is used to define quality care, data is collected to inform quality improvement initiatives, identify gaps in quality care delivery, or benchmark quality achievement.

Quality is a critical outcome sought and measured in the transition to value-based healthcare. Care coordination is vital to producing quality outcomes on an organizational and individual patient level. Integrating care coordination into healthcare delivery across the continuum provides for seamless care transitions and assists with the identification of social and support needs that the care plan can address, such as financial concerns or caregiving issues (Harkness, 2020). Deficient care coordination leads to poor patient outcomes, health deterioration, and ineffective resource management (Möckli et al., 2021).

Elliot et al. (2021) found that integration of care coordination was positively correlated to clinical performance and meeting 9 of 13 Healthcare Effectiveness and Data Information Set (HEDIS) quality indicators of healthcare and service. Knowing that care coordination is central

Quality and Resource Use Outcomes of Nurse Case Management

- Quality Outcomes
  - Patient adherence to the plan of care and treatment plan
  - Continuity of care
  - Improved follow-up and outpatient appointment attendance
  - Patient self-management of health
  - Prevention of delays in care
- Resource Use Outcomes
  - Patient cost savings
  - Decreased emergency room visits
  - Prevention of admission or readmission to acute care setting (Garnett et al., 2020, p. 68)

to quality healthcare requires the nurse to understand the components that create quality care coordination and contribute to resource and cost management. Quality care coordination requires focused attention concerning barriers to accessible and equitable care, proactive education, and management of potential health symptoms and conditions.

Knowledge, skills, and attitudes are required to coordinate high-quality healthcare. These are represented in current care coordination quality measures and in the **care coordination measurement framework** developed by The Agency for Healthcare Research and Quality (AHRQ). This framework uses an indexing system of available measures and measurement gaps to identify crucial domains for measuring care coordination efforts and their measurable effects.

The care coordination measurement framework consists of the following nine domains:

1. Establish accountability or negotiate accountability.
2. Communicate.
3. Facilitate transitions.
4. Assess needs and goals.
5. Create a proactive plan of care.
6. Monitor, follow up, and respond to change.
7. Support self-management goals.
8. Link to community resources.
9. Align resources to patient and population needs (McDonald et al., 2014).

These care coordination domains are supported by nursing knowledge and skills encompassing all aspects of nursing practice, such as holistically addressing patient needs through the inclusion of interprofessional teamwork, understanding the value of the PCP as the focal point for coordination of care, embracing the importance of disease and self-management of health, promoting the need for medication reconciliation in transitions of care, and comprehending that use of health information technologies (HIT), such as the electronic health record (EHR), supports quality information transfer and data maintenance (McDonald et al., 2014). When reviewing these domains, a picture of what constitutes quality care coordination emerges. See Table 6.1—Care Coordination Measure Mapping Table

TABLE 6.1 Care Coordination Measure Mapping Table

	Measurement Perspective		
	Patient/Family	**Health Care Professional(s)**	**System Representative(s)**
Care Coordination Activities			
Establish accountability or negotiate responsibility			
Communicate			
Interpersonal communication			
Information transfer			
Facilitate transitions			
Across settings			
As coordination needs change			
Assess needs and goals			
Create a proactive plan of care			
Monitor, follow up, and respond to change			
Support self-management goals			
Link to community resources			
Align resources with patient and population needs			

(Continued)

TABLE 6.1 *(Continued)*

Broad Approaches Potentially Related to Care Coordination
Teamwork focused on coordination
Healthcare home
Care management
Medication management
Health IT-enabled coordination

Source: K.M. McDonald, et al, "Chapter 3. Care Coordination Measurement Framework," *Care Coordination Measures Atlas Update*, p. 318. 2014.

Quality Measures Sets and Care Coordination

Quality measure sets are groups of meaningful core measures that measure the quality of care provided and can be used to improve healthcare quality. These measure sets are developed with stakeholders such as patients, providers, and payers and vary depending on the type of healthcare being delivered and the patient population. Quality measures in care coordination promote the development and sustainability of valuable care coordination systems to support quality healthcare (Girmash & Honsberger, 2022). The purpose of quality measure sets is to promote quality in care coordination delivery, reduce waste in the healthcare system, and improve the ability of patients to make informed healthcare decisions (CMS, 2021a).

Several data sources can be used to determine whether quality care coordination has been delivered. Each specific quality measure developed in a measure set consists of several parts to ensure it encompasses the various aspects of quality in that measure and translates into a measurable aspect of health. For example, a quality measure will have a description such as "connection and follow-up with community resources to help the patient take care of themselves or someone in their family." Then, the measure will have a numerator and a denominator. This would be the number of patients during the measurement period that reported "yes" they did receive "connection and follow-up with community resources to help them take care of themselves or a family member" (the numerator) divided by the total number of patients surveyed in the measurement period (the denominator).

The quality measure may also have exclusion criteria such as age group or what other types of healthcare services they are receiving. So in the example of "connection and follow-up with community resources to help them take care of themselves or a family member," potential exclusion criteria may be patients who report they are receiving hospice services, as the hospice service provider would likely be the agency accountable for resource connections. Lastly, the quality measure will have a brief rationale identifying why it is a measure and how it links to outcomes or management of resources (CMS, 2021a).

Quality measure set data analysis, evaluation, and application are used to design interventions that promote positive health outcomes, coordinate care, and connect specific measures and regulations to quality healthcare delivery. A common source of quality measure data is the use of a quality measure set such as a patient survey examining their care coordination experience, for instance the Care Coordination Quality Measure for Primary Care or the Consumer Assessment of Healthcare Providers and Systems (CAHPS® or HCAHPS® for hospital-based care). These surveys solicit important data concerning whether patients received timely care, how communication was provided, and if their care was coordinated. Specific questions related to care coordination include whether follow-up was provided, medication education was given, and if their providers knew important aspects of their health and medical history (AHRQ, 2023a).

The hospital version of the CAHPS® or HCAHPS® asks additional questions concerning transitions of care, such as "did doctors, nurses, or other hospital staff talk with you about whether you would have the help you needed when you left the hospital?" (CMS, 2021b, Appendix A, p. 3). These types of surveys are also available for special populations, such as children with medical complexity. The Family Experiences with Care Coordination (FECC) survey includes a 20-quality measure set related to care coordination for children with complex medical conditions and their families (Gidengil et al., 2017). See Table 6.2 for the FECC quality measure set.

TABLE 6.2 Family Experiences with Care Coordination Quality Measure Set

Care Coordination Services
Has care coordinator
Access to care coordinator
Care coordinator helped to obtain community services
Care coordinator contact in last 3 months
Care coordinator asked about concerns and health changes
Care coordinator assisted with specialist service referrals
Care coordinator was knowledgeable, supportive, and advocated for child's needs
Caregiver has access to a medical interpreter when needed
Messaging
Appropriate written visit summary content
Written visit summary was useful and easy to understand
Invited to join hospital rounds
Appropriate written hospitalization summary content
Written hospital summary was easy to understand
Caregiver has access to electronic health record
Electronic health record has immunization and medication information
Healthcare provider communicated with school staff about child's condition

(Continued)

TABLE 6.2 ***(Continued)***

Protocols/Plans
Child has a shared care plan
Child has a written transition plan
Child has emergency care plan

Source: Agency for Healthcare Research and Quality, "Measures: Family Experiences with Care Coordination Measure Set (FECC)," Measure Fact Sheet – The AHRQ-CMS Pediatric Quality Measures Program (PQMP), p. 4, Agency for Healthcare Research and Quality, 2015.

Another predominant way to gain data concerning care coordination quality is to examine organizational measures such as the ones included in HEDIS. Example measures that are part of HEDIS and directly relate to care coordination include the following:

1. use of opioids from multiple providers—multiple prescribers and multiple pharmacies
2. plan all-cause readmissions—observed-to-expected ratio—18–64 years
3. follow-up after emergency department visit for mental illness, 7-day total
4. transitions of care
   a. notification of inpatient admission—65+ years
   b. receipt of discharge information—65+ years
   c. patient engagement after inpatient discharge—65+ years
   d. medication reconciliation post-discharge—65+ years
5. hospitalization following discharge from a skilled nursing facility 30-day total (NCQA, 2021, pp. 6–10).

This type of quality measure data is often collected through EHRs, which points to the importance of documentation in healthcare. Suppose a follow-up call is made or a visit is arranged for a patient after an emergency room visit for a mental health issue, and it is not documented. In that case, it will not be counted toward meeting the quality measure of emergency department mental illness-related visit follow-up. The Centers for Medicare and Medicaid Services (CMS) provide an annual report of quality measures across settings that serve Medicare beneficiaries as well as identified **measurement gaps**, which are gaps in a type of measure or concept that is missing or reflects something that is not measured or not adequately measured and affects the ability to measure that quality area or indicator (Waddill, 2022). These gaps are essential to understand because if there are gaps in measurement, the care coordination offered may not be meeting patient and organizational needs and not be contributing to quality healthcare delivery. See Table 6.3 for a sample listing of measurement gaps found in 2021.

TABLE 6.3 Sample Communication and Care Coordination Measurement Gaps by Clinical Setting

	Setting			
Measurement	**Acute**	**Post-Acute**	**Clinician/ Accountable Care Organization**	**Managed Care**
Care transitions and transfers: Quality and Safety across facilities and Settings	X	X		
Care coordination and hand-offs using electronic clinical quality measures (eCQMs)			X	
Communication and care coordination including rural populations	X		X	X
Dialysis: Coordination for transient patients		X		
Medication review and reconciliation: discharge and transfers	X	X	X	X
Readmission: condition-specific, 7-day time frame, interaction with mortality	X			
Timely exchange of clinical information		X	X	
Transitions of care for cancer patients across facilities and outpatient settings	X	X	X	X

"X" indicates a gap in one or more programs within a setting from key sources published from January 1, 2018, to March 31, 2020 (CMS Center for Clinical Standards & Quality, 2021, p. 16)

As quality measures are reviewed, there are consistencies in what quality looks like concerning care coordination delivery. Quality care coordination includes accountability, communication, interprofessional practice, facilitation of transitions, proactive coordination and care management, monitoring, follow-up, community resource linkages, referral facilitation, assessing needs and goals of care, supporting patient self-management of health, leveraging HIT for care coordination, resource management, health education, and advocacy. Care coordination is a comprehensive and encompassing nursing role based on delivering interventions that can positively impact long-term health behaviors, patient self-management of health, continuity of care, and resource use (Garnett et al., 2020). Quality measures of care coordination contribute to recognizing the critical role nurses have in the successful coordination of care and informing the role of, and incentives to, the integration of care coordination services for quality healthcare delivery (ANA, 2021).

Quality Care Coordination Documentation

Quality care coordination is offered in multiple ways across settings and addresses global patient needs. These care coordination interventions must be measured and documented clearly in the organization's documentation system. This may be an EHR, utilization management software, free text notes, or other third-party documentation systems. Quality measure data is usually retrieved from electronic documentation systems, and the care coordinating nurse must diligently document care coordination interventions for quality measure data retrieval. High-quality documentation is accessible, accurate, complete, timely, and reflective of the nursing process (ANA, 2010). The care coordinating nurse can follow the **FACT** (factual, accurate, complete, timely) acronym to guide quality documentation that assists in identifying and retrieving quality measure data. See Figure 6.1—Quality Care Coordination Documentation: FACT.

It is essential for successful coordination and care transitions that communications across settings and the results of those interactions are promptly documented. Suppose an issue becomes evident with coordinating care, such as the inability to schedule follow-up care appointments or meetings. In that case, this does need to be documented, as well as why the issue

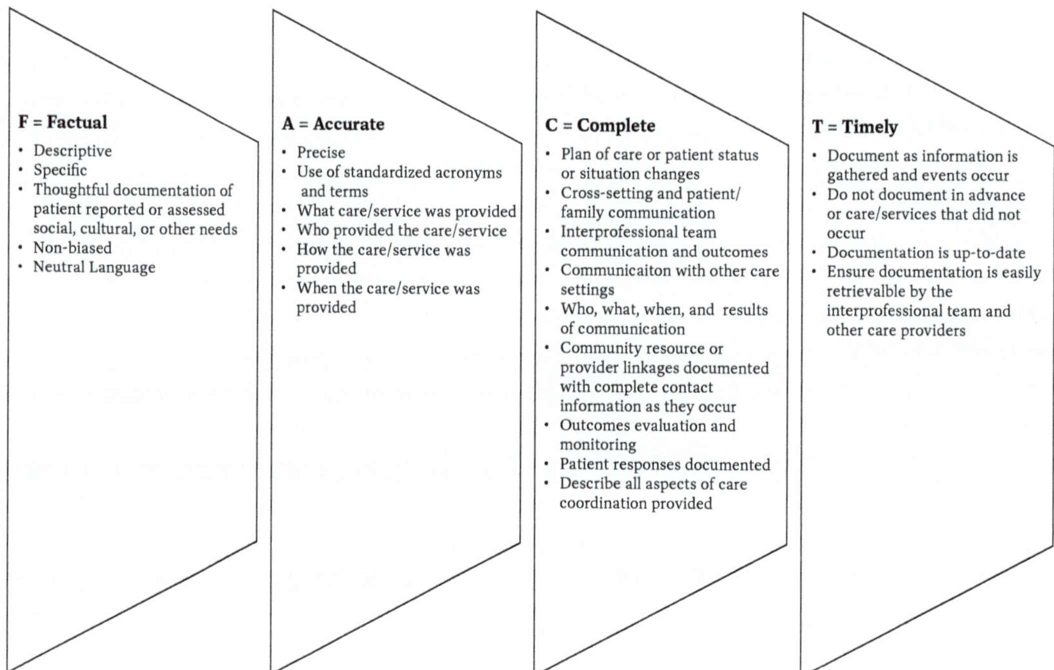

FIGURE 6.1 Quality Care Coordination Documentation: FACT

occurred, what was done to mitigate the issue, and what education or support was given to the patient or family/caregiver concerning the issue. In this way, another nurse care coordinator will know what was done, what was effective, and what care coordination barriers still exist. This information can be used to compare with previous patient status and contexts, providing a solid baseline of patient data to inform care coordination practices. Properly documented information can also inform quality improvement initiatives concerning care coordination practices on an individual, departmental, or organizational level, enhancing the ability to meet system-level care coordination-related quality measures.

Value-Based Healthcare Quality Measures

Value-based healthcare promotes quality outcomes by identifying meaningful quality measures that indicate that quality care has been provided. Sometimes, the care coordinating nurse may need help understanding why the measures are in place or how they connect to nursing practice. A shift in perspective or understanding of quality measures' vital role in ethical nursing practice may be needed. Quality measures are fundamental to integrating patient advocacy and nursing ethical practice skills like collaboration and promoting a culture of safety and accountability into healthcare transformation and value-based quality care delivery (ANA, 2015). The professional nurse's role in promoting a culture of quality and safety mirrors care coordination practice through the need to reduce errors and waste and advocate for system-level changes, if needed, to promote quality care delivery to support positive patient outcomes.

Quality measures are integrally connected to financial performance, reimbursement, and organizational ratings, which affect healthcare financing and health outcomes. Care coordination is critical to the organization's work to link healthcare to quality delivery, measures, and resource management, creating a value-based system. These goals are the foundation of care coordination, working to achieve value and quality in the care provided, managing costs, and ensuring that patients can engage in the best quality of health and life possible through addressing issues such as social determinants of health, accessibility, and equity in healthcare. This brings the definition of value to the forefront. Value is often considered the quality of care divided by the cost. But how do we know we have provided quality care?

The Institute of Medicine (IOM, 2001) defines quality as "the degree to which health services for individuals and populations increase the likelihood of desired health outcomes and are consistent with current professional knowledge" (p. 232). This perspective of quality in healthcare adds a pivotal aspect to the definition of value in healthcare and includes services, which are defined as satisfaction and effective relationships. In this view, value equals "resources (funds and labor and supplies) + quality (appropriateness of interventions) + service (satisfaction and effective relationships)" (Porter-O'Grady & Malloch, 2018, p. 375). Measures of patient knowledge of their health, satisfaction, and engagement may not appear to point to quality care delivery. Still, measures of this type indicate the system's ability to deliver a framework of relevant and preventative care, which ultimately decreases cost and enhances patient quality of life and wellness and job satisfaction for nurses.

Ultimately, ensuring coordination and continuity of care occurs in every patient interaction and that the service provided supports patient and relationship-centered care, good patient outcomes, and positive health results will lead to the appropriate use of resources, cost management, proper nursing interventions, effective interprofessional collaboration, and patient satisfaction. The opposite is just as true. Fragmented or nonexistent coordination and continuity of care produce adverse patient outcomes and health results, ineffective interprofessional collaboration and relationships, and dissatisfaction among patients and nurses. See Figure 6.2 for a diagram of how care coordination contributes to value in healthcare.

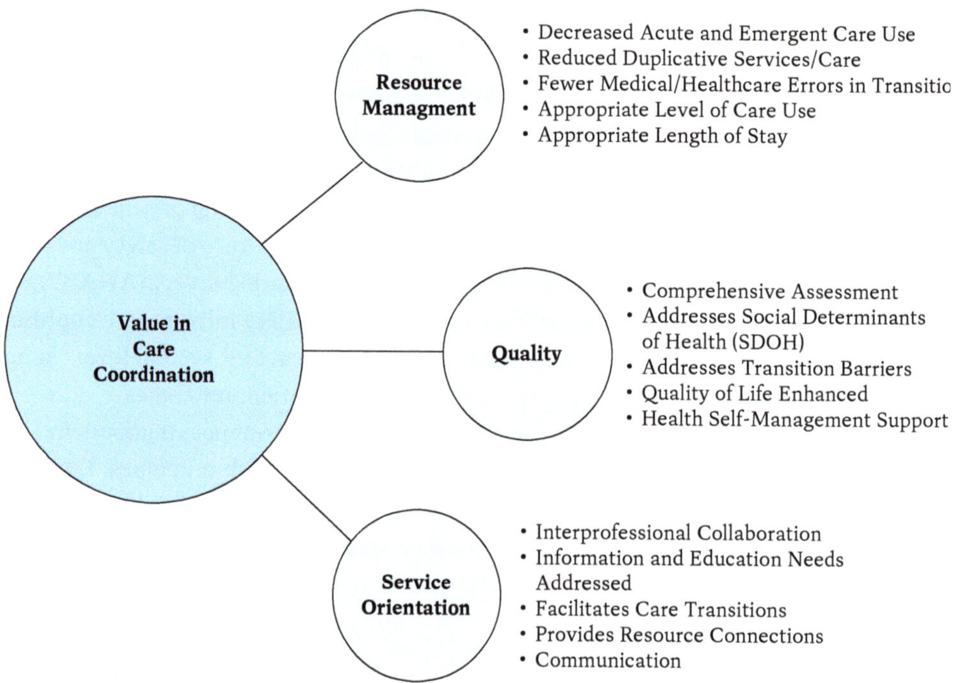

FIGURE 6.2 Value in Care Coordination

"Finding the value of a healthcare service requires healthcare leaders and care providers to ask the following questions:

What is the actual service provided?

How do organizational processes support this service?

What are the interactions between these processes?

What impact does the service have on patients and the community?" (Porter-O'Grady & Malloch, 2018, p. 375)

Meaningful Quality Measures

Various quality measure sets are available, depending on the healthcare organization's focus and population served. The healthcare organization may use the data generated by the quality measure set to direct quality improvement efforts, adding to the value of the care delivered. Home health organizations may use the OASIS (Outcome and Assessment Information Set), a hospital or clinic may use HEDIS, and a skilled nursing facility may use MDS (Minimum Data Set). Each of these different quality measure sets is designed to collect data about the value and quality of care the organization provides to improve the quality of the care delivered. Each measure set focuses on a different aspect of healthcare delivery. Still, the measures provided relate to the Institute of Medicine's six domains of quality healthcare—safe, efficient, effective, patient-centered, equitable, and timely care (AHRQ, 2022).

CMS is working to streamline these various quality measure sets through its Universal Foundation initiative. CMS has developed the **Meaningful Measures 2.0** initiative as part of its National Quality Strategy and Universal Foundation initiative. This initiative promotes value in healthcare by focusing on high-impact quality areas that are meaningful to patients and are person-centered. Meaningful Measures 2.0 is based upon nine domains to build value-based care and promote health equity. The domains of quality healthcare have been expanded to specify areas of prevention, chronic conditions, and behavioral health, including patient and caregiver voices as key stakeholders, and solidify the need for care coordination in quality healthcare. The nine domains include (a) person-centered care, (b) safety, (c) chronic conditions, (d) seamless care coordination, (e) equity, (f) affordability and efficiency, (g) wellness and prevention, (i) behavioral health, and (j) individual and caregiver voice (CMS, 2023). With the development of Meaningful Measures 2.0, CMS will be moving toward determining measures to assess healthcare quality across the lifespan and continuum of care (Jacobs et al., 2023). See Figure 6.3 for a visual—CMS Building Value-Based Care and Promoting Health Equity Domains.

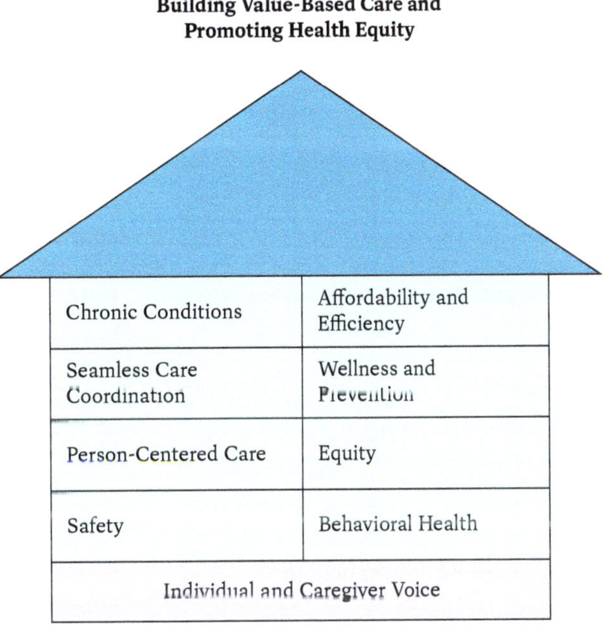

FIGURE 6.3 CMS Building Value-Based Care and Promoting Health Equity Domains

Quality measures are connected to reimbursement in several value-based payment and purchasing models and are also used to collect population-level data concerning health outcomes and equity. These quality measure sets are used to incentivize and promote the transition to value-based healthcare delivery and system, leading to quality healthcare and sustainability of the healthcare system (CMS, 2021a). The nine value-based care and health equity domains identified by CMS will be used to determine quality in healthcare. These domains likely will use a variety of measures focusing on different aspects of quality health, such as composite score measures, which combine two or more measures to create a single measure and score; a cost/resource use measure; an efficiency measure; an outcome measure, patient-reported outcome-based measures, process measures, and structure measures. See Table 6.4 for an example of how care coordination contributes to meeting types of quality measures.

TABLE 6.4 Relationship of Care Coordination to Quality Measures Attainment

Quality Measure Type	Measure Description	Care Coordination Example	CMS Healthcare Domain
Composite	A measure that uses two or more measures to create a single measure and score.	The *CMS PSI 90 measure* is used in the *BPCI Advanced* value-based payment program, which relies heavily upon care coordination. The CMS PSI 90 measures 10 indicators, including pressure ulcers, falls, and post-operative conditions such as post-operative sepsis. CMS calculates the measure on a hospital level and calculates a weighted average based on the indicators. This score is then included in a composite quality score that is used to adjust reimbursement positively or negatively (CMS, 2019).	Safety
Cost/Resource Use	A measure that examines health services in dollars spent or units/frequency of a resource. This type of measure may be applied to a specific diagnosis or to a population.	The Hospital Readmissions Reduction Program relies on effective care coordination and transition management. The *Excess Days in Acute Care (EDAC) after Hospitalization for Acute Myocardial Infarction (AMI)* measure indicates if care coordination and transition management were effective in managing costs and resources.	Seamless Care Coordination

Efficiency	A measure of the cost of care associated with a specific health outcome.	The measure of *Screening for Social Determinants of Health (SDOH)* is a kind of preliminary risk assessment used in the care coordinators comprehensive assessment process. Identification of SDOH that may cause barriers or challenges to transitions and health outcomes are crucial for successful care coordination and if neglected, may lead to increased costs of care and lack of health equity related to SDOH.	Equity
Outcome	A measure of the health status of a patient after receiving healthcare—could be a positive or negative change in health status.	The *Resolution of At Least 1 Health-Related Social Need* measure identifies the need for care coordination, comprehensive assessment, and person-centered care practices to affect health outcomes positively. When resolution of health-related social needs does not occur, this can result in negative health status changes.	Equity
Process	A measure that identifies steps to follow for quality care provision.	The *Connection to Community Service Provider* measure is essential for quality healthcare, follow-up, prevention of negative health outcomes, and inappropriate resource use. Care coordination is a critical piece of meeting this measure and ensuring positive health outcomes.	Equity

(CMS, 2021a, p. 9; Measures Management System, 2023)

Currently, CMS quality measures are monitored and reviewed at least annually. This may include a basic review or a comprehensive reevaluation to ensure the measures contribute to the value and quality of healthcare. The monitoring and review process includes periodic literature surveillance for new research, data analysis of the measure for attainment and unintended consequences that the measure may have on practice or outcomes, and response to and solicitation of questions and input from stakeholders about the measure (CMS, 2021a).

Role of the Care Coordinating Nurse in Quality Improvement

Care coordination is delivered across a system and continuum of healthcare involving various stakeholders, with often differing perspectives and priorities for quality improvement strategies. For quality outcomes to be met on the patient level, some systems-level initiatives will likely need to be developed and implemented. Nurses are integral to the coordination and continuity of care, bringing systems-level knowledge concerning patient goals and priorities of care to system-wide quality improvement initiatives. The nurse is in a key position to advocate for the patient's perspective and that of the nursing discipline, identifying barriers or issues to effective care coordination implementation and care transitions. To do this, the nurse must understand the healthcare system, the community, the resources available, common health issues, the patient population served, and comprehensive knowledge of the continuum of care (Lamb, 2013).

The nurse must also understand that the interpersonal aspects of the patient–nurse partnership are the basis of quality care delivery and identifying quality improvement issues (Lamb, 2013). The foundation of relationship and person-centered care delivery opens an opportunity for dialogue about patient priorities of care, barriers to care, health literacy needs, social determinants of health issues that may offer challenges to the patient in being engaged in their healthcare, and an opportunity to provide essential health education and promotion. This dialogue and collaboration are crucial in achieving quality care as they contribute to identifying relevant system issues, nurse advocacy needs, and system-level needs related to quality improvement in the organization and nursing practice (Haas et al., 2014).

Through engaging with patients and their families/caregivers, nurses can advocate for patients and their families/caregivers to become actively involved in quality improvement initiatives, supporting the development of culturally and patient-relevant strategies. Patients and their families/caregivers are critical stakeholders in quality healthcare delivery. It is essential that patients, nurses, providers, organizations, and systems work collaboratively to identify quality improvement needs and develop implementation strategies for quality and value-based healthcare delivery.

Any quality improvement strategy must ultimately adapt to patient, community, and organizational needs. The nurse care coordinator has a central role in constructing and implementing quality care coordination practices by offering insight into the characteristics of the patient population through a comprehensive assessment of challenges and barriers to care and integrating the context of the local community and resources into identifying priority issues and improvement designs (Garber, 2023). Care coordinating nurses also have core knowledge concerning the stakeholders involved in the patient's healthcare and the number and variety of interprofessional team members who may contribute to the quality improvement initiative. The care coordinator's knowledge of evidence-based practice guidelines, national standards of care coordination practice, and an understanding of current care coordination processes and outcomes are critical for identifying, developing, and implementing quality improvement strategies that support and surround patients with coordinated care delivery and quality outcomes.

Continuous Quality Improvement (CQI)

Continuous quality improvement (CQI) is a systematic, ongoing improvement approach to develop processes, safety, or care delivery, leading to enhanced quality measure attainment by optimizing processes and procedures in definable and repeatable pathways. Often, organizational improvement processes can begin with a **workaround** or an initial one-off approach that is difficult to define, repeat, and optimize. Workarounds are temporary fixes or responses to a process, policy, or healthcare problem that does not eliminate the original problem. Organizations engage in CQI to improve their processes and procedures into an optimized format for the best return on investment of resources and to engage in best practices. So relying on a workaround or one-off solution does not lead to quality healthcare delivery and can often lead to further difficulties in the long term.

Quality measurement has been integrated into healthcare processes, collecting data and tracking outcomes with the goal of quality care delivery. Many organizations run quality measure data regularly, such as length of stay or immunization rates, to inform the application of the measure and use this information to address opportunities for improvement in processes and outcomes. This may be in the form of a "**report card**," where a report is constructed from several data sources that contain quality scores related to care coordination interventions or other quality measures that can be made public and are used to promote accountability, transparency, and healthcare quality. Then, this data is compared across the health care system or other organizations to develop best care coordination practices (Evidence-Based Practice Centers®, 2023). The organization may also use this data to mitigate risk or address system-level goals of equitable and accessible care (Finkelman, 2016).

CQI is integral to care coordination and nursing practice and is based on the identification and prioritization of improvement opportunities on a continual basis (CSSC, 2018). CQI involves identifying and defining a process or patient care problem, using data to benchmark or compare current quality measure scores to scores representing best practices, designing improvement goals, and engaging in an iterative improvement process. The iterative approach ensures that identified problems are not changed into different issues and do not create new problems (O'Donnell & Gupta, 2023).

The care coordinator uses data daily, applying it to the nursing process to direct care and intervention planning. Through processes of pacing the case, collaboration with the interprofessional team, and individualized person-centered care planning, the care coordinator continuously monitors data and outcomes and makes changes as needed to promote quality and safety in the healthcare system and patient outcomes. This means the care coordinating nurse must understand organizational benchmarks and quality measures and align their practice to ensure these outcomes are met (Haas et al., 2014).

The nurse care coordinator must have knowledge related to common potential threats to the successful coordination of care, such as communication barriers, patient education needs, and authorization processes, as well as knowledge concerning processes and procedures that must be followed to ensure these threats are mitigated. The nurse must also understand the impact of these types of risks to successful care coordination, organizational initiatives, quality measures being applied, financial outcomes, and patient outcomes.

To apply CQI to their practice, the care coordinating nurse must also possess the skills of communication, critical analysis, and synthesis of available data and resources. Communication is a paramount skill as the nurse must proactively communicate potential or actual barriers to meeting quality measures and work to develop an individualized plan to address the barrier and potentially longer-term processes to guide other care-coordinating nurses in the future. Additionally, the nurse must communicate effectively when providing patient education and health promotion to mitigate any potential quality or safety issues throughout the continuum of care.

The nurse must also be able to engage in self-reflective analysis of their practice when issues arise to analyze whether there are needed improvements in their knowledge base or approach to implementing coordination of care. In this way, the nurse can access available resources in their organization, the community, or through national organizations to address gaps in knowledge or skills, engage in CQI for their professional development, and address organizational processes or resources that may need refinement or initiation. Engagement in the CQI process on an organizational or professional development level requires the nurse to value the role of improving the care coordination process through meeting quality measures and identified organizational and patient outcomes (Haas et al., 2014).

Continuous Quality Improvement (CQI) Model: Lean

When considering continuous quality improvement (CQI) in care coordination practice, the nurse needs to understand the CQI model used in their organization. This will assist in identifying appropriate CQI opportunities to enhance quality in care and attainment of measures. A variety of CQI models are frequently used in the healthcare setting, such as Lean. Healthcare transformation to value-based healthcare lends itself to the use of Lean, as the Lean philosophy adapts well to the need for rapid changes and addressing complex and multidimensional social issues and patient needs (Morell-Santandreu et al., 2021). Lean is a CQI methodology leading to value and quality in healthcare through ongoing process improvement that focuses on efficiency and effectiveness by eliminating waste and non-value-added activities.

> Lean aims to create a culture of continuous improvement while standardizing best practices to address healthcare-specific challenges, including rising costs, concerns about patient safety and care quality, and wasted time or resources. (Hung et al., 2022, p. 503)

The Lean CQI philosophy mirrors the goals and principles of care coordination in healthcare.

Lean focuses on waste or muda in the healthcare system, which could be waiting times, errors in care, duplicative care, or the inappropriate use of resources. The goal is to identify and reduce non-value-added work and activities, thereby opening the amount of time and effort available for value-added or quality-added work and activities (O'Donnell & Gupta, 2023). The application of Lean is evident when considering the goal of care coordination, which is to manage resources and costs and provide seamless care transitions. Care coordination relies on work processes and policies that provide effective continuity of care and care transitions. Removing wasted actions and resources reduces the opportunity for errors, gaps in care, and unneeded costs.

Lean has a foundation of focusing on the customer/patient to create value, engaging in continuous quality improvement (Kaizen), data-driven decision-making, structured problem-solving, and standardization (Porumboiu, 2023). This philosophical framework supports value-based healthcare and the use of quality measures that examine the patient experience. It also supports the need for data collection of measures to identify quality gaps or improvement opportunities in processes and procedures. **Data-driven decision-making** is a central component of Lean. It supports using data, information, or other metrics, such as report cards, to inform decision-making that aligns with quality measures and healthcare.

Kaizen is a CQI strategy foundational to Lean that uses proactive, small, targeted strategies at all system levels, focusing on where the work occurs and the processes used. The Kaizen concept embraces incremental changes to enhance processes and services, such as the "just-in-time" (JIT) approach. JIT typically applies to inventory processes, but in care coordination, this method can also apply when looking at the efficiency of processes and managing resources because inefficient care coordination ultimately generates increased costs to the patient or the healthcare system.

When a quick response, change in process, or focused education is needed, the nurse may consider a JIT intervention. Once implemented, the JIT intervention needs monitoring and evaluating to determine whether it met goals and outcomes such as patient satisfaction, and whether the organization has the capacity and readiness to implement the JIT intervention on a longer-term basis (Balkhi et al., 2022). By using JIT, the care coordinator can address needed support or changes in processes to provide quality care coordination (Nahum-Shani et al., 2018; CSSC, 2018).

Eight waste or muda types have been identified when applying Lean to healthcare. These include (a) waiting times, (b) excessive inventory or supplies, (c) defects in the quality of care and reimbursement, (d) unnecessary transportation of supplies and patients between floors and settings, (e) movement that does not add value to patient care, (f) overproduction (e.g., duplicate testing, redundancy in care), (g) overprocessing (i.e., when time, effort, and resources do not improve quality of care), and (h) wasted human potential (i.e., when nurses are wasting energy and effort on non-value-added actions they have limited time for person and relationship-based care or professional development (NEJM Catalyst, 2018, para. 5).

Just-in-Time Advantages

"When you have every staff member making 'seemingly small' improvements every day, what you end up with is a fully engaged workforce committed to improvement and together over time that can add up to significant organizational improvements in patient care and outcomes" (Kelly et al., 2018, p. 394).

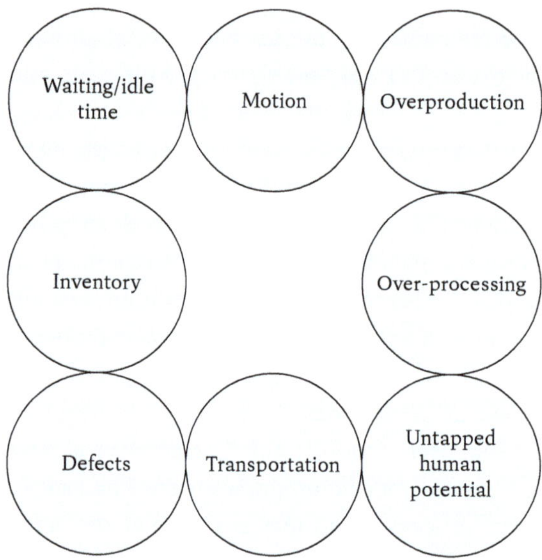

FIGURE 6.4 Lean Waste in Healthcare

These eight types of waste can be mitigated with the integration of quality care coordination into the healthcare system. For example, when continuity and coordination of care are the center of healthcare delivery, waiting times can be decreased through effective follow-up management. Defects in the quality of care and reimbursement, overprocessing, and overproduction can be reduced through implementating appropriate healthcare services and understanding value-based care reimbursement strategies. See Figure 6.4 for a visual of Lean waste in healthcare.

Lean Implications for Care Coordination

As the healthcare system has been and will become more accountable for quality care delivery and seamless transitions of care across the continuum, there is great application for Lean methodologies to ensure quality healthcare and care coordination practices. For example, specific quality care coordination measures include effective patient education, improved communication with the patient and across settings, and efficient and timely follow-up. Suppose Lean methodology was applied to quality care coordination for acute care readmissions, which cost approximately 12.4% more than the original admission (AHRQ, 2023b). In that case, it might

Application of Lean: Readmissions

A Lean project was developed to redesign the discharge process at an acute care system with the goal of reducing readmission rates for three diagnoses: heart failure, acute myocardial infarction, and pneumonia. Readmissions were seen as costly and largely avoidable; therefore, there was a need for a Lean quality intervention. Financial data, the number of readmissions, and financial penalties for readmission data were examined, showing an excess cost of approximately $360,000 for readmissions (Breslin et al., 2014, p. 79). A flow diagram was used to delineate the steps in the discharge process from admission to discharge, with cause and effect and relationships between processes, policies, and people identified, locating potential areas for improvement. The redesigned discharge plan focused on post-discharge service arrangement, testing and results, equipment, medication reconciliation, teach-back education, and cross-setting communication. Key focus areas included identifying/arranging for a PCP and arranging a PCP follow-up appointment pre-discharge. The redesigned discharge process met recognized principles of care coordination, such as person-centered care, an accessible PCP, seamless care transitions across the continuum, and assuring that cost and quality benchmarks are met (Breslin et al., 2014).

mean making process improvements in the implementation of quality assessment of discharge needs at admission, engaging in clear and complete communication concerning the discharge plan with the patient and family/caregivers, and delivering timely post-acute care follow-up to positively impact the number of readmissions (Breslin et al., 2014). Lean quality improvement methods have been shown to reduce errors, improve quality of care, produce financial savings, and improve care coordination practices (Graig & Perosino, 2011).

Several factors can affect quality care coordination practice, each of which can be addressed with Lean. Using Lean, standardized processes can be developed to decrease variation in the quality of care coordination delivered. This also can contribute to accessibility and equity in healthcare services by addressing social determinants and influencers of health. Furthermore, the Lean approach can leverage data-informed decision-making and process improvements to address duplicative or inappropriate care delivery, decreasing resource use and costs and meeting the seven rights of care coordination. Lean quality improvement strategies can also assist in identifying and addressing preventable patient injuries and readmissions, such as improving medication reconciliation processes and teach-back practices and integrating evidence-based practice guidelines into care coordination services offered. Ultimately, Lean strategies address the inherent waste and non-value-added or inefficient services in the healthcare system that contribute to increased costs and resource use and decreased patient outcomes (HealthCatalyst, 2018). See Figure 6.5—The Value of Lean in Care Coordination.

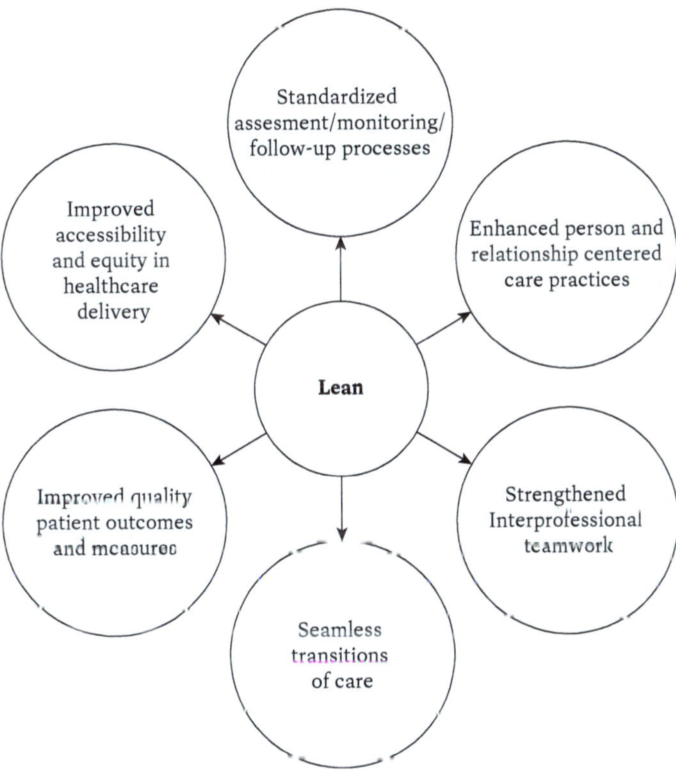

FIGURE 6.5 The Value of Lean in Care Coordination

Integrating the structured quality approach of Lean into care coordination practices has significant benefits, such as improving the patient experience through better communication and person-centered care delivery. Additionally, resources and costs are managed by ensuring that resources are effectively allocated and minimizing inefficient care transitions and costs. Furthermore, successful care coordination minimizes errors in care delivery, medication adherence, and safety, thus effectively managing costs and resources and promoting positive health outcomes (Socconini, 2023). Lastly, the integration of Lean quality improvement strategies and data-informed methods into care coordination practices can assist with developing policies and decision-making processes that are consistent and evidence-based, leading to quality care coordination (Socconini, 2023).

Lean methodology contributes to standardizing processes and procedures, managing resources, and eliminating waste, such as duplicative efforts or engaging in processes that do not produce the desired results. Standardization and streamlining of care coordination activities result in fewer delays in care transitions, decreased length of stays, patient needs being met, and increased nurse and patient satisfaction. Collaborative practices are strengthened and interprofessional teamwork and communication processes across settings are improved. Seamless and coordinated care provides for enhanced accessibility and equity in healthcare through appropriate follow-up care, health promotion and education, and empowering patients in the self-management of their own health (Singer & Porta, 2022). All of these potential improvements in care coordination practices through the use of Lean in the healthcare system can ultimately lead to quality improvement changes that positively impact the quality of care, better use of resources, and excellence in person-centered care delivery.

CHAPTER SUMMARY

Care coordination is critical to the value and quality of healthcare, supporting cost and resource management, continuity and follow-up of care, and timely and equitable access to care (Elliott et al., 2021). Integration of care coordination into healthcare delivery across the continuum provides seamless care transitions, increased positive health outcomes, and effective cost and resource management. It is estimated that fragmented care coordination and transitions resulted in $27 to $78 billion in unnecessary spending in 2019 (Shrank et al., 2019). The healthcare system is compelled to improve the quality of care and care coordination to meet patients' needs and deliver quality, value-based healthcare (NCQA, 2023). Healthcare transition to value-based reimbursement and purchasing translates to the need to collect quality measure data, identify gaps in quality care delivery and measurement, and benchmark quality achievement.

Several quality measure sets and specific quality measures or indicators apply to care coordination practice, all of which promote quality in care coordination delivery, including accountability, interprofessional practice, transition facilitation, and supports for patient self-management of health. To retrieve quality measure data, the care coordinating nurse must leverage HIT and electronic documentation systems to ensure that care coordination interventions are appropriately documented and retrievable for data generation purposes. Quality measure data informs quality improvement initiatives and care coordination practices. This includes utilizing CQI processes like Lean to examine care coordination processes and procedures, lowering risks for patients through comprehensive assessment and analyzing quality measures and health outcomes data to inform quality practices.

Although measuring care coordination can be challenging at times due to documentation issues or lack of processes or procedures, it is essential to understand the role of quality measures in informing quality improvement strategies and enhancing healthcare quality (Mockli et al., 2023). The nurse plays a crucial role in ensuring quality healthcare is provided through advocacy, a broad knowledge of the healthcare system and the patient perspective, and knowledge of current care coordination processes and outcomes. This may take the form of engaging in "just-in-time" improvements, identifying muda in care coordination processes, or using data-informed decision-making in daily care coordination practice.

In whatever setting nurses may work, they must be prepared to provide for coordination and continuity of care. By meeting quality care coordination measures, such as effective cross-setting communication and patient engagement, the nurse contributes to a culture of quality healthcare (Harkness, 2020). This contributes to the value of healthcare through managing resources appropriately, ensuring quality care and care coordination is provided, and maintaining a service orientation toward each encounter with patients, their families/caregivers, and the interprofessional team. In this way, the knowledge, skills, and attitudes the nurse employs will provide for fewer delays in care, efficient resource use, and increased patient and nurse satisfaction.

CHAPTER 6 GLOSSARY

Care Coordination Measurement Framework: A framework developed by the Agency for Healthcare Research and Quality (AHRQ) using an indexing system of available measures and measurement gaps to identify crucial domains for measuring care coordination efforts and their measurable effects.

Continuous Quality Improvement (CQI): A systematic approach of ongoing improvement to improve processes, safety, or care delivery, leading to enhanced quality measure attainment through optimizing processes and procedures in definable and repeatable pathways.

Data-Driven Decision-Making: Using data, information, or other metrics, such as report cards, to inform decision-making that aligns with quality measures and healthcare.

FACT: An acronym to guide quality documentation, assisting in identifying and retrieving quality measure data. FACT stands for Factual, Accurate, Complete, and Timely.

Kaizen: A continuous quality improvement strategy foundational to Lean that uses proactive, small, targeted strategies, focusing on where the work occurs and the processes used.

Lean: A continuous quality improvement methodology leading to value and quality in healthcare through ongoing process improvement that focuses on efficiency and effectiveness through eliminating waste and non-value-added activities.

Meaningful Measures 2.0: A Center for Medicare and Medicaid Services (CMS) initiative that promotes value in healthcare by focusing on high-impact quality areas that are meaningful to patients and are person-centered.

Measurement Gaps: An identified gap in a type of measure or concept; something that is missing or reflects something that is not measured or not adequately measured and affects the ability to measure the focus or quality area.

Quality Measure: A standard designed to measure a specific performance area to monitor, evaluate, and improve healthcare quality.

Quality Measure Sets: Quality measure sets are groups of meaningful core measures that measure the quality of care provided and can be used to improve healthcare quality. Quality measure sets are developed with stakeholders such as patients, providers, and payers and vary depending on the type of healthcare being delivered and the patient population. Example quality measure sets are the AHRQ quality indicators or the Consumer Assessment of Healthcare Providers and Systems (CAHPS®).

Report Card: A report constructed from several data sources that contain quality scores of a healthcare system or provider compared to other healthcare systems or providers. Report cards can be made public and are used to promote accountability, transparency, and healthcare quality.

Workaround: A temporary fix or response to a process, policy, or healthcare problem that does not eliminate the original problem.

DISCUSSION QUESTIONS AND ACTIVITIES

Discussion Questions

1. Create a definition of quality care coordination. Then identify one scope or standard of nursing practice and one nursing code of ethics that form the foundation of your definition and how your definition supports meeting quality care coordination measures.
2. Discuss the connection between quality measures and value-based healthcare. Provide an overview of how quality measures are designed to assist in quality healthcare delivery, and identify one nursing intervention that you have used or seen used in your clinical experiences that supports the use of quality measures in transforming to a quality value-based healthcare system.

3. Choose one of the nine domains of the care coordination measurement framework. Define what the domain is, what it means to care coordination practice, and how the domain affects quality, equity, and accessibility in healthcare.
4. Look up/access a healthcare patient satisfaction survey such as the "Care Coordination Quality Measure for Primary Care," the CAHPS® or HCAPHS®, or the "Family Experience with Care Coordination" survey. Review the questions in the survey and discuss how the data from the survey could be used to design care coordination interventions that promote quality care delivery.
5. Service is considered a part of quality healthcare. Discuss how the concept and provision of service promote meeting quality measures concerning coordinated and continuity of care.

Activities

1. Directions for affinity diagram exercise:

   a. As a group (no more than six people in each group), choose a quality measure set, such as the OASIS (Outcome and Assessment Information Set), HEDIS (Healthcare Effectiveness Data and Information Set), or the MDS (Minimum Data Set).

   b. Review the quality measure set, choose three quality measures from the set, and create an affinity diagram for each one (a total of three).

   c. To create an affinity diagram, you will identify the three quality measures and put them at the top of a whiteboard or flip chart page. Each quality measure will have its own whiteboard space or flip chart page.

   d. Then pass out sticky notes to each group member. Each group member will record on a sticky note how they believe care coordination can meet the quality measure. Ask participants to use a noun, a verb, and no more than seven words.

   e. You can create as many sticky notes as you want. Usually, affinity diagrams will have many sticky notes.

   f. When you are done creating sticky notes and brainstorming ideas, look at all of the notes under the quality measure and create groupings of sticky notes where there is a connection or commonality among the notes. Some sticky notes may not fit in a group, and that is okay.

   g. Then, for each grouping, create a header or phrase that describes the theme of the group of sticky notes.

h. Place all the sticky notes that connect to the header or phrase beneath that header. A lone sticky note without a header is designated a "loner" but may be as important as those that belong under a header.

i. The final affinity diagram can follow the template below or another template.

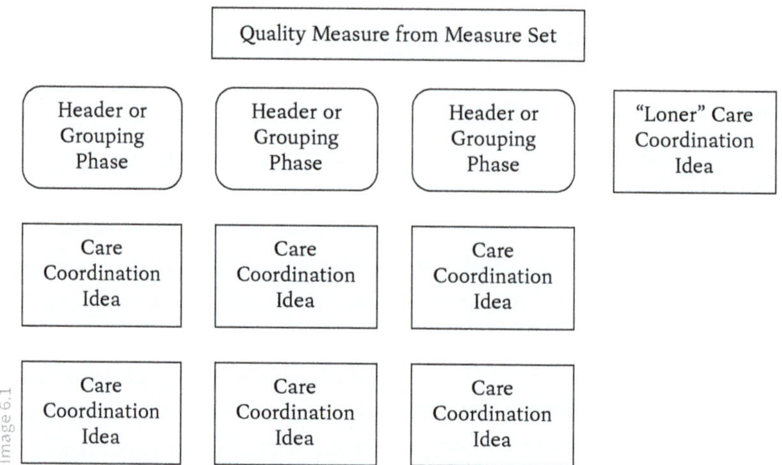

2. Select one of the eight identified areas of waste or muda when applying Lean to healthcare from the list below:

   a. Waiting or idle times

   b. Inventory (e.g., excess inventory or supplies)

   c. Defects (e.g., in quality of care and reimbursement)

   d. Transportation (e.g., unnecessary transportation of supplies and patients)

   e. Motion (e.g., movement that does not add value to patient care)

   f. Overproduction (e.g., duplicate testing, redundancy in care)

   g. Overprocessing (e.g., when time, effort, and resources do not improve the quality of care)

   h. Untapped human potential (e.g., nurses wasting energy on non-value-added actions, limiting time for person- and relationship-centered care or professional development)

   Then write an essay discussing the nurse's role in addressing this type of waste in healthcare and identifying two specific actions the nurse can use to decrease the type of waste and how this contributes to quality healthcare delivery. The essay must be at least two pages long, in APA format, and cite at least two references.

3. Case Study:

A 38-year-old male patient named Roy was brought into the emergency room by the local police department for a mental health evaluation. Roy has a history of being in and out of the emergency room and having multiple medical and psychiatric hospital admissions. The last time Roy was admitted inpatient was for dehydration. He has a mental health diagnosis of schizoaffective bipolar disorder and has currently been diagnosed with rhabdomyolysis and admitted to inpatient hospitalization for medical stabilization. Roy is treated with intravenous (IV) fluids and then cleared for admittance to the local psychiatric hospital for continued treatment of his schizoaffective bipolar disorder, which at times leads Roy to periods of mania where he exercises excessively, exhibits unusual behaviors, and has difficulty communicating and managing his personal care.

Roy has been hospitalized at the psychiatric hospital for 2 weeks, has had his medications adjusted, is appropriately participating in the therapeutic milieu, and has been cleared for discharge to the community with outpatient follow-up. The care coordinating nurse at the psychiatric hospital recently graduated and has been studying for the NCLEX in every spare moment. The new nurse received 3 weeks of orientation to general hospital procedures and practices, rotating on each unit and the admissions center for a few days each. Since the previous care coordinating nurse had retired and was unavailable to orient the new nurses, they were given a handbook on the specific care coordination policies and procedures to review and told to ask the charge nurse on duty if they had questions. The care coordinating nurse has developed a discharge plan, set a follow-up appointment for Roy with an outpatient psychiatrist in 3 days, and phoned his new prescriptions into his pharmacy. Roy is discharged, tells the care coordinating nurse he will pick up his medications the next day, and walks to the nearest bus stop to go home.

Seven days later, Roy arrives at the local emergency room unresponsive and is admitted to the intensive care unit with an intracranial hemorrhage. Upon investigation, it was found that Roy did not have a copy of his discharge summary, so he did not know which medications were new or who to contact with questions or for follow-up. Because of this, he had taken both his old, prescribed medications, which included nefazodone, and his newly prescribed medications, which included lumateperone. This medication interaction caused severe hypotension and loss of consciousness. When Roy fell, he hit his head on his fireplace mantle, causing an intracranial hemorrhage.

The care coordinating nurse did not provide medication education, as the nurse believed the pharmacist would provide medication education when Roy picked up his new medications the day after discharge, but Roy had sent his brother to pick up the medications because he did not have a car and felt too tired to take the bus to the pharmacy. The care coordination nurse did not print out and give Roy the discharge summary because an assessment found that he had difficulty reading, so it was mailed to his brother, who is Roy's healthcare power of attorney. Furthermore, the discharge summary was not forwarded to the outpatient psychiatrist, so when Roy did not show up for the appointment, the psychiatrist's scheduler put another patient into that time slot. No follow-up was provided, as the psychiatrist did not know what the appointment was for and thought that Roy would call to reschedule later.

1. Create a cause-and-effect fishbone diagram about this case study. Place the problem (Roy's fall or other problem you identify) in a box to the right. Then identify the major causes contributing to the problem at the top of the fishbones. This could be people, processes, materials, or any other major cause that contributed to the problem. Then identify specific possible causes in the major cause areas, such as Process → lack of discharge summary. Some potential causes may fit more than one major cause fishbone.
2. You may want to ask yourself questions such as these to prompt brainstorming on causes of the identified problem: How did this happen? What could have happened differently? What is an identified major cause area likely to have contributed to the problem?
3. You may make your fishbone cause-and-effect diagram using the template below or use another fishbone cause-and-effect template.

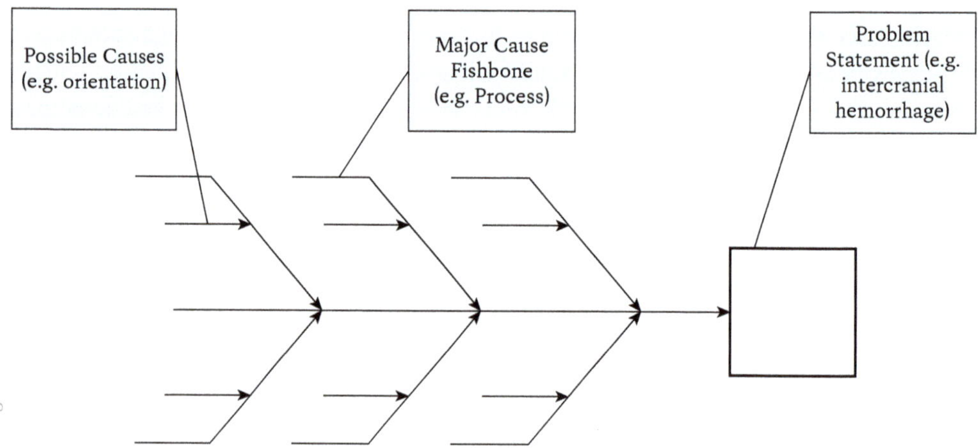

NCLEX STYLE QUESTIONS

1. Which of the following is a common result for patients who receive fragmented care coordination practice? (Select all that apply.)

   a. Misunderstanding follow-up directions

   b. Lack of information about the care needed after leaving the clinic or hospital

   c. Knowing about when follow-up appointments are

   d. Engaging in a medication reconciliation process

2. Which of the following is true about quality measures?

    a. A quality measure is used to improve healthcare delivery
    b. A quality measure is used to measure patient acuity
    c. A quality measure, if used correctly, can increase siloed care
    d. A quality measure only applies to hospital reimbursement

3. Collected data is used in continuous quality improvement to inform which of the following? (Select all that apply.)

    a. Quality care delivery
    b. Gaps in quality
    c. CQI projects
    d. Service charges

4. Matching question: Match the following care coordination outcomes to whether it is a quality or resource outcome.

    Continuity of care
    Improved follow-up
    Decreased emergency room visits
    Prevention of delays in care
    Prevention of admission to acute care

    Questions 5 to 6 are related to the following scenario:

    Jordan Knox is a 72-year-old female with a history of smoking for 50 years and a COPD (chronic obstructive pulmonary disorder) diagnosis. Jordan has a history of regularly missing follow-up, specialist, and primary care appointments due to lack of transportation, and she has told the nurse care coordinator that she likes smoking and doesn't want to receive information about smoking cessation programs.

5. The nurse care coordinator is considering how to best support Jordan in getting to her appointments so that her COPD can be managed. Which of the following domains of the care coordination measure framework should the nurse focus their care coordination efforts on to meet this goal? (Select the most appropriate.)

    a. Assess needs and goals
    b. Link to community resources
    c. Negotiate accountability
    d. Align resources to the patient

6. The nurse care coordinator knows that there is a clinic quality measure related to offering smoking cessation to patients identified as smokers but does not want to keep "bothering" Jordan with smoking cessation program pamphlets. Which of the following domains of the care coordination measure framework should the nurse focus their care coordination efforts on to meet this goal? (Select the most appropriate.)

   a. Communicate
   b. Support self-management goals
   c. Assess needs and goals
   d. Create a proactive plan of care

7. Which of the following is a quality measure set commonly used in skilled nursing facilities?

   a. HAVEN
   b. FACT
   c. MDS
   d. HCPDS

8. You are precepting a new nurse and explaining the quality measures your clinic uses to determine if quality healthcare has been delivered. You know the new nurse understands the nurse's role in quality measures in healthcare when they tell you which of the following?

   a. Quality measures add much work but are needed for reimbursement, so they are important.
   b. Quality measures are not related to nursing practice but help the patients have a voice when they get a post-visit survey.
   c. Quality measures are needed for a culture of quality and safety, and it is the role of leadership to ensure that culture is in place.
   d. Quality measures are an opportunity to integrate advocacy, ethical practice, and accountability into quality nursing care delivery.

9. Service has been introduced as a component of quality and value in healthcare. Which of the following is the "formula" for value in healthcare that includes service?

   a. Value = Supplies + Quality + Customer Focus
   b. Value = Resources +Service + Relationships

c. Value = Resources + Quality + Service

d. Value = Quality + Service + Cost

10. You are a newly graduated nurse working in the intensive care unit. The provider has ordered a medication for one of your patients. Upon review of the electronic health record (EHR), you see the patient is receiving another medication that might cause an adverse effect if the two medications interact. You contact the provider with your concerns. The provider becomes upset and tells you the medication is correct, they know what the patient should get, and that you are wasting their time. You decide to consult with the unit charge nurse before giving the medication. Which domains of value-based care and health equity are you following by contacting the provider and then consulting with the charge nurse?

   a. Individual and caregiver voice

   b. Behavioral health

   c. Safety

   d. Equity

11. Which of the following describes the foundation of the Lean continuous quality improvement methodology? (Select all that apply.)

   a. Kaizen

   b. Standardization

   c. Creative problem-solving

   d. Team decision-making

12. You are working with a team of care coordinators from the hospital on a Lean improvement project to decrease 30-day all-cause readmission rates. You are collecting information from various sources, such as pulling readmission percentages from the electronic health record (EHR) system and looking at your organization's past "report cards" to decide what the focus of your improvement project should be. Which of the following describes this type of decision-making?

   a. Metric-based decision-making

   b. Health information technology decision-making

   c. Just-in-time decision-making

   d. Data-driven decision-making

13. You are the nurse care coordinator on the medical floor of the local acute care hospital. A patient has been admitted for pneumonia with potential sepsis after being transferred from a critical access hospital 90 miles away. The patient had a chest x-ray and labs performed at the critical access hospital this morning before being transferred to your hospital. However, the hospital uses a different electronic health record (EHR) system, so this information cannot be accessed and the results were not included in the hard copy packet sent with the patient. The admitting hospitalist orders a new chest x-ray and labs to be drawn. You know that this duplicative testing order represents which type of waste or muda in the healthcare system?

    a. Overproduction
    b. Overprocessing
    c. Transportation
    d. Inventory

14. Fill in the blank:

    Meaningful measures 2.0 is an initiative to promote ______ in healthcare by focusing on high-impact ______ areas that are meaningful to ______ and are ______.

15. Which nursing actions include essential nursing knowledge, skills, and attitudes supporting quality measure attainment and quality healthcare delivery? (Select all that apply.)

    a. Accurate and timely documentation
    b. Interprofessional teamwork
    c. Medication reconciliation by the pharmacist
    d. Leveraging health information technologies for information transfer and maintenance

REFERENCES

Agency for Healthcare Research and Quality (AHRQ). (2021). *Family experiences with coordination of care (FECC) measure: Has care coordinator.* Author. https://www.ahrq.gov/pqmp/measures/fecc-care-coordination.html

Agency for Healthcare Research and Quality (AHRQ). (2022). Six *domains of healthcare quality.* Author. https://www.ahrq.gov/talkingquality/measures/six-domains.html

Agency for Healthcare Research and Quality (AHRQ). (2023a). *CAHPS clinician & group survey.* Author. https://www.ahrq.gov/cahps/surveys-guidance/cg/index.html

Agency for Healthcare Research and Quality (AHRQ). (2023b). *Hospital admission versus readmission costs, 2020.* Author. https://www.ahrq.gov/data/infographics/hospital-readmission-costs.html

American Nurses Association (ANA). (2010). *Principles for nursing documentation: Guidance for registered nurses.* https://www.nursingworld.org/~4af4f2/globalassets/docs/ana/ethics/principles-of-nursing-documentation.pdf

American Nurses Association (ANA). (2015). *Code of ethics for nurses with interpretive statements.* American Nurses Association.

American Nurses Association (ANA). (2021). *Care coordination and registered nurses' essential role* (ANA position statement). https://www.nursingworld.org/practice-policy/nursing-excellence/official-position-statements/id/care-coordination-and-registered-nurses-essential-role/

Balkhi, B., Alshahrani, A., & Khan, A. (2022). Just-in-time approach in healthcare inventory management: Does it really work? *Saudi Pharmaceutical Journal, 30*(12), 1830–1835, https://doi.org/10.1016/j.jsps.2022.10.013.

Breslin, S. E., Hamilton, K. M., & Paynter, J. (2014). Deployment of Lean Six Sigma in care coordination: An improved discharge process. *Professional Case Management, 19*(2), 77–85. https://doi.org/10.1097/NCM.0000000000000016

Centers for Medicare and Medicaid Services (CMS). (2019). *Quality measures fact sheet.* https://www.cms.gov/priorities/innovation/files/fact-sheet/bpciadvanced-fs-psi90.pdf

Centers for Medicare and Medicaid Services (CMS). (2021a). *Quality measures: How they are developed, used, and maintained.* https://www.cms.gov/sites/default/files/2021-09/Quality-Measures-How-They-Are-Developed-Used-Maintained.pdf

Centers for Medicare and Medicaid Services (CMS). (2021b). *CAHPS® hospital survey (HCAHPS): Quality assurance guidelines* (v 16.0). https://www.cms.gov/files/document/hcahps-qag-v160.pdf

Centers for Medicare and Medicaid Services (CMS). (2023). *Meaningful measures 2.0: Moving to measure prioritization and modernization.* https://www.cms.gov/medicare/quality/meaningful-measures-initiative/meaningful-measures-20

Centers for Medicare and Medicaid Services (CMS) Center for Clinical Standards & Quality. (2021). *2021 national assessment of the Centers for Medicare and Medicaid Services (CMS) quality measures report.* https://www.cms.gov/files/document/2021-national-impact-assessment-report.pdf

Council for Six Sigma Certification (CSSC). (2018). *Six Sigma a complete step-by-step guide: A complete training and reference guide for white belts, yellow belts, green belts, and black belts.* Harmony Living.

Elliott, M. N., Adams, J. L., Klein, D. J., Haviland, A. M., Beckett, M. K., Hays, R. D., Gaillot, S., Edwards, C. A., Dembosky, J. W., & Schneider, E. C. (2021). Patient-reported care coordination is associated with better performance on clinical care measures. *Journal of General Internal Medicine, 36*(12), 3665–3671. https://doi.org/10.1007/s11606-021-07122-8

Evidence-Based Practice Centers®. (2023). *Use of report cards and outcome measurements to improve the safety of surgical care rapid response* (Pub. No. 23(4)-EHC019-4). The Agency for Healthcare Research and Quality. https://effectivehealthcare.ahrq.gov/sites/default/files/related_files/mhs-IV-rapid-response-surgical-report-cards.pdf

Finkelman, A. (2016). *Leadership and management for nurses: Core competencies for quality care* (3rd ed.). Pearson.

Garber, J. (2023). *An ethical imperative: How nurses can be leaders in reducing overuse.* Lown Institute. https://lowninstitute.org/an-ethical-imperative-how-nurses-can-be-leaders-in-reducing-overuse/

Garnett, D., Hardy, L., Fitzgerald, E., Fisher, T., Graham, L., & Overcash, J. (2020). Nurse case manager: Measurement of care coordination activities and quality and resource use outcomes when caring for the complex patient with hematologic cancer. *Clinical Journal of Oncology Nursing, 24*(1), 65–74. https://doi.org/10.1188/20.CJON.65-74

Gidengil, C., Parast, L., Burkhart, Q., Brown, J., Elliott, M. N., Casey Lion, K., C., McGlynn, E. A., Schneider, E. C., & Mangione-Smith, R. (2017). Development and implementation of the family experiences with coordination of care survey quality measures. *Academic Pediatrics, 17*(8), 863–870, https://doi.org/10.1016/j.acap.2017.03.012

Girmash, E., & Honsberger, K. (2022). *Aligning quality measures with the National Care Coordination Standards for children and youth with special health care needs (CYSHCN).* https://nashp.org/aligning-quality-measures-with-the-national-care-coordination-standards-for-children-and-youth-with-special-health-care-needs-cyshcn/

Graig, L., & Perosino, K. (2011). *Applying Lean to improve the patient visit process at three Federally Qualified Health Centers.* Altarum Institute. https://altarum.org/sites/default/files/uploaded-related-files/Applying-Lean-Report_FINAL.pdf

Haas, S. A., Swan, B. A., & Haynes, T. S. (2014). *Care coordination and transition management core curriculum.* American Academy of Ambulatory Care Nursing.

Harkness, T. (2020). Effective care coordination and transition management for older adults. *Nursing Made Incredibly Easy! 18*(5), 26–32. https://doi.org/10.1097/01.NME.0000694184.27758.b9

HealthCatalyst. (2018). *Lean healthcare: 6 methodologies for improvement from Dr. Brent James*. https://www.healthcatalyst.com/insights/lean-healthcare-methodologies-improvement

Hung, D. Y., Kim, P., Li, M., Huang, Q., Cantril, C., Colocci, N., & Dillon, E. C. (2022). Lean practices for resource use, timeliness, and coordination of care in breast cancer navigation. *Clinical Journal of Oncology Nursing, 26*(5), 503–509. https://doi.org/10.1188/22.CJON.503-509

Institute of Medicine (IOM). (2001). *Crossing the quality chasm: A new health system for the 21st century*. National Academies of Science.

Institute of Medicine (IOM). (2011). *The future of nursing: Leading change, advancing health*. The National Academies Press.

Jacobs, D. B., Schreiber, M., Seshamani, M., Tsai, D., Fowler, E., & Fleisher, L. A. (2023). Aligning quality measures across CMS—The Universal Foundation. *The New England Journal of Medicine, 388*(9), 776–779. https://doi.org/10.1056/NEJMp2215539

Kelly, P., Vottero, B. A., & Christie-McAuliffe, C. A. (Eds.). (2018). *Introduction to quality and safety education for nurses: Core competencies for nursing leadership and management* (2nd ed.). Springer Publishing Company.

Lamb, G. (2013). *Care coordination: The game changer. How nursing is revolutionizing quality care*. American Nurses Association.

McDonald, K. M, Schultz, E., Albin, L., Pineda, N., Lonhart, J., Sundaram, V., Smith-Spangler, C., Brustrom, J., Malcolm, E., Rohn, L., & Davies, S. (2014). *Care coordination atlas version 4* (Prepared by Stanford University under subcontract to American Institutes for Research on Contract No. HHSA290-2010-00005I). AHRQ Publication No. 14-0037-EF. Agency for Healthcare Research and Quality.

Measures Management System. (2023). *2023 measures under consideration list now available!* https://mmshub.cms.gov/news-events/2023-measures-under-consideration-list-now-available

Möckli, N., Simon, M., Denhaerynck, K., Martins, T., Meyer-Massetti, C., Fischer, R., & Zúñiga, F. (2023). Care coordination in homecare and its relationship with quality of care: A national multicenter cross-sectional study. *International Journal of Nursing Studies, 145*,104544. https://doi.org/10.1016/j.ijnurstu.2023.104544.

Möckli, N., Simon, M., Meyer-Massetti, C., Pihet, S., Fischer, R., Wächter, M., Serdaly, C., & Zúñiga, F. (2021). Factors associated with homecare coordination and quality of care: A research protocol for a national multi-center cross-sectional study. *BMC Health Services Research, 21*(1), 306. https://doi.org/10.1186/s12913-021-06294-7

Morell-Santandreu, O., Santandreu-Mascarell, C., Garcia-Sabater, J. J. (2021). A model for the implementation of lean improvements in healthcare environments as applied in a primary care center. *International Journal of Environmental Research and Public Health, 18*(6), 2876. https://doi.org/10.3390/ijerph18062876

Nahum-Shani, I., Smith, S. N., Spring, B. J., Collins, L. M., Witkiewitz, K., Tewari, A., & Murphy, S. A. (2018). Just-in-time adaptive interventions (JITAIs) in mobile health: Key components and design principles for ongoing health behavior support. *Annals of Behavioral Medicine: A Publication of the Society of Behavioral Medicine, 52*(6), 446–462. https://doi.org/10.1007/s12160-016-9830-8

National Committee for Quality Assurance (NCQA). (2021). *Required HEDIS® and CAHPS® measures for HEDIS reporting year 2022*. https://www.ncqa.org/wp-content/uploads/2021/02/20210709_2022_List_of_Required_Performance_Measures.pdf

National Committee for Quality Assurance (NCQA). (2023). *Transitions of care (TRC)*. https://www.ncqa.org/hedis/measures/transitions-of-care/

NEJM Catalyst. (2018). *What is lean healthcare?* Massachusetts Medical Society. https://catalyst.nejm.org/doi/full/10.1056/CAT.18.0193

O'Donnell, B., & Gupta, V. (2023). *Continuous quality improvement*. StatPearls Publishing. https://www.ncbi.nlm.nih.gov/books/NBK559239/

Porter-O'Grady, T., & Malloch, K. (2018). *Quantum leadership: Creating sustainable value in health care* (5th ed.). Jones & Bartlett Learning.

Porumboiu, D. (2023). *Demystifying Lean Six Sigma: A continuous improvement framework*. https://www.viima.com/blog/lean-six-sigma

Shi, L., & Singh, D. (2019). *Essentials of the U.S. health care system* (5th ed.). Jones & Bartlett Learning.

Shrank, W. H., Rogstad, T. L., & Parekh, N. (2019). Waste in the US health care system: Estimated costs and potential for savings. *JAMA, 322*(15), 1501–1509. https://doi.org/10.1001/jama.2019.13978

Singer, C., & Porta, C. (2022). Improving patient well-being in the United States through care coordination interventions informed by social determinants of health. *Health & Social Care in the Community, 30*(6), 2270–2281. https://doi.org/10.1111/hsc.13776

Socconini, L. (2023). *Lean Six Sigma in healthcare: Improving patient care and efficiency.* Lean Six Sigma Institute. https://leansixsigmainstitute.org/lean-six-sigma-in-healthcare-improving-patient-care-and-efficiency/

Waddill, K. (2022). *CQMC finds quality measurement gaps, supports digital measures.* Xtelligent Healthcare Media. https://healthpayerintelligence.com/news/cmqc-finds-quality-measurement-gaps-including-in-equity-measures

Wells, R., Breckenridge, E. D., Siañez, M., Tamayo, L., Kum, H. C., & Ohsfeldt, R. L. (2020). Self-reported quality, health, and cost-related outcomes of care coordination among patients with complex health needs. *Population Health Management, 23*(1), 59–67. https://doi.org/10.1089/pop.2019.0007

Credits

Fig. 6.3: Centers for Medicare & Medicaid Services, https://www.cms.gov/medicare/quality/meaningful-measures-initiative/meaningful-measures-20, 2023.

Fig. 6.4: Source: NEJM Catalyst; https://catalyst.nejm.org/doi/full/10.1056/CAT.18.0193.

CHAPTER 7

Innovative Healthcare Delivery Models

LEARNING OBJECTIVES

1. Differentiate various innovative healthcare delivery models.
2. Analyze how care coordination is promoted in each healthcare delivery model.
3. Consider each model's connection with the goals of the Quintuple Aim.
4. Recognize the role of care coordination in healthcare system transformation.

KEY TERMS

- Accountable Health Communities (AHC)
- advanced primary care or patient-centered medical home (PCMH)
- change drivers
- collaborative care model (CoCM)
- demonstration project
- digital literacy
- downstream healthcare
- federally qualified health center (FQHC)
- health related social need (HRSN)
- home-based primary care (HBPC)
- patient panel
- substance use disorder (SUD)
- teamlet
- telehealth
- transitional care programs (TCPs)
- upstream healthcare

Introduction

Healthcare delivery models and designs will continue to evolve and adapt, moving the focal point of healthcare from the acute care setting to community-based settings such as primary care clinics and health systems offering a preventative and cohesive approach to healthcare. Integrated care coordination will be central to these new models and delivery systems. There are many reasons for these changes in healthcare delivery, such as the need to manage resources and costs and to meet aspects of the Quintuple Aim, like the aims of better health and improved patient experience.

Several additional change drivers are prompting the development and introduction of healthcare delivery models outside traditional care practices and settings. **Change drivers** can include external factors such as the growth in technologies or changes in reimbursement methods. They also can consist of internal factors, such as workforce burnout or patient satisfaction rates. These external and internal forces affect the healthcare system and delivery of care.

One significant change driver in today's healthcare system is the growth and need for patient engagement in healthcare. Patients are now more than ever able to easily access information concerning their health conditions, and if they are to effectively self-manage their health, they must be actively engaged. The development of accessible health information and digital technologies, such as patient portals, smartwatches, and wellness apps, will continue to drive design changes in healthcare delivery. Since the COVID-19 pandemic, there has been a growth in telehealth care delivery, and this has also been the impetus for changes in healthcare financing regarding this type of healthcare. Furthermore, between 2015 and 2050, the percentage of the world's population over 60 years is expected to increase from 12% to 22% (WHO, 2022, Key Facts). As the United States population ages, there are rising rates of chronic diseases, contributing to the historical need to manage costs and resources and address workforce shortages while ensuring healthcare needs are met (Edelmann, 2023; Zimlichman et al., 2021).

Due to these many change drivers of healthcare delivery and design, we will see more healthcare offered in innovative settings and the development of healthcare system designs that integrate care coordination and address healthcare holistically across illness, wellness, the lifespan, and continuum of care. This will require a shift in perspective, viewing healthcare from a coordinated systems level to best utilize and leverage resources, services, and infrastructure on a community and organizational level to provide for good patient outcomes and resource and cost management. See Table 7.1 for an example of some external and internal drivers of healthcare system change.

TABLE 7.1 Example Healthcare System Change Drivers

Example Change Drivers	
External	**Internal**
Need to address social determinants of health (SDOH) in the healthcare system	Workforce shortages
Rise of consumerism in healthcare	Workforce burnout
Need to address health inequity and accessibility issues	Organizational transitions to accountable care organizations (ACOs) or other value-based healthcare delivery models
Value-based reimbursement strategies	Retirement of nurses or those leaving the discipline leading to a knowledge and practice experience gap
Expansion of health information and digital technologies	Organizational policies that support the healthcare workforce working to their full scope of practice or licensure

Fragmented and siloed care being delivered without a focus on continuity and care coordination will need to decrease significantly to address these healthcare change drivers. Value-based healthcare and reimbursement programs aim to reduce costs and increase positive patient outcomes. This will require a shift in perspective to preventative and community-based services and care that will meet patients where they live, providing relevant care that can be integrated into the context of the patient's daily life. We have seen some of this transformation already with reimbursement strategies and quality measures calling for care coordination to be integrated into care provided, as well as measures on transitions of care and risk screenings and the development of professional practice standards that include interprofessional practice across disciplines.

We have also seen the development of new roles in healthcare, such as community health workers, medical scribes, care navigators, and health coaches. The roles of pharmacists have expanded, and there has been a continued call for nurses to practice to their full scope of licensure (Zimlichman et al., 2021). "If health care systems are to evolve, they must shift both operations and leadership out of the hospital" (Zimlichman et al., 2021, p. 4). The future of healthcare will need to embrace a healthcare system that integrates continuous quality improvement and dynamic innovation, addressing change drivers and offering coordinated healthcare that meets not only patients' medical needs but also their holistic needs in various settings (Zimlichman et al., 2021).

Innovative Healthcare Delivery Models

Several healthcare delivery systems that embrace this need for innovative healthcare design have been developed. Some of these are based in hospitals, clinics, or across settings. A few of these leading-edge models include the collaborative care model (CoCM), advanced primary care or patient-centered medical home (PCMH), the federally qualified medical center (FQHC), home-based primary care (HBPC) or house calls, transitional care programs (TCPs), telehealth/telemedicine/virtual healthcare, and Accountable Health Communities (AHC). Each of these models provides a glimpse into what is needed on a health systems level to meet the Quintuple Aim and the multidimensional healthcare needs of the United States population.

Collaborative Care Model (CoCM)

The **collaborative care model (CoCM)** is a cohesive healthcare model providing integrated team-based primary medical care and mental health (MH) and/or **substance use disorder (SUD)** care and services, often with services co-located. The model aims to improve outcomes and resource utilization by integrating robust care coordination and an interprofessional approach to meet patient needs holistically (Edelmann, 2023). CoCM involves integrating MH/SUD services with primary care services for patients with both medical and MH/ SUD conditions. SUD is a disorder that affects the brain and behavior, with varying levels of severity, that leads to the inability of a person to control their use of substances, including medications, alcohol, and illegal substances (NIMH, 2023).

A team-based approach to care is offered by co-locating MH/SUD providers on the primary care clinic site or by having partnerships between primary care providers (PCP) and clinicians that treat those with MH/SUD so that patients can have their health needs met collaboratively. Core principles of this model include strong team-based care and collaboration with the PCP, integration of care management, psychiatric consultation access, and a focus on population-based care by identifying those most at risk for poor outcomes and providing coordinated and comprehensive care to address medical as well as MH/SUD needs (Jackson-Triche et al., 2020).

The population of patients with medical and comorbid MH/SUD conditions has increased levels of healthcare costs and resource use. Healthcare costs for this population of patients with dual medical and MH/SUD conditions have been shown to be two to three times higher than those populations with a medical condition only. In 2017, this dual-needs population was estimated to incur an additional $406 billion in healthcare costs, most of which were for medical services (Melek et al., 2018). It has been estimated that up to 17% of these additional healthcare costs could be mitigated by integrating medical and mental health/SUD services (Melek et al., 2018). Several chronic health conditions have been associated with increased medical costs for those patients with comorbid MH/SUD. These include anemia, liver disease, epilepsy, congestive heart failure (CHF), and osteoporosis. It is projected that through the CoCM, approximately $1,040 per patient/member per month (PMPM) or $12,480 per patient/member per year could be saved (Melek et al., 2018, p. 10).

One example of a CoCM is a program that utilized specialized nurses to deliver a depression treatment program over 12 months for those patients with a comorbid condition of diabetes. This program saved $46 PMPM over two years, for approximately 5% savings for this group of patients (Melek et al., 2018). Another example would be a health system that offered an integrated team-based care approach and found that this change in practice from traditional care practices led to 11% fewer hospital admissions, 23% fewer emergency room visits, and 3% lower healthcare costs (Melek et al., 2018). Furthermore, a primary care clinic provided CoCM for those identified as having depression in the clinic's panel and found that the model reduced racial and ethnic disparities in outcomes. This CoCM intervention targeted geographic locations in the **patient panel** (the population of patients assigned to or associated with the clinic). It ensured that significant numbers of African American and Latinx patients with a diagnosis of depression received the intervention, resulting in improved mental health-related quality of life in both years the program was offered (Jackson-Triche et al., 2020).

CoCM Support of the Quintuple Aim

CoCM has excellent value in addressing healthcare equity and accessibility. By integrating medical, mental health, and/or SUD services, the patient's holistic needs can be addressed, and overall health treatment can be improved. Supporting medical providers in integrating MH/SUD conditions into treatment plans and care delivery can assist in meeting multidimensional needs related to social determinants of health (SDOH) or accessibility and health equity issues, mitigating the risks of poor MH or SUD. Through interprofessional integrated care and treatment across settings, the CoCM supports better outcomes (Schraeder & Shelton, 2011). The CoCM is an essential part of a healthcare delivery system that can individualize and tailor interventions and care to meet the needs of underserved and at-risk patient populations, improving access to care and health outcomes (American Psychiatric Association, n.d.).

CoCM Support of Coordinated Care

Many aspects of CoCM support care coordination rights and guiding principles. Most significantly, the CoCM is an integrated care model based on collaboration and communication, ensuring that the right transition is made when transitions in care are needed. Furthermore, CoCM promotes proactive advocacy and care delivery through the foundation of integrated care, providing a person- and relationship-based model of interprofessional care and ensuring the care delivered is right for the patient. Most importantly, CoCM ensures that care is delivered at the right time with the right resources. Through this integrated care model, care is provided proactively to address potential medical and MH/SUD conditions with the accountability of the interprofessional team. This ensures that any gaps in care or barriers to care and the patient's holistic needs are addressed, monitored, and followed up, leading to appropriate resource use and cost management.

Advanced Primary Care: The Patient-Centered Medical Home (PCMH)

Advanced primary care, also known as the patient-centered medical home (PCMH), utilizes the PCP clinic to focus on comprehensive, quality, safe, person-centered, and coordinated care and provides accessible services. The use of comprehensive and coordinated care contributes to good outcomes, patient engagement, and improved access to healthcare. This model focuses on preventive care and wellness and is provided through interprofessional teams to meet patient needs in a relevant and culturally sensitive approach (Edelmann, 2023). The designation of "home" in the PCMH acronym can cause confusion, thinking that the PCMH is a specific place, which is not always the case. The PCMH often offers comprehensive services, including mental health, dental, social work, etc., all under one roof. Other times, the PCMH may be offered as part of a system where the comprehensive patient needs are met, but may be offered in various places throughout the healthcare system and through relationships with community resources and services. The goal of the PCMH is to provide coordinated care that will address barriers and issues with health to meet needs quickly and effectively through the interprofessional team approach (Grys, 2022).

The PCMH healthcare delivery model often utilizes a PCP as the lead of a "teamlet." The **teamlet** is typically made up of one provider and one or two other healthcare workers (e.g., MA, RN, LPN, SW, etc.) that work together daily, usually in a primary care setting. The teamlet may vary in makeup depending on workforce availability, system and community needs, and reimbursement structures used (Mason et al., 2021). Often the teamlet consists of the PCP, a medical assistant (MA), a primary care registered nurse (RN), a licensed professional nurse (LPN), or a social worker (SW). The teamlet concept, with various scopes of practice and

The Implications of Home

"Not only does 'patient-centered' place the importance directly on the patient but using 'home' implies comfort and wholeness" (Grys, 2022, p. 41).

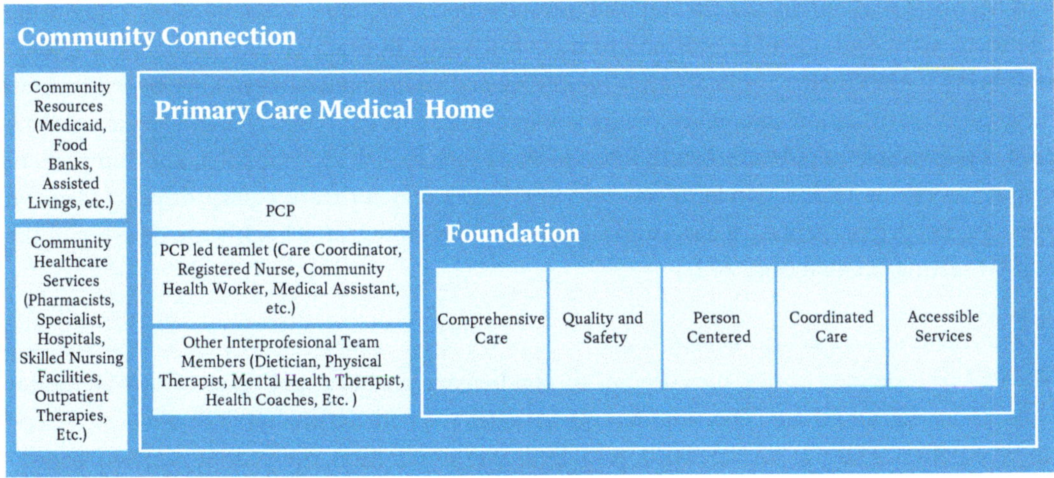

FIGURE 7.1 Patient-Centered Medical Home (PCMH) Model

training levels, allows flexibility in the delivery of screenings, chronic care management, and care coordination in a timely and resource-efficient manner (Mason et al., 2021).

Currently, there are approximately 13,000 PCP practices and more than 67,000 clinicians recognized as PCMHs by the National Council for Quality Assurance (NCQA) in the U.S. (NCQA, 2024). In studies, PCMHs have been found to have some positive effects, causing a decrease in emergency room use, an increase in the use of primary care services, and increases in patient satisfaction and the use of preventative care services (Veet et al., 2020). See Figure 7.1 for a visual of the foundation and framework of the PCMH.

PCMH Support of the Quintuple Aim

The foundation of the PCMH focuses on "upstream" healthcare services, prevention, care coordination, and primary care provision to reduce "downstream" healthcare use, such as hospital admission or emergency room visits. **Upstream healthcare** seeks to address the root causes of healthcare issues rather than focusing on disease or symptom management, aiming to improve long-term health outcomes and manage resources and costs of healthcare (James, 2020). **Downstream healthcare**, such as chronic disease management, is delivered after a medical event or need occurs. Focusing on upstream healthcare ultimately lowers care costs (Maeng et al., 2016). The PCMH framework is based on comprehensive care, quality and safety, person-centered care, coordinated care, and accessible services (AHRQ, 2022). With this framework, the model addresses all aspects of the Quintuple Aim, offering improved patient experience through coordinated care and engagement. Better health outcomes can offset any initial costs associated with PCMH implementation by delivering better preventative care, resulting in longer-term cost and resource savings through potential decreases in unmanaged health conditions, hospital admissions, and emergency room use.

The PCMH accomplishes its goals of comprehensive, quality, safe, coordinated, and person-centered care by having each healthcare team member work to their full scope of practice and licensure and enhancing patient and family/support system engagement. By integrating the team, with each member working to their full scope of practice and licensure, clinician well-being is enhanced, as collaborative teamwork and staff empowerment have been shown to increase job satisfaction among healthcare workers (Karaferis et al., 2022). Lastly, by integrating care coordination, population-health interventions such as risk stratification, and comprehensive services, the PCMH can address areas and issues of healthcare equity, offering targeted services, needed preventative care, and support to direct integrated healthcare delivery in the PCMH setting (Itchhaporia, 2021).

PCMH Support of Coordinated Care

The PCMH is defined as the "provision of comprehensive primary care services that facilitates communication and shared decision-making between the patient, his/her PCP, other providers, and the patient's family" (AHA, 2010, p. 2). By its very definition, the PCMH supports coordinated care principles and rights. Relationship-centered care can be provided through actions like shared decision-making and patient autonomy, which ensure the right care is provided and respects the patient's goals of care. The focus on communication and collaborative practice ensures seamless transitions in care. Furthermore, through person-centered education and coordinated care planning, gaps and barriers to care are addressed, costs are managed, and patient self-management of health is supported for long-term better health outcomes.

Federally Qualified Health Center (FQHC)

The **Federally Qualified Health Center (FQHC)** provides a critical healthcare delivery model that meets the needs of some of the most vulnerable patients. The FQHC is a federally funded outpatient clinic or health center that provides comprehensive services for all age groups, offers after-hours access, and bases charges on a sliding scale in medically underserved areas or with healthcare provider shortages. FQHCs provide a safety net of providers that offer outpatient services to vulnerable populations or areas and qualify for specific types of reimbursement from Medicare and Medicaid (RHIHub, 2023). The FQHC can be a community health clinic, a migrant health center, or an outpatient clinic operated by a tribal organization. For FQHC certification, the clinic or organization must be a grantee of specific types of federal grants, provide comprehensive services, participate in ongoing quality assurance, and meet safety requirements (Medicare Learning Network, 2023). "Over 9.6 million rural residents were served by the Health Center Program in 2022, according to the Health Resources and Services Administration (HRSA)" (RHIHub, 2023, para. 2).

Comprehensive services include physicians, nurse practitioners, physician assistants, certified nurse midwives, clinical psychologists, and social workers. The FQHC may also offer visiting nurse services for homebound patients and training and nutrition therapy for patients with diabetes or renal disease. The FQHC often provides chronic care management services for Medicare beneficiaries with two or more chronic conditions. Transitional care coordination, chronic pain care management, and behavioral health integration are offered in the FQHC model of care (Medicare Learning Network, 2023). These comprehensive services seek to meet the holistic needs of the patient. If the clinic does not offer preventive, dental, pharmacy, mental health, substance use services, health education, and necessary transportation and translation services, the FQHC is expected to arrange with other organizations or clinicians to offer this care (FQHC Associates, n.d.; RHIHub, 2023). See Table 7.2 for a list of requirements for FQHCs.

TABLE 7.2 Federally Qualified Health Center (FQHC) Requirements

Federally Qualified Health Center (FQHC) Requirements	
Facility Type	Public or nonprofit
Age Groups Served	Must provide care for all age groups.
Location	Must be in an urban or nonurban area with a medically underserved population or a shortage of healthcare providers.
Board of Directors	Must have a board of directors of which at least 51% are patients of the FQHC.
Services Offered	At a minimum, but not limited to, maternity and prenatal care, preventative care, dental services, emergency care, and pharmacy services.
Charges	Must offer care to all residents in the service area with charges based on a sliding fee scale. Cannot deny patients care due to inability to pay.
After-Hours Care	Must provide after-hours services to respond to patient emergencies by phone, face-to-face, or by arrangement with another provider.
Quality Assurance	Must have a continuous quality assurance program in place.

(RHIHub, 2023, Table 1)

FQHC Support of the Quintuple Aim

The FQHC is required to serve medically underserved populations—those that have been underrepresented in the healthcare system design or delivery. Because the mission of the FQHC is to address healthcare equity, it is a key to this goal of the Quintuple Aim. Delivering healthcare in the FQHC model removes obstacles to receiving and accessing care (Farrell et al., 2023). Additionally, the requirement that the FQHC board have 51% membership from patients who receive care at the FQHC assists the clinic in delivering culturally relevant care that represents the patient population being served.

Health Equity

"Health equity should involve everyone experiencing a fair opportunity to be as healthy as possible" (Farrell et al., 2023, p. 563).

The FQHC model contributes to better outcomes and lower costs by providing an integrated and comprehensive approach to care delivery for all ages and across health needs, such as medical, dental, and pharmacy care. This meets the patient's needs on a holistic level. This, paired with accessible and affordable healthcare, can improve short- and long-term patient outcomes. By being a point of contact for emergent conditions, the FQHC can also address health concerns at the lowest level and appropriate level of care, addressing care needs promptly and preventing unneeded emergency room visits and hospital admissions. This assists in managing resources and costs and improves the patient experience.

FQHC Support of Coordinated Care

The FQHC model supports the use of care coordination to meet the healthcare needs of medically underserved and underrepresented populations (Dickson et al., 2022). FQHC reimbursement strategies also support integrated care coordination services. FQHCs can bill for chronic care management and transitional care management services, including care coordination and patient and family/caregiver engagement (Medicare Learning Network, 2022). Through the integration of care coordination in the FQHC, healthcare delivery and transition of care needs are met based on the communication of essential information and collaboration with other healthcare and community resource partners. This dynamic coordination of care and care planning addresses potential barriers to care and ensures that resources are utilized to support positive outcomes. By being the point of contact for emergent conditions and offering after-hours support, the FQHC provides accessible and equitable care. The FQHC model ensures that all care coordination patients' rights are met and that care coordination guiding principles are a foundational part of healthcare delivery.

Home-Based Primary Care (HBPC): House Calls

Home-based primary care (HBPC) is also often called "house calls." HBPC is comprehensive primary healthcare delivered in a patient's home or residence for those with difficulty leaving their home. It frequently utilizes an interprofessional team-based approach and follows the patient to the end of their life. This is usually delivered to patients who are frail or isolated (Cornwell, 2019; Totten et al., 2016). HBPC services are also offered in skilled living or assisted living facilities, with a specific HBPC agency agreeing to provide these services to the facility's residents. A benefit to this type of primary care is that once a relationship is started with the patient, the provider in the HBPC can provide ongoing care through end-of-life care, contributing to continuity and coordination of care.

House calls used to be standard practice for a PCP but had become almost nonexistent by the 1980s (Totten et al., 2016). Healthcare delivery has become more fragmented, with hospitalists managing and delivering care in the hospital setting and the PCP providing care in the community clinic setting, leading to siloed care and communication and coordination issues. The HBPC model solves this dilemma, ensuring continuity of care across transitions and care coordination. With the development of portable x-ray and ultrasound equipment and other modern technologies, the HBPC program can include most diagnostic or monitoring testing needed. This contributes to decreased costs, as the HBPC provider can order these diagnostic tests to be delivered in the home or residential setting, reducing the need for an emergency room visit or hospital admission (Cornwell, 2019).

HBPC healthcare models have been shown to increase patient satisfaction and decrease costs. The Veteran's Health Administration HBPC was found to provide "a remarkable 59% reduction in hospital days, an 89% reduction in nursing home days, and a 21% reduction in 30-day readmissions" (Cornwell, 2019, p. 3). In addition, the HBPC model can offer appropriate end-of-life care in the person's home or place of residence, rather than hospitalization at the end of life. This is an important outcome as most people indicate they would prefer to die at home. An example of this person-centered outcome is from an HBPC that had 1,022 deaths between 2014 and 2018, with 76% of these people dying at home. Most were in hospice care and not hospitalized in their last three months of life (Cornwell, 2019, p. 4).

Some barriers to this model include financial reimbursement, EHR transfer and linkage of patient information, and the time it takes to travel from home to home to provide the healthcare service (Mason et al., 2021). HBPC typically sees between five and seven patients per day, a much different experience from a PCP in a clinic setting. This allows time to perform a comprehensive assessment of needs, coordinate care, and make needed connections and referrals. However, this does limit reimbursement if a fee-for-service model is utilized. There are also issues concerning the safety of the provider or interprofessional team member, requiring additional training in de-escalation techniques, environmental scanning, emergency response planning, and integration of security escorts if needed. There may also be patient safety concerns related to the physical environment, such as infection control or barriers to communication, education, and training for the patient or their family/caregiver. Additionally, some patients may not want to participate in HBPC due to privacy concerns, not feeling comfortable having others in their living environment, or preferring to have treatments or diagnostics offered in the acute care setting (Chandrashekar et al., 2019).

HBPC Support of the Quintuple Aim

HBPC supports better outcomes and decreased overall costs, as the house call approach delivers coordinated and comprehensive care and services to those who are frail, chronically ill, or medically complex. Patients receive care and diagnostic tests in the comfort of their home or residence, improving the patient experience and reducing the costs of potential emergency room or urgent care visits. HBPC provides "convenience and comfort" for patients and a "rewarding care experience" for clinicians, as through the model, clinicians can develop meaningful relationships with patients and their families/support systems (HCCI, 2020, p. 7). HBPC meets all aspects of the Quintuple Aim by reducing costs of preventable acute care admissions, improving patient satisfaction, providing greater clinician job satisfaction, supporting a better quality of life for the population served, and addressing the accessibility of healthcare for the frail, medically complex, and home limited patients, improving health equity. "Missed medical appointments, fragmented care, and poor control of chronic conditions—the factors most frequently cited for emergency room visits, acute hospitalizations, and institutionalization for this population—can be reduced through HBPC" (HCCI, 2020, p. 4).

HBPC Support of Coordinated Care

There are many benefits to the HBPC model concerning coordination of care. By nurturing a strong provider and patient relationship and delivering relationship-centered care, the care planning is right for the patient and delivered in the least restrictive environment—their home or residence. Patients receive high-quality care in the safety of their own homes, with HBPC often being available in the evenings and on weekends as needed. By offering more frequent and flexible visits, with the ability to order diagnostic tests to be conducted in the home setting for quick results and data to direct diagnosis, treatment, and monitoring interventions, the patient receives care in the least resource-intensive setting in an accessible and timely manner. The patient can "age in place" in the comfort of their home, preventing complications of acute care admissions, such as delirium and functional or cognitive decline, and increasing patient engagement and person-centered care (Totten et al., 2016). Ultimately, the HBPC healthcare model meets all patient care coordination rights and decreases costs and resource use through fewer acute incidents requiring hospitalization and reduced use of emergency or urgent care services.

Transitional Care Programs (TCPs)

Transitional care programs (TCPs) are designed to provide follow-up and support for patients with moderately complex transition of care needs due to health conditions, social determinants of health, or other issues. TCPs offer a range of time-limited services that assist patients with complex conditions or situations to transfer between settings in a timely, quality, and safe manner (Naylor et al., 2011). These types of patients can have higher healthcare costs and rates of emergency room use or readmissions. "Research indicates that one in five readmissions could have been avoided with proper transitional care management" (Marder, 2022, Article Summary). Additionally, hospitalized patients who lack the medical, health, and social support needed for post-acute care often may have delayed discharges while these barriers and gaps in care are addressed. This can lead to higher incidences of functional decline or health complications, such as infections or delirium. Ultimately, this contributes to system-level resource issues like emergency room overcrowding, increased costs, and overall poorer health outcomes for the patient (McGilton et al., 2021).

There are several types of TCPs, yet all have the goal of providing the support and resources needed for patients to be able to self-manage their health and providing timely, quality, and safe continuity of care as patients move from one setting to another (Welkin, 2021; Wong, 2023). TCPs all have similar components, including comprehensive assessment, care plan development, monitoring, treatment (including medication reconciliation and case management), interprofessional discharge planning, and patient and family education. However, each also has some unique features to meet the needs of the population served. Most TCPs focus on organizational, system, and patient outcomes of cost and resource use, better medical outcomes, quality of life, and well-being (McGilton et al., 2021). See Table 7.3 for common TCPs, settings used, and unique components.

TABLE 7.3 Common Transitional Care Programs

Transitional Care Program	Setting Used	Selected Components
Transitional Care Model (TCM) https://hign.org/consultgeri/try-this-series/transitional-care-model-tcm	Hospital-to-Home Transitions	• Home Visits • Hospital Screening Tool for High-Risk Older Adults
Care Transitions Intervention (CTI) https://caretransitions.health	Hospital-to-Home Transitions	• Transition Coach • Red Flags
Better Outcomes for Older Adults Through Safe Transitions (BOOST) https://psnet.ahrq.gov/innovation/project-boost-increases-patient-understanding-treatment-and-follow-care	Hospital-to-Home Transitions	• Risk Specific Interventions • Technical Assistance
Project Re-engineered Discharge (RED) https://www.ahrq.gov/patient-safety/settings/hospital/red/toolkit/index.html	Hospital-to-Home Transitions	• Discharge Plan Reconciliation with National Guidelines/Clinical Pathways • Emergency Plan
Chronic Care Model (CCM) https://www.act-center.org/application/files/1616/3511/6445/Model_Chronic_Care.pdf	Clinic to Home Transitions	• Decision Support • Self-Management Support
INTERACT™ https://pathway-interact.com/interact-tools/interact-tools-library/	Skilled Nursing Facility to Home Transitions	• Advanced Care Planning Tools • Care Path and Change in Condition Cards

(Enderlin et al., 2013, p. 49)

Some TCPs may not follow a specific model or tool kit but focus on particular settings or populations that are vulnerable or at higher risk for healthcare complications or costs. An example of this might be an elder-friendly emergency room that implements transitional care interventions because older adults account for up to 15% of all emergency room visits (Ukkonen et al., 2019). Many of these older adults have chronic health conditions such as congestive heart failure (CHF) or diabetes that can be exacerbated if not managed well at home. Specific interventions shown to reduce return emergency room visits are comprehensive needs assessment, caregiver involvement, self-management of health education, telephone call visits, and discharge planning (Jehloh et al., 2022). Transitional care interventions in this example might be offered to all elderly patients who visit the emergency room and may include an assessment at admission for potential barriers to discharge, self-management of health education, coordination of care with the PCP, and timely follow-up from the emergency room staff across settings and with the patient to ensure questions and potential safety issues or barriers are addressed.

TCPs Support of the Quintuple Aim

TCPs support better outcomes, lower costs, and improved patient experience by offering education for patients and their families/support systems, collaborative care planning, and face-to-face, telephone, and virtual support services. These essential services strengthen patients' ability to self-manage and monitor their health, leading to fewer emergency room visits and readmissions, lower costs, and improved outcomes (Wong, 2023). TCPs are delivered through various settings, including hospitals, skilled nursing facilities, and clinics. Due to the system-wide reach of TCPs, costs are managed in the acute care setting and across the continuum of care.

Each setting may offer slightly different TCPs, but all programs contribute to the goals of the Quintuple Aim. Health equity is addressed by meeting patients in the context of their lives and offering relevant and individualized support and resources that contribute to their being able to self-manage their health in the long term. Shared decision-making, care planning tools, and other interventions are offered to ensure continuity and care coordination across settings. Through a coordinated framework, TCPs work through steps of comprehensive assessment, education, medication reconciliation, follow-up, monitoring, and connecting needed resources, referrals, and support services to ensure a successful transition. By doing this, TCPs also contribute to clinicians' well-being by delivering quality care, enabling them to find value, meaning, and purpose in their work (Mehta et al., 2021).

TCPs Support of Coordinated Care

TCPs are based on efficient and effective care coordination. Proactive education is provided to ensure that health self-management goals and strategies are appropriate. The use of coordinated care planning, monitoring, and follow-up ensures that the right resources are used and costs are managed. The basis of a TCP is timeliness—to assess, plan for, and make needed connections to resources and services so that care is delivered in a timely manner in the right setting and at the least restrictive level of care.

Through advocacy and person-centered care, the right transition is made that meets patient needs, preferences, and outcomes. TCPs are designed to create the best possible transition plan, empower patients and their families/support systems, provide additional support and resources, ensure adequate monitoring and follow-up, and provide appropriate and relevant education. TCPs provide a time-limited bridge between one setting and another based on collaborative communication, with the goal of preventing poor outcomes and providing safe and quality care transition (NACNS, n.d.). "Transitional care interventions show the most promise for reducing hospitalizations and costs enough to generate net savings" (Schraeder & Shelton, 2011, p. 58).

Telehealth/Telemedicine/Virtual Healthcare

Although the terms "**telehealth**" "telemedicine" and "virtual healthcare" are often used interchangeably, they represent different aspects and focuses of digital healthcare delivery. The term "telehealth" indicates healthcare that is delivered virtually or digitally, which supports nonclinical health needs, links the patient with the provider, or allows remote delivery of clinical care. "Virtual healthcare" refers to healthcare offered through digital communication. This could be a real-time consultation via Zoom, a phone app that reminds patients to refill their medications, or an artificial intelligence (AI)-generated virtual assistant on a health-systems web page. Virtual healthcare links the patient and their provider for various purposes from any location with an internet connection, such as a provider messaging feature embedded in a patient's electronic health portal (Rajaee, 2023). "Telemedicine" is a type of virtual healthcare and refers to the use of technology to provide healthcare remotely, such as diagnosis and treatment. Telemedicine is delivered in real time through video conferencing or phone links (Rajaee, 2023). This could be a telemedicine specialist consultation, where the patient can receive specialist care and advice without attending an in-person appointment. It could also be the use of remote patient monitoring (RPM), where a patient's vital signs or other data are collected and sent to the patient's provider for review.

The differences between virtual healthcare and telemedicine relate to the scope and focus of the use of technology. Telemedicine focuses solely on clinical care, whereas virtual healthcare could also support nonclinical healthcare needs (Rajaee, 2023). Telemedicine is used for clinical outcomes such as diagnosis, treatment, and monitoring, using technology like video conferencing and RPM. Meanwhile, virtual healthcare may use more global technological applications such as AI-generated virtual assistance or mobile apps that support patient activation, engagement, and self-management of their health. See Figure 7.2 for a visual of the connection between telehealth, virtual health, and telemedicine.

Although about 60% of healthcare consumers are reported to expect telehealth availability for their healthcare appointments and to monitor items like lab results or medication renewals,

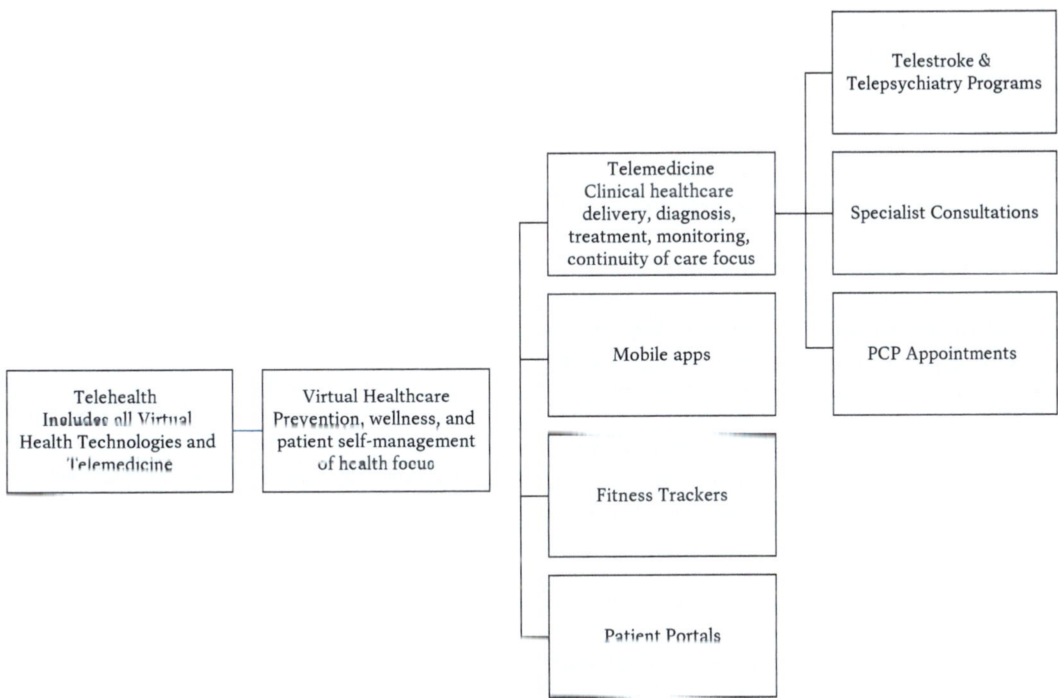

FIGURE 7.2 Telehealth, Virtual Healthcare, and Telemedicine Flowchart

there are some issues with telehealth (Edelmann, 2023). For it to be used effectively, the patient must be digitally literate, have internet connectivity for most applications, and some uses require specialized equipment, such as RPM devices. The need for these items for effective telehealth delivery may contribute to some healthcare equity issues. For example, "over one-quarter of the US population lacks broadband in their homes, concentrated among individuals with annual incomes less than $30,000" (Tilhou et al., 2024, p. 2). Those in areas without internet connectivity, without insurance coverage or the ability to privately purchase RPM devices, or the inability to participate in telehealth due to digital illiteracy will not be able to benefit from telehealth care, although they may need this type of healthcare delivery.

Digital literacy is a crucial requirement for effective use of telehealth. Digital literacy is the ability of a patient to "seek, find, understand, and appraise health information from electronic sources and apply the knowledge gained to addressing or solving a health problem" (Seidel et al., 2023, para. 1). About one-third of US residents lack basic digital skills, with Black and Hispanic populations being overrepresented in this group (Kendall et al., 2023, Takeaways). Additionally, about one-third of the 32 million Americans who cannot use a computer are seniors (TEC, 2021, para. 1). This can be problematic, as digital literacy is required for communication and collaboration with providers via telehealth systems and involves both cognitive and technical skills.

Patients must be able to retrieve and find information online and access and manage telehealth technologies (Seidel et al., 2023). Patients may have difficulty managing the technology, such as turning on cameras or sending messages electronically; they may not have the software needed to complete forms before an appointment, such as a PDF reader; or they may be uncomfortable communicating remotely (Telehealth.HHS.gov, 2023). Although telehealth improves convenience, access, patient engagement, and health equity issues, it is essential to be aware of and proactively address potential barriers to effective telehealth care delivery. This points to the importance of a comprehensive assessment by the care coordinating nurse to ensure that if telehealth interventions are in the care plan, they are appropriate for the patient or that proper education and training are provided for effective care coordination and positive patient outcomes and experiences.

Telehealth Support of the Quintuple Aim

Whether you are considering virtual healthcare or telemedicine specifically, these healthcare delivery models offer patients better accessibility to care, lower costs, and enhanced continuity of care. Barriers such as geographical area are overcome through the ability to attend consultations and other appointments without the need to participate face-to-face. This addresses the Quintuple Aim of equity by overcoming the barrier to access (Tilhou et al., 2024). Technology use reduces costs through timely healthcare delivery, which decreases emergency room visits and transportation costs for the patient. They also provide a convenient way to provide follow-up services, such as necessary referrals, support, and progress monitoring with the treatment plan, with the ability to make real-time changes as needed (Rajaee, 2023). Furthermore, "a majority of clinicians agreed or strongly agreed that telehealth gives them an opportunity to build rapport with patients (67–88%) and they are able to treat their patients' needs well through telehealth

(71–88%)" (Sugarman et al., 2021, p. 1401). In turn, use of virtual healthcare or telemedicine supports clinician well-being and sense of meaning and professional satisfaction.

Telehealth Support of Coordinated Care

Telehealth is a valuable tool for supported coordinated care in populations that may have issues with access to care, have social or mental health care needs, or have chronic conditions (Davidson et al., 2020). Telehealth care and services facilitate the engagement of the patient and their families/support systems in healthcare delivery and outcomes, can reduce acute care visits and manage costs. Telehealth supports care in the least restrictive environment and the lowest level of care by helping patients remain in their homes as they recover or receive continued treatment and monitoring. Telehealth services support interprofessional practice by simplifying needed transitions, meetings, or consultations with multiple providers and the patient, ensuring that the patient receives the right care. Moreover, telehealth services lend themselves to the immediacy of information and education that proactively addresses healthcare issues in a timely and accessible manner. Telehealth can be used to support all care coordination rights and guiding principles.

Accountable Health Communities (AHC)

The **Accountable Health Communities (AHC)** model was a **demonstration project** launched by the Centers for Medicare and Medicaid Services (CMS) in 2017 to test specific changes to the healthcare system, evaluating potential improvements in care quality, efficiency, and resource management across the system before permanent resource investment or infrastructure changes. The AHC utilized a systems-based care approach to the integration of public health and healthcare delivery with the goal of improving health outcomes and decreasing healthcare utilization through proactively addressing **health-related social needs (HRSNs)**, which are circumstances or needs that affect the capacity of a person to sustain health or well-being.

The focus on HSRNs in the AHC demonstration project was identified due to the estimation that up to "60% of preventable deaths are rooted in modifiable behaviors and exposures that occur in the community" (Alley et al., 2016, p. 8). It required a multisystem partnership between organizations that served the community and emphasized the shared accountability for the health of the community and making population-level changes in health and outcomes (NACO, n.d.). The AHC proactively connected patients with community resources to address any HRSNs to reduce costs and utilization

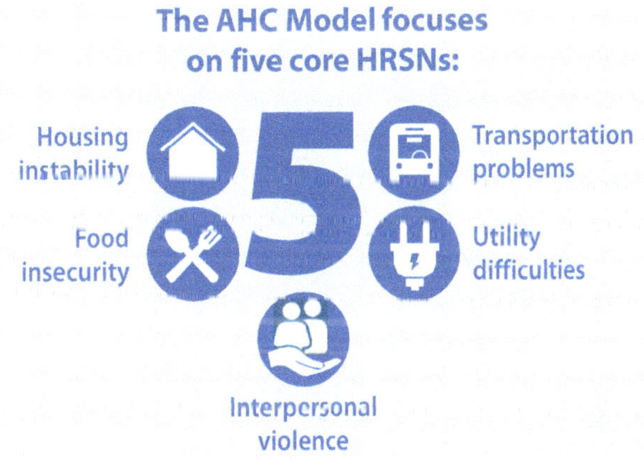

FIGURE 7.3 The AHC Model Focuses on Five Core HRSNs

of healthcare services and improve health outcomes (CMS, 2023a). Five core HRSNs were addressed in the AHC model: (a) housing, (b) food, (c) interpersonal violence, (d) transportation, and (e) utilities. See Figure 7.3 for the HRSN model.

The AHC offered screening for Medicare and Medicare recipients related to HRSNs and then connected the patient to community resources needed to support positive health outcomes. The screenings occurred across settings, and it was found that approximately 35% of patients screened reported at least one HRSN (Johnson et al., 2022). Navigation services were also offered in this model if the patient had one identified HRSN and two or more emergency room visits in the last year. A designated navigator followed up with patients concerning their HRSNs and worked with the patient to develop a plan to resolve the needs identified through connection with community resources (Johnson et al., 2022).

The AHC model has been shown to decrease emergency room visits, and patients reported being more engaged and proactive in seeking healthcare through the connection with community resources (CMS, 2023a; Health Affairs, 2023). Furthermore, it was found that respiratory illness exacerbations decreased among patients who received support for housing conditions and issues. The connection between environmental conditions and exacerbations is believed to have led to this decrease (CMS, 2023b).

Other studies have shown that system and community-level issues such as the lack of community resource infrastructure and reliable patient contact information (e.g., the housing insecure population, those without an address or contact phone number) decreased the efficacy of the AHC model (Health Affairs, 2023). Food insecurity was found to be the most prevalent HRSN in the AHC demonstration, and the most common infrastructure barriers identified in accessing community services were transportation, ineligibility for the service, wait lists, and the lack of resources in the community (CMS, 2023a).

The demonstration project for the AHC has ended with CMS. However, many participating organizations still use the systems and structures developed through their demonstration project to scale the model and expand HRSN across their health systems. CMS will likely continue to build on the AHC and integrate lessons learned into accountable care organizations (ACOs) or other initiatives, such as the Accountable Care Organization Realizing Equity, Access, and Community Health (ACO REACH) model, which requires ACOs to collect data concerning HRSNs for their patient populations to inform and advance health equity initiatives (CMS, 2022). Additionally, the AHC model can inform best practices for health systems, organizations, and communities nationwide concerning strategies that may assist in meeting patients' HRSNs that contribute to poor health outcomes.

Benefits of the AHC Model

"The AHC model reflects a growing emphasis on population health in CMS payment policy, which aims to support a transition from a health care delivery system to a true health system" (Alley, 2016, p. 11).

AHC Support of the Quintuple Aim

With the addition of health equity in the Quintuple Aim, nurses will see more population-level strategies implemented to address social, community, and system issues that contribute to a lack of equitable health resources and outcomes. The AHC model offers a valuable template for ways to contribute to better outcomes, lower costs, improve patient experience, and address health equity. Achieving better outcomes and costs will only be attainable by addressing healthcare inequity and addressing satisfaction and retention of the healthcare workforce (Mate, 2022). All parts will be needed to create a better healthcare system.

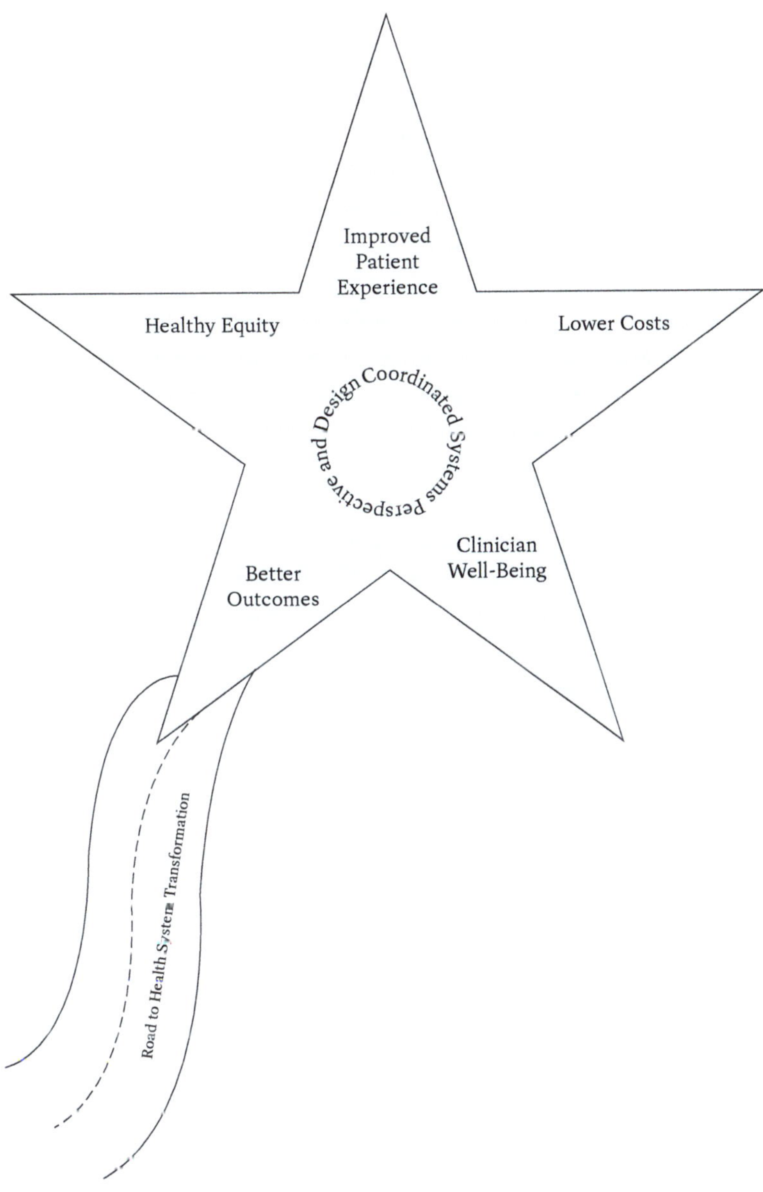

FIGURE 7.4 Health System Transformation Guiding Star

The Quintuple Aim can be viewed as a guiding star, rather than in a linear progression, pointing the way to the healthcare system transformation. The AHC model gives guidance on how to address patients' needs holistically and identifies needed system-level infrastructure development for an effective healthcare system that can meet HRSNs through a coordinated systems perspective design. See Figure 7.4 for a visual of the health system transformation guiding star, based upon the Quintuple Aim.

AHC Support of Coordinated Care

The AHC framework and acknowledgment of the extensive impact of HRSNs on health, patient experience, and resource use calls for all healthcare workers to engage in coordinated care across the continuum. When HRSNs can be addressed effectively, it has been shown to decrease healthcare utilization. However, this will require nurses to engage in effective interprofessional teamwork and collaborative practice and be knowledgeable concerning community resources. AHC delivers a person- and relationship-centered care model that promotes the patient receiving the right care and offers coordination of referrals and resources so the patient can receive care at the lowest level of care required, allowing for decreased resource use. Through screening for HRSNs, the right resources can be provided and monitored for effectiveness, assisting in long-term health outcomes and offering needed education on accessing resources, information, and self-management of health. Although many areas of the nation may need more community resource infrastructure to implement the AHC fully, the model offers a vision of where the healthcare system can evolve and the importance of coordinated care holistically meeting the patient's needs.

CHAPTER SUMMARY

As healthcare evolves and develops new healthcare delivery models, the need to integrate systems-level continuity of care and care coordination and management will be essential. The use of value-based healthcare strategies and reimbursement brings to the forefront how all the parts of the healthcare system work together (Young, 2022). We can think of a car and how it gets us from one place to another, but it will not get us to our endpoint if the radiator is not working (Mate, 2022). All parts of the car, just like the healthcare system, need to work together for the outcome of coordinated, quality, safe, cost-effective, and value-added care delivery.

Healthcare systems and models must provide clinical integration across the continuum of care, including management and transfer of patient information and data for seamless care transitions. Specific programs must be integrated to address those with chronic health conditions or other population-health needs, including assessing and addressing any HRSN barriers or challenges. These programs must be designed and delivered with a framework of continuous quality improvement and leveraging health information technologies that can be used across healthcare systems, generate data concerning quality measures and at-risk patients, and facilitate closed-loop communications, transitions, and referrals (AHA, 2019). See Figure 7.5 for a visual of what care coordination practices and services will need to be offered to integrate a coordinated systems perspective and design into a transformed healthcare system.

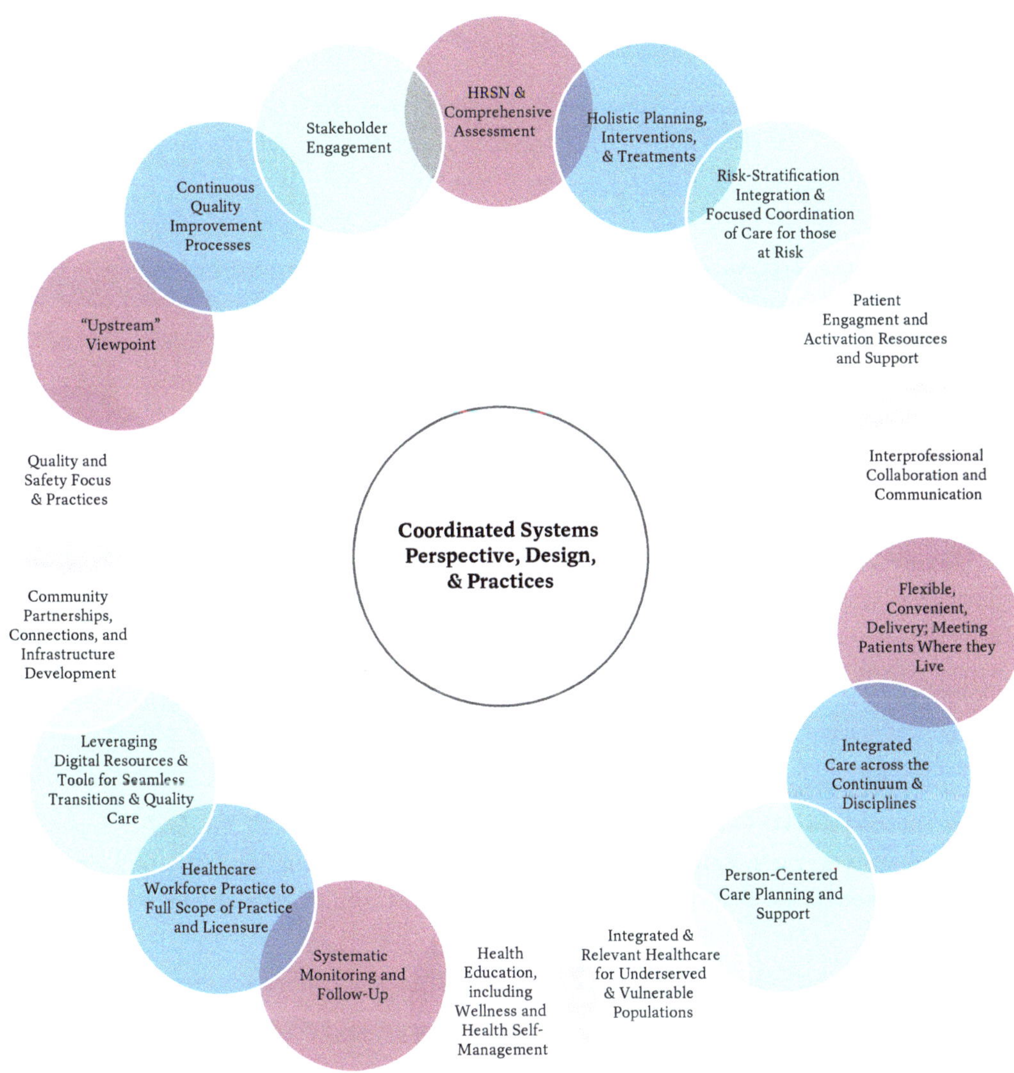

FIGURE 7.5 Health System Transformation: Coordinated Systems Perspective, Design, and Practices

Healthcare transformation, integration, and financial support of coordinated and innovative healthcare delivery designs will require governmental, payer, organizational, and health system support that streamlines processes and regulations. Through innovative care delivery designs that integrate coordinated systems of care level perspectives and infrastructures, meaning and purpose in the work nurses and other healthcare providers deliver can be sustained. The quality and effectiveness of care can be enhanced, and barriers to providing person- and relationship-centered care can be alleviated. Ultimately, this ensures successful transitions, care coordination, better outcomes, cost and resource management, and sustainability of the healthcare system.

New Models Are Hard Work

"Health system leaders reported that adopting a new care model is **hard, time-consuming work** because it redefines the responsibilities of providers who provide the care and how they do it" (AHA, 2019, p. 5).

CHAPTER 7 GLOSSARY

Accountable Health Communities (AHC): A systems-based care approach integration of public health and healthcare delivery with the goal of improving health outcomes and decreasing healthcare utilization through proactively addressing HRSNs.

Advanced Primary Care (PCMH): A comprehensive primary care model that focuses on quality, safe, person-centered, and coordinated care, and provides accessible services.

Change Drivers: External (e.g., technology development, reimbursement processes) or internal factors (e.g., workforce shortages, patient satisfaction) that affect the healthcare system and how care is delivered.

Collaborative Care Model (CoCM): A cohesive healthcare model providing integrated team-based primary medical care and mental health and/or substance use disorder care and services, often with services co-located.

Demonstration Project: Centers for Medicare and Medicaid projects that test changes to the healthcare system, evaluating potential improvements in care quality, efficiency, or resource management across the health system before permanent resource investment or infrastructure changes.

Digital Literacy: The cognitive and technical skills needed to retrieve and find information electronically, access and utilize telehealth technologies, and communicate and collaborate with healthcare providers.

Downstream Healthcare: Healthcare delivered after a medical event or need occurs, such as chronic disease management.

Federally Qualified Health Center (FQHC): A federally funded outpatient clinic or health center that provides comprehensive services for all age groups, offers after-hours access, and bases charges on a sliding scale in medically underserved areas or with healthcare provider shortages.

Health Related Social Need (HRSN): Circumstances or needs that affect the capacity of a person to sustain health or well-being, including housing instability, food insecurity, interpersonal violence, or transportation or utility difficulties.

Home-Based Primary Care (HBPC): Primary healthcare delivered in a patient's home or residence for those who have difficulty leaving their home, often utilizing an interprofessional team-based approach and following the patient through end of life.

Patient Panel: The population of patients assigned to or associated with a provider or clinic.

Substance Use Disorder (SUD): A disorder that affects the brain and behavior, with varying levels of symptoms that lead to the inability of a person to control their use of substances, including medications, alcohol, and illegal substances.

Teamlet: A team of one provider and one or two other healthcare workers (e.g., MA, RN, LPN, SW, etc.) that work together daily, usually in a primary care setting.

Telehealth: Healthcare that is delivered virtually or digitally, which supports nonclinical health needs, links the patient with the provider, or allows remote delivery of clinical care.

Transitional Care Programs (TCPs): Healthcare that provides time-limited services, follow-up, and support during transitions between settings for patients with a moderately complex transition due to health conditions, social determinants of health, or other issues.

Upstream Healthcare: Healthcare that seeks to address root causes of healthcare issues, rather than focus on disease or symptom management, to improve long-term health outcomes and manage resources and costs of healthcare.

DISCUSSION QUESTIONS AND ACTIVITIES

Discussion Questions

1. Identify one current change driver in the healthcare system and discuss how it promotes the development of innovative healthcare delivery models. Describe how a healthcare model could integrate addressing the identified change driver in their innovative delivery designs.
2. Discuss how HRSNs can contribute to poor health outcomes and how integrated care delivery models such as the CoCM can address these issues.
3. Discuss the teamlet concept and how the teamlet can assist in meeting the Quintuple Aim and care coordination rights.
4. Home-based primary care (HBPC) is a person-centered approach to healthcare delivery, yet there are several barriers to its implementation on a large scale. Identify two changes that need to happen in the healthcare system to address these barriers, and explore what might be required to make those changes.
5. For healthcare transformation to occur and innovative models of healthcare delivery to evolve, responsibilities, roles, priorities of care, and how nurses provide care will need to be reenvisioned. Discuss how you see the responsibilities, roles, and how nurses do their work evolving in these innovative healthcare delivery designs.

Activities

1. In teams (of no more than six), work together to create ideas, connect ideas, or combine ideas to describe how you would design a new innovative healthcare delivery model that would support care coordination and continuity of care.

   a. Each participant will initially generate their own ideas using the template below. Each participant will write three ideas within 5 to 10 minutes.

How to design a new innovative healthcare delivery model			
	Idea 1	**Idea 2**	**Idea 3**
Participant 1			
Participant 2			
Participant 3			
Participant 4			
Participant 5			
Participant 6			

   b. Once everyone has completed their template, do the following as a team:

      - Review all the ideas.
      - Delete duplicates, combine similar ideas, or connect more than one idea to make a cohesive new idea encompassing all those connected.
      - Decide upon your top idea as a team.

   c. As a team, complete a SWOT (strengths, weaknesses, opportunities, and threats) analysis concerning the implementation of your team idea. A strength would reflect what your idea would do well or offer or what resources it would provide. A weakness would concern what other stakeholders might see as an issue with your design idea or barriers to implementation. An opportunity might be what change drivers your idea takes advantage of or how your idea can contribute to a robust health system. A threat might be something that would derail your idea from implementation or other competing innovative designs.

      - You may use the template below for your SWOT analysis. Identify at least one strength, one weakness, one opportunity, and one threat.

2. Choose two different innovative healthcare delivery models presented and compare and contrast the models. Include how each model addresses coordination and continuity of care, what patient and system outcomes the model focuses upon, the commonalities between the models, and how they differ.

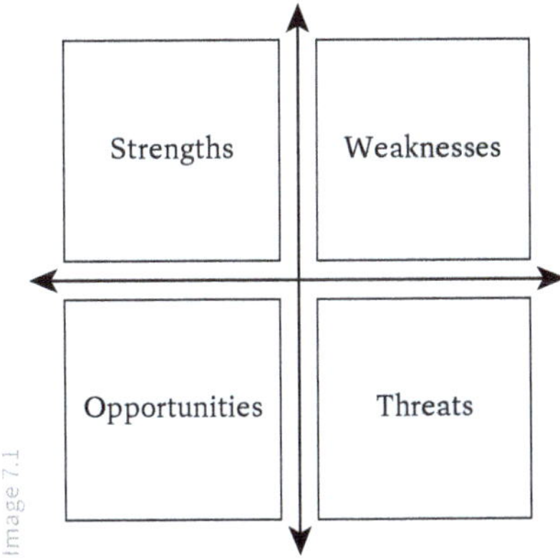

3. Transitional Care Program (TCP) Case Study

   Mr. Martin is a 72-year-old retired carpenter who lives alone in a long-term stay motel room in a rural area. He has a grandson who lives about 15 miles away and assists him to the grocery store and laundromat once a week. Mr. Martin has hypercholesteremia and hypertension and will be discharged in the next couple of days from the hospital following a coronary artery bypass (CABG) surgery. The cardiovascular intensive care unit (CVICU) nurse knows that Mr. Martin meets the hospital transitional care program criteria, so he has notified the transition case manager of Mr. Martin's admission. The transitions case manager met with Mr. Martin to explain the transitions program and noticed that Mr. Martin had several discharge teaching information sheets on his bedside table under his lunch tray. The transitions case manager also noticed Mr. Martin seemed very fatigued, often closing his eyes. Mr. Martin says he is waiting for the pharmacist to come by and tell him about all his new medications and that his girlfriend will be by later to take all of this "stuff" to her place, as he will stay there for a couple of days post-discharge.

   - Identify two areas concerning this interaction that must be addressed in the transition care plan. How should the transitional case manager address these issues using the nursing process?

   The transitional case manager arrived at Mr. Martin's residence for a home visit two days post-discharge. The transitional case manager asks Mr. Martin to gather all his medications and paperwork so they can review them together. Mr. Martin indicates that he no longer has any paperwork; he thinks it is still at his girlfriend's house. He does gather his prescribed and over-the-counter medications but says he is still waiting for one that his grandson was supposed to pick it up but has yet to get. Mr. Martin then asks why the transitional case manager is there.

   - How would you describe the role of the transitional care program case manager to Mr. Martin?

   - What barriers have been discovered in the visit that may contribute to poor patient outcomes? How should the transitional care manager address these barriers?

   Mr. Martin has been discharged for two weeks, and the transitional care manager is doing a follow-up virtual visit. Mr. Martin joins the virtual call and says he is feeling better, but the transitional care manager notices he is disheveled, and it looks like he hasn't had a shower for several days.

- What types of questions should the transitional care manager ask to determine if Mr. Martin is doing well?
- Are there things in the environment the transitional care manager should look for?

The follow-up virtual visit is ending.

- How should the transitional care manager end this interaction to ensure that the patient has positive outcomes and successfully transitions to his residence and community?

NCLEX STYLE QUESTIONS

1. You are a transitional program care manager meeting with a patient hospitalized for surgical intervention of a bowel obstruction. The patient will be discharged home later in the day with home health nursing to monitor surgical wound healing and physical therapy for mobility and strengthening. As you meet with the patient to discuss the transitional care program, which of the following should you include in your teaching? (Select all that apply.)

   a. Discuss with the patient any questions or concerns about the new medications prescribed.

   b. Review and provide a written follow-up plan, including names to contact with questions.

   c. Indicate to the patient that prior to the patient leaving the hospital, they will want to ask the physical therapist any questions they might have.

   d. Suggest the patient collect all their discharge information and paperwork and give it to the home health nurse.

2. A patient was sent home with instructions to request their medication refills in their patient portal, as this will make the request easy and keep a record of it, so the patient portal system will send a text message reminder when a refill is due. The patient attempts to request the refill but has difficulty finding where to do this in the patient portal. This represents which of the following barriers to using virtual healthcare services.

   a. Connectivity

   b. Specialized Equipment

   c. Digital Literacy

   d. Software

3. Several change drivers affect how healthcare delivery models are evolving. Some of these are internal drivers and others are external drivers. Which of the following is an external change driver? (Select all that apply.)

a. Rise of consumerism

b. Workforce shortages

c. Organizational policies

d. Expansion of digital technologies

4. You are precepting a student nurse in your CoCM clinic and explaining to the student the benefits of the integrated CoCM. The student understands how this care integration benefits the patient when they say the following to you: (Select all that apply.)

   a. Your clinic offers services for those with medical and mental health needs in the same spot because people with both these conditions can't manage their care effectively.

   b. Your clinic uses population-based care for those at most risk of poor outcomes by integrating medical and mental health care needs in one location.

   c. Your clinic offers integrated care so providers can quickly see more patients, enhancing accessibility.

   d. Your clinic offers comprehensive medical and mental health care to address patients' holistic needs.

5. Advanced primary care is also known as which of the following.

   a. House Calls

   b. AHC

   c. PCMH

   d. FQHC

6. You are explaining the concept of the PCMH and what it can offer to a new patient in your PCMH clinic. The patient understands the education provided during teach-back when they tell you which of the following: (Select all that apply.)

   a. The PCMH is in a central location, just like a house, where all my care needs can be provided.

   b. The PCMH will offer me comprehensive care services with coordinated care using an interprofessional team.

   c. The PCMH will help me get more downstream services and care.

   d. The PCMH might assign me to a teamlet that will include my primary care provider.

7. You are the discharge planner at the regional trauma center. You are meeting with a patient who had been life-flighted to the trauma center after a farm tractor accident. While meeting with the patient to discuss the discharge plan, you find that the patient does not have a primary care provider, is a migrant farmworker, does not have insurance, and lives in an area with a primary care provider shortage. You know which of the following models is the best healthcare delivery system for this patient when they return home:

   a. PCMH
   b. AHC
   c. FQHC
   d. CoCM

8. You are working with a patient who is being discharged to an assisted living facility (ALF). They do not have a primary care provider, but you know that the ALF has a provider that will take on patients who are residents of the ALF. You are explaining this to the patient and describing which of the following healthcare models?

   a. AHC
   b. TCP
   c. Telehealth
   d. HBPC

9. The HBPC, although an innovative healthcare model, has several barriers to delivery. These barriers include which of the following:

   a. Potential provider and patient safety issues
   b. Lack of financial reimbursement
   c. Travel time between patients
   d. All of the above

10. Using the HBPC model can reduce several issues related to fragmented care. These include which of the following: (Select all that apply.)

   a. Emergency room visits
   b. Missed medical appointments
   c. Self-management of health
   d. Psychiatric hospital admissions

11. You are a nurse care coordinator for a rural clinic. Your clinic has just opened a telemedicine room that patients can use for their appointments. You are designing an educational flyer to inform your clinic's panel of patients about this new service. Which of the following sentences would you include in the service description?
    a. The new telemedicine room will be available for real-time virtual consultations or appointments, decreasing your need to drive into town for clinical care.
    b. The new telemedicine room will provide an artificial intelligence virtual assistant to help you search for health information related to your health conditions.
    c. The new telemedicine room will download remote patient monitoring device data.
    d. The new telemedicine room will only be available to those who show digital literacy competency.

12. Which of the following does HRSN stand for?
    a. Health-related substance needs
    b. Health-related shared needs
    c. Health-related system needs
    d. Heath-related social needs

13. The Accountable Health Community model has been shown to do which of the following: (Select all that apply.)
    a. Decrease emergency room visits
    b. Decrease respiratory illness exacerbations
    c. Increase community resources
    d. Increase reliable patient contact information

14. Healthcare that seeks to address the root causes of health issues is called what type of healthcare?
    a. Downriver healthcare
    b. Root cause healthcare
    c. Upstream healthcare
    d. Social needs-based healthcare

15. The foundation of the PCMH has five components, including which of the following: (Select all that apply.)

    a. Quality and safety and accessible services

    b. Focused assessment and coordinated care

    c. Population-health and person-centered care

    d. Comprehensive care and continuous services

REFERENCES

Agency for Healthcare Research and Quality (AHRQ). (2022). *Defining the PCMH.* https://www.ahrq.gov/ncepcr/research/care-coordination/pcmh/define.html

Alley, D. E., Asomugha, C. N., Conway, P. H., & Sanghavi, D. M. (2016). Accountable health communities—addressing social needs through Medicare and Medicaid. *The New England Journal of Medicine, 374*(1), 8–11. https://doi.org/10.1056/NEJMp1512532

American Hospital Association (AHA). (2010). *Patient-Centered Medical Home (PCMH): AHA research synthesis report.* https://www.aha.org/system/files/2018-02/patient-centered-medical-home-aha-research-synthesis-report-2010.pdf

American Hospital Association (AHA). (2019). *Evolving care models: Aligning care delivery to emerging payment models.* https://www.aha.org/system/files/media/file/2019/04/MarketInsights_CareModelsReport.pdf

American Psychiatric Association. (n.d.). *The role of collaborative care in reducing mental health inequities.* https://www.psychiatry.org/getmedia/e24b9d4f-df28-43a1-8359-25cc4f9de661/APA-Role-CoCM-Reducing-Mental-Health-Inequities.pdf

Centers for Medicare and Medicaid Services (CMS). (2022). *ACO realizing equity, access, and community health (REACH) model: Request for applications.* https://www.cms.gov/priorities/innovation/media/document/aco-reach-rfa

Centers for Medicare and Medicaid Services (CMS). (2023a). *Accountable health communities' model 2018–2021: Findings at a glance.* https://www.cms.gov/priorities/innovation/data-and-reports/2023/ahc-second-eval-rpt-fg

Centers for Medicare and Medicaid Services (CMS). (2023b). *Accountable health communities (AHC) model evaluation: Second evaluation report.* https://www.cms.gov/priorities/innovation/data-and-reports/2023/ahc-second-eval-rpt

Chandrashekar, P., Moodley, S., & Jain, S. H. (2019). 5 obstacles to home-based health care, and how to overcome them. *Harvard Business Review.* https://hbr.org/2019/10/5-obstacles-to-home-based-health-care-and-how-to-overcome-them

Cornwell, T. (2019). Home-based primary care's perfect storm. *Home Centered Care Institute.* https://www.hccinstitute.org/app/uploads/2020/03/Perfect-Storm_200302.pdf?x18749&x31299

Davidson, R., Barrett, D. I., Rixon, L., Newman, S., & ACT Program (2020). How the integration of telehealth and coordinated care approaches impact health care service organization structure and ethos: Mixed methods study. *JMIR Nursing, 3*(1), e20282. https://doi.org/10.2196/20282

Dickson, K. S., Holt, T., & Arredondo, E. (2022). Applying implementation mapping to expand a care coordination program at a Federally Qualified Health Center. *Frontiers in Public Health, 10,* 844898. https://doi.org/10.3389/fpubh.2022.844898

Edelmann, S. (2023). *The innovative healthcare delivery models that will drive patient-centered care.* https://healthcaretransformers.com/value-based-healthcare/innovative-healthcare-delivery-models-driving-patient-centered-care/

Enderlin, C. A., McLeskey, N., Rooker, J. L., Steinhauser, C., D'Avolio, D., Gusewelle, R., & Ennen, K. A. (2013). Review of current conceptual models and frameworks to guide transitions of care in older adults. *Geriatric Nursing, 34*(1), 47–52. https://doi.org/10.1016/j.gerinurse.2012.08.003

Farrell, T., Greer, A., Bennie, S., Hageman, H., & Pfeifle, A. (2023). Academic health centers and the Quintuple Aim of health care. *Academic Medicine, 98* (5), 563–568. https://doi.org/10.1097/ACM.0000000000005031.

FQHC Associates. (n.d.). *What is an FQHC?* https://www.fqhc.org/what-is-an-fqhc

Grys, C. A. (2022). Digital health: The next evolution of healthcare delivery. *Nursing, 52*(10), 40–43. https://doi.org/10.1097/01.NURSE.0000872464.40584.87

Health Affairs. (2023). *Ahead of print: Evaluating CMS's accountable health communities' model's effectiveness.* https://www.healthaffairs.org/content/forefront/ahead-print-evaluating-cms-s-accountable-health-communities-model-s-effectiveness

Home Centered Care Institute (HCCI). (2020). *The future of healthcare is in the home.* https://www.hccinstitute.org/app/uploads/2020/10/HCCI-Prospectus_201001_Final.pdf?x32444

Itchhaporia, D. (2021). The evolution of the Quintuple Aim: Health equity, health outcomes, and the economy. *Journal of the American College of Cardiology, 78*(22), 2262–2264. https://www.jacc.org/doi/10.1016/j.jacc.2021.10.018

Jackson-Triche, M. E., Unützer, J., & Wells, K. B. (2020). Achieving mental health equity: Collaborative care. *The Psychiatric Clinics of North America, 43*(3), 501–510. https://doi.org/10.1016/j.psc.2020.05.008

James, T. (2020). *What is upstream healthcare?* Boston Medical Center Health System. https://healthcity.bmc.org/population-health/upstream-healthcare-sdoh-root-causes

Jehloh, L., Songwathana, P., & Sae-Sia, W. (2022). Transitional care interventions to reduce emergency department visits in older adults: A systematic review. *Belitung Nursing Journal, 8*(3), 187–196. https://doi.org/10.33546/bnj.2100

Johnson, K. A., Barolin, N., Ogbue, C., & Vaerlander, K. (2022) Lessons from five years of the CMS accountable health communities model. *Health Affairs.* https://www.healthaffairs.org/content/forefront/lessons-five-years-cms-accountable-health-communities-model

Karaferis, D., Aletras, V., & Niakas, D. (2022). Determining dimensions of job satisfaction in healthcare using factor analysis. *BMC Psychology, 10*(1), 240. https://doi.org/10.1186/s40359-022-00941-2

Kendall, J., Colavito, A., & Moller, Z. (2023). America's digital skills divide. *Third Way.* http://thirdway.imgix.net/pdfs/americas-digital-skills-divide.pdf

Maeng, D. D., Sciandra, J. P., & Tomcavage, J. F. (2016). The impact of a regional patient-centered medical home initiative on cost of care among commercially insured population in the US. *Risk Management and Healthcare Policy, 9*, 67–74. https://doi.org/10.2147/RMHP.S102826

Marder, K. S. (2022). Improving transitional care management: A five-step framework. *HealthCatalyst.* https://www.healthcatalyst.com/insights/improving-transitional-care-management-five-steps

Mason, L., Perez, D., McLemore, A., Monica R., & Dickson E. (2021). *Policy & politics in nursing and health care* (8th Ed.). Elsevier Health Sciences.

Mate, K. (2022). On the Quintuple Aim: Why expand beyond the triple aim? *Institute for Healthcare Improvement.* https://www.ihi.org/insights/quintuple-aim-why-expand-beyond-triple-aim#:~:text=Cooper%2C%20MD%2C%20MPH%2C%20and,all%20without%20these%20additional%20aims.

McGilton, K. S., Vellani, S., Krassikova, A., Robertson, S., Irwin, C., Cumal, A., Bethell, J., Burr, E., Keatings, M., McKay, S., Nichol, K., Puts, M., Singh, A., & Sidani, S. (2021). Understanding transitional care programs for older adults who experience delayed discharge: A scoping review. *BMC Geriatrics, 21*(210), 1–18. https://doi.org/10.1186/s12877-021-02099-9

Medicare Learning Network. (2022). *Chronic care management services.* https://www.cms.gov/outreach-and-education/medicare-learning-network-mln/mlnproducts/downloads/chroniccaremanagement.pdf

Medicare Learning Network. (2023). *Federally Qualified Health Center.* https://www.cms.gov/files/document/mln006397-federally-qualified-health-center.pdf

Mehta, L. S., Elkind, M. S. V., Achenbach, S., Pinto, F. J., & Poppas, A. (2021). Clinician well-being: Addressing global needs for improvements in the health care field: a joint statement from the American College of Cardiology, American Heart Association, European Society of Cardiology, and World Heart Federation. *Global Heart, 16*(1), 1–5. https://doi.org/10.5334/gh.1067

Melek, S. P., Norris D. T., Paulus, J., Matthews, K., Weaver, A., & Davenport S. (2018). *Potential economic impact of integrated medical-behavioral healthcare: Updated projections for 2017.* Milliman. https://www.milliman.com/-/media/milliman/importedfiles/uploadedfiles/insight/2018/potential-economic-impact-integrated-healthcare.ashx

National Association of Clinical Nurse Specialists (NACNS). (n.d.). *Definitions of transitional care.* https://nacns.org/resources/toolkits-and-reports/transitions-of-care/definitions-of-transitional-care/#:~:text=Transitional%20Care%20Definition%3A&text=Transitional%20Care%3A%20is%20a%20set,care%20within%20the%20same%20location.

National Association of Counties (NACO). (n.d.). *Profiles of county innovations in health care delivery: Accountable care communities.* https://www.naco.org/sites/default/files/documents/Accountable-Care-Communities.pdf

National Council for Quality Assurance. (2024). *Patient-centered medical home recognition.* https://www.ncqa.org/employers/ncqa-programs-of-interest-to-employers/patient-centered-medical-home-recognition/

National Institute of Mental Health (NIMH). (2023). *Substance use and co-occurring mental disorders.* https://www.nimh.nih.gov/health/topics/substance-use-and-mental-health#:~:text=Substance%20use%20disorder%20(SUD)%20is,most%20severe%20form%20of%20SUD.

Naylor, M. D., Aiken, L. H., Kurtzman, E. T., Olds, D. M., & Hirschman, K. B. (2011). The care span: The importance of transitional care in achieving health reform. *Health affairs (Project Hope), 30*(4), 746–754. https://doi.org/10.1377/hlthaff.2011.0041

Rajaee, L. (2023). Virtual care vs telehealth: Understanding the distinctions. *Elation.* https://www.elationhealth.com/resources/blogs/virtual-care-vs-telehealth-understanding-the-distinctions

Rural Health Information Hub (RHIHub). (2023). *Federally Qualified Health Centers (FQHCs) and the health center program.* https://www.ruralhealthinfo.org/topics/federally-qualified-health-centers

Schraeder, C., & Shelton, P. (Eds.). (2011). *Comprehensive care coordination for chronically ill adults.* Wiley-Blackwell.

Seidel, E., Cortes, T., & Chong, C., (2023). Digital health literacy. *The PSNet Collection.* https://psnet.ahrq.gov/primer/digital-health-literacy#:~:text=Examples%20of%20digital%20health%20literacy,communicate%20with%20healthcare%20providers%20electronically.

Sugarman, D. E., Horvitz, L. E., Greenfield, S. F., & Busch, A. B. (2021). Clinicians' perceptions of rapid scale-up of telehealth services in outpatient mental health treatment. *Telemedicine Journal and E-health: The Official Journal of the American Telemedicine Association, 27*(12), 1399–1408. https://doi.org/10.1089/tmj.2020.0481

Telehealth Equity Coalition (TEC). (2021). *Improving digital literacy to improve telehealth equity.* https://www.telehealthequitycoalition.org/improving-digital-literacy-to-improve-telehealth-equity.html

Telehealth.HHS.gov. (2023). *Improving access to telehealth.* https://telehealth.hhs.gov/providers/health-equity-in-telehealth/improving-access-to-telehealth#telehealth-for-patients-with-low-digital-literacy

Tilhou, A. S., Jain, A., & DeLeire, T. (2024). Telehealth expansion, internet speed, and primary care access before and during COVID-19. *JAMA Network Open*, 7(1), e2347686. https://doi.org/10.1001/jamanetworkopen.2023.47686

Totten, A. M., White-Chu, E. F., Wasson N., Morgan, E., Kansagara, D., Davis-O'Reilly, C., Goodlin, S. (2016). Home-based primary care interventions. *Agency for Healthcare Research and Quality.* https://www.ncbi.nlm.nih.gov/books/NBK356253/pdf/Bookshelf_NBK356253.pdf

Ukkonen, M., Jämsen, E., Zeitlin, R., & Pauniaho, S. L. (2019). Emergency department visits in older patients: A population-based survey. *BMC Emergency Medicine, 19*(20), 1–8. https://doi.org/10.1186/s12873-019-0236-3

Veet, C. A., Radomski, T. R., D'Avella, C., Hernandez, I., Wessel, C., Swart, E. C. S., Shrank, W. H., & Parekh, N. (2020). Impact of healthcare delivery system type on clinical, utilization, and cost outcomes of patient-centered medical homes: A systematic review. *Journal of General Internal Medicine, 35*(4), 1276–1284. https://doi.org/10.1007/s11606-019-05594-3

Welkin. (2021). *Transition care management: Transitioning patients to a new care setting.* https://welkinhealth.com/transition-care/

Wong, C. (2023). The 5 transitional care models and their impact on patient outcomes. *Experience.care.* https://experience.care/blog/5-transitional-care-models/

World Health Organization (WHO). (2022). *Aging and health.* https://www.who.int/news-room/fact-sheets/detail/ageing-and-health

Young, M. (2022). Focus on Quintuple Aim to address workforce burnout and equity. *Relias Media.* https://www.reliasmedia.com/articles/149298-focus-on-quintuple-aim-to-address-workforce-burnout-and-equity#:~:text=Focus%20on%20Quintuple%20Aim%20to%20Address%20Workforce%20Burnout%20and%20Equity,-May%201%2C%202022&text=By%20Melinda%20Young-,If%20there%20is%20anything%20the%20COVID%2D19%20crisis%20has%20shown,to%20improve%20value%2Dbased%20care.

Zimlichman, E., Nicklin, W., Aggarwal, R., & Bates, D. (2021, March 3). Health care 2030: The coming transformation. *NEJM Catalyst.* https://catalyst.nejm.org/doi/full/10.1056/CAT.20.0569

Credits

Table 7.2: Jayne Josephsen, "Federally Qualified Health Centers (FQHCs) and the Health Center Program," RHIhub. Copyright © 2023 by Rural Health Information Hub.

Fig. 7.3: CDC, https://www.cms.gov/priorities/innovation/data-and-reports/2023/ahc-second-eval-rpt-fg, 2023.

Fig. 7.4: D. Itchhaporia, "The Evolution of the Quintuple Aim: Health Equity, Health Outcomes, and the Economy," *Journal of the American College of Cardiology*, vol. 78, no. 22. Copyright © 2021 by American College of Cardiology Foundation.

CHAPTER 8

Healthcare Financing and Value-Based Payment Models

LEARNING OBJECTIVES

1. Examine healthcare financing models.
2. Identify key components of value-based payment models.
3. Understand how healthcare financing models may impact care coordination practice.
4. Recognize the benefits and limitations of various healthcare financing models.

KEY TERMS

- Accountable Care Organization (ACO)
- ambulatory payment classifications (APC)
- capitated payment
- case mix index (CMI)
- critical access hospitals (CAH)
- diagnostic-related group (DRG)
- dual-eligible
- episodic payment/bundled payment
- fee-for-service
- healthcare financing
- length of stay (LOS)
- Medicaid
- Medicare
- Medigap Plan
- prospective payment
- retrospective payment
- rural emergency hospital (REH)
- self-funded insurance
- shared savings
- third-party payer
- value-based healthcare

Introduction

In the United States, healthcare financing and payment models can be as complicated as the healthcare system. This makes navigating and understanding the payment models confusing for patients and nurses. **Healthcare financing** concerns how the healthcare organization or setting gets reimbursed or paid for services and supplies provided. In the United States, this is done mainly through third-party payers or commercial insurance providers that pay for much of the healthcare

Third Party
Payer Insurance
Provider
Co-Pays,
Deductibles
Premiums
Utilization
Review
Charges
for
Services
Pre-
Authorization &
Authorization of
Services
Coding for
Supplies and
Services
Billing
Insurance
Claims
Identified
Third Party
Healthcare Quality
Measures Met or
Not Met
Payer Denials
and Provider
Appeals
?

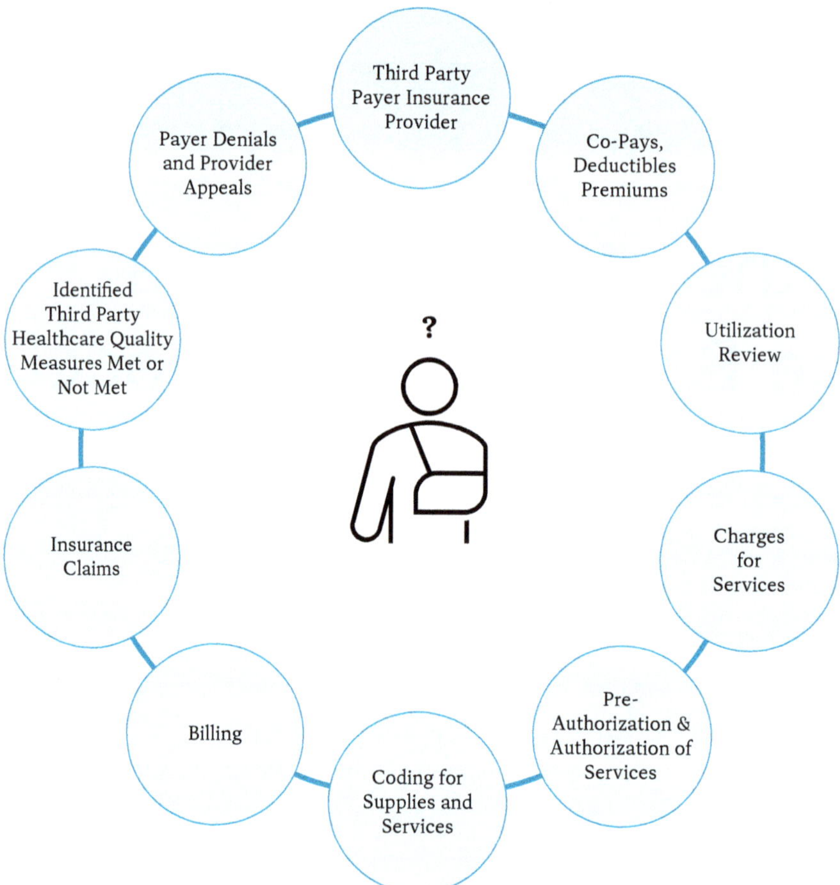

FIGURE 8.1 Healthcare Financing System Components

patients receive (Finkler et al., 2019). However, sometimes patients pay out of pocket for healthcare services. The use of third-party payers contributes to a complex system of payment that requires coding of services and billing for services, as well as a utilization review, insurance claims, and collection of quality benchmark data that may affect reimbursement rates. This often leaves the patient in the middle of a system in which there may be a lack of price transparency, and patients may not understand how services are authorized and recommended or how costs, co-pays, and deductibles are determined. See Figure 8.1—Healthcare Financing System Components.

Healthcare reimbursement and payment systems are further complicated by several differing payment models designed to assist in healthcare transformation and bring value to the healthcare delivered. The advent of value-based payment structures, such as the Medicare Improvements for Patients and Providers Act in 2008 and the Affordable Care Act in 2010, has set the tone for healthcare transformation from a **fee-for-service** payment model to a focus on value and quality in care received (CMS, 2023a, September 6). Over the years, several more programs have been introduced, and legislation continues to promote connecting value and quality with healthcare delivery. As a result of this, many third-party payers connect reimbursement rates to clinical quality measures, and several different healthcare financing models have been developed. See

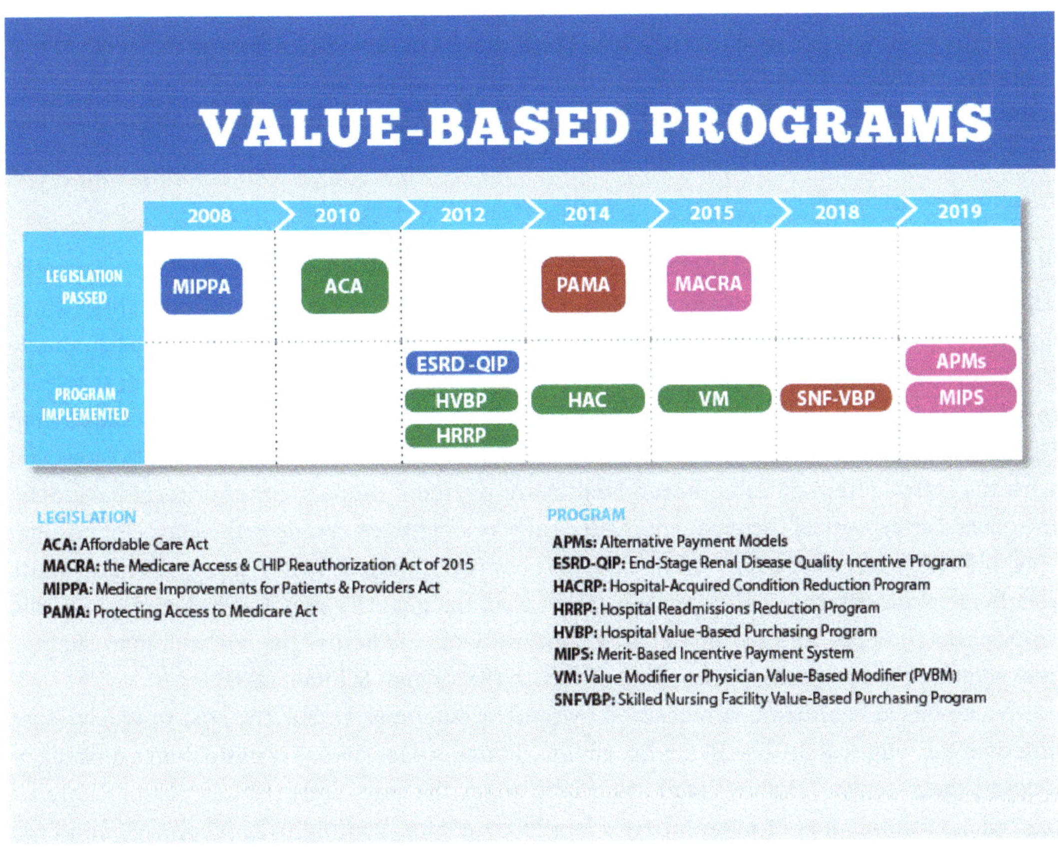

FIGURE 8.2 Value-Based Programs Timeline

Figure 8.2 for a timeline of legislation passed and value-based programs implemented by the Centers for Medicare and Medicaid Services (CMS).

Value-based healthcare on an individual level aims to assist patients in attaining better health outcomes and managing their healthcare costs while improving satisfaction with care received. On a larger community level, value-based healthcare focuses on building healthier communities through preventative care, patient engagement, promotion of health self-management, and reduction of overall healthcare spending (NEJM Catalyst, 2017). The care coordinating nurse must recognize the need for value-based payment structures to promote better health outcomes. In addition, the nurse must understand the various healthcare payment models used to promote outcomes while assisting resource and cost management, as these are also central goals of care coordination. These goals are often strategically achieved through an in-depth understanding of payment sources and models and how these can most cost-effectively assist in meeting patient goals.

Additionally, the nurse has an ethical obligation to support self-determination and the interests of the patients they care for, which requires the patient to be given the information needed to make informed decisions regarding their health and plan of care and to understand how to navigate the healthcare payer system to access care options and resources required (ANA, 2015). Furthermore, in the nursing scope of practice, the nurse is called to support resource stewardship, which includes securing appropriate resources to address patient needs across the continuum of care (ANA, 2019). This requires nurses to understand the benefits and limitations of value-based payment and healthcare financing models to provide appropriate patient advocacy, education, and resources and to support the development of legislation and payment models that address the Quintuple Aim.

Value-Based Healthcare Payment Models

The United States healthcare system has primarily been a fee-for-service model of care in which a provider or organization is paid for each episode of care delivered. This led to some healthcare providers and organizations being incentivized to provide volume-based care rather than care focused on prevention or patient outcomes (Lewis et al., 2023). Many components of the current healthcare system continue to be reimbursed in the fee-for-service payment model. However, with the introduction of value-based healthcare payment models, other criteria have been introduced as aspects of the payment model, such as incentives to reduce the length of hospital stay, reduction of emergency room visits, and improved patient health outcomes. This pairs reimbursement with the quality of care, rather than the quantity or volume of care given, and emphasizes the need for coordinated and continuity of care across the continuum to support preventative care and self-management of health (Knickman & Elbel, 2019).

Value-based healthcare is measured by patient outcomes versus the cost to receive that outcome. See Figure 8.3—The Value-Based Care Formula. However, it is more than a formula or a cost/benefit analysis. Value-based healthcare aligns the care delivered to a person-centered approach with the goal of overall better health outcomes, leading to reduced costs and the need for ongoing care (Teisberg et al., 2020). This is closely connected to the Quintuple Aim and the philosophy of optimizing and investing in health, prioritizing health, and promoting preventative care, and proactive disease treatment and management (Itchhaporia, 2021). Value-based healthcare involves ensuring the seven rights of care coordination are met, that quality measurements such as patient satisfaction and health outcomes are met, and that the organization supports this through a culture of quality care delivery. There are several value-based payment models, including those of Accountable Care Organizations, hospital-value-based purchasing, capitated payments, and episodic payments. This is not an all-inclusive listing of value-based payment models, but each one has coordinated care as a central aspect of the model.

$$\text{Value} = \frac{\text{Quality}}{\text{Cost}}$$

FIGURE 8.3 The Value-Based Care Formula

Accountable Care Organizations (ACO)

An **Accountable Care Organization** (ACO) is a group of providers or organizations that take responsibility and accountability for the cost of healthcare for the population of patients served. Ideally, the ACO includes hospitals, providers, and care delivery facilities commonly used for post-acute discharge care. The ACO assists with the potential fragmentation of care as it maintains accountability for the care of the patients it serves across the care continuum (Young & Kroth, 2018). Case management, chronic disease management, care coordination, and health information technology are used to ensure that patients receive appropriate care, and that duplicate or unnecessary services are eliminated within the ACO (Shi & Singh, 2019). The ACO model strongly supports and utilizes care coordination, collaborative and person-centered care, and the sharing of essential information to achieve quality benchmarks and identified patient outcomes. ACOs provide a high-level systems approach to managing costs, increasing quality, and meeting the objectives of the Quintuple Aim.

Medicare is a large payer for ACOs, and to be an ACO, the organization or group of providers needs to serve at least 5,000 Medicare beneficiaries for at least 3 years (Knickman & Elbel, 2019, p. 216). Medicare not only reimburses the ACO for care delivered through a fee-for-service model but also offers **shared savings** programs. This means that the ACO gets paid to keep the patient healthy. The payer makes a payment to the ACO, usually annually and in proportion to savings seen, based on lower costs evidenced by successfully managing avoidable use of healthcare and offering coordinated care. This saves Medicare money, which passes on these savings to the ACO through this annual shared savings payment (CMS, 2023, November 2).

To participate, the ACO must meet identified clinical quality benchmarks, such as decreased repeat emergency room visits. This incentivizes the ACO to provide quality healthcare. ACOs have been found to improve quality and reduce costs, leading to value-based healthcare delivery. The reductions in costs are typically seen in reduced emergency room visits, reduced inpatient admissions, and reductions in outpatient care spending. ACO programs have also seen improvements in preventative care, wellness strategies, and chronic disease management (Dreyer & Maddox, 2023). In 2022, Medicare saved $1.8 billion in shared savings programs, generating value-based healthcare through cost management and enhancing the delivery of quality healthcare (HHS, 2023).

Implementing the ACO model involves some challenges, including the potential lack of ability to share vital patient information needed for care coordination due to interoperability issues between settings in the ACO and their respective electronic health record systems (EHR). In addition, the ACO model requires person-centered and interprofessional practice to ensure that patient needs are met across the continuum and that tools such as shared decision-making and collaborative care planning are utilized to effectively manage costs and ensure patients receive the most appropriate care. The ACO organization may need to do some initial organizational work to ensure policies and processes are in place to support the model of care and interprofessional practices. Depending on the ACO model, there may also be restrictions on specialist referrals, which may incentivize referrals within the ACO and potentially limit patient choice for referrals outside the ACO (Tretina, 2021).

Medicare Shared Savings Programs

"The Medicare Shared Savings Program helps millions of people with Medicare experience coordinated health care while also reducing costs for the Medicare program," said CMS Administrator Chiquita Brooks-LaSure (HHS, 2023, para. 3).

Hospital Value-Based Purchasing

The hospital value-based purchasing program (VBP) sponsored by CMS focuses on the quality of care delivered by hospitals, linking reimbursement and payment rates to clinical outcomes (NEJM Catalyst, 2017). This payment model is also used by many third-party payers and excludes hospitals that have low patient volume or are specialty hospitals, such as psychiatric hospitals. The goal is to de-incentivize the hospital from providing inappropriate, unnecessary, or duplicative care and services. The hospital receives a total performance score (TPS) that identifies how well the hospital met clinical outcome benchmarks. It may earn financial incentives if the hospital exceeds outcome benchmarks (Young & Kroth, 2018).

The participating hospital's performance is determined by meeting clinical outcomes such as healthcare-associated infection rates, patient satisfaction, patient safety issues (e.g., falls, wrong-site surgeries, medication errors), and cost reductions. Medicare uses a **prospective payment** model or a set predetermined amount for inpatient hospital stays based on the patient's diagnosis and severity of illness, which is identified by the patient's diagnostic-related group code (DRG). VBP is funded through a 2% reduction in these prospective payments in all Medicare payments for participating hospitals. The withheld monies are redistributed to the hospital through "a value-based incentive payment with a percentage payment that may be less than, equal to, or more than the reduction in payment" (CMS, 2023b, September 6, para. 9). VBP links payment to healthcare quality in the inpatient setting through tying "a portion of payments to performance on certain quality measures such as death within 30 days after a heart attack and patient experience of care" (DiChiara, 2015, para. 4). Patients can access the rating for hospitals in their community by going to the Care Compare website sponsored by CMS (https://www.cms.gov/medicare/quality/physician-compare-initiative).

Capitated Payment Model

Capitated payment models offer fixed payments per patient served. In this model, a health organization or provider receives a set amount in advance for each patient, determined by the number of patients, the time in which services are to be provided, and the healthcare service. For example, CMS offers a capitated model for dual Medicare and Medicaid beneficiaries in which CMS and the state pay each health plan in the program a prospective capitation payment (CMS, 2023c, September 6). Usually, capitated payment models are in a per member per month model (PMPM), and the provider or organization assumes the financial risk of caring for the patient population and potentially exceeding the PMPM rate or payment (Cleverley & Cleverley, 2018).

Capitation models are primarily funded by insurance premiums received by third-party payers from their members. Some capitation payment programs may involve a risk pool where some monies are held until the end of the program year. If the provider or organization does well in managing costs and resources and coordinating care, the provider or organization may have the risk-pool monies paid to them; if not, the funds may be held by the third-party payer to cover the deficit or costs of care (Alguire, n.d.). This incentivizes resource and cost management by delivering appropriate, coordinated, and preventative care for the patient.

Capitated Payment Model Example

A capitation payment model example would be a third-party payer negotiating a rate of $40 PMPM with a PCP for healthcare services. So the PCP receives $480 per year for each patient utilizing that third-party payer. If a single patient only uses $200 of healthcare services from the allocated $480, then the PCP would make a profit of $280 for that patient. If that patient utilized $1,500 of healthcare services from the PCP in a year, then the PCP would lose $1,020 on that patient. This can incentivize the PCP to offer preventative care and wellness services to ensure the patient will not need frequent high-cost healthcare from their clinic.

Capitated payment models can benefit payers, as they share the financial risk concerning patient care costs for their members. However, many providers may only be willing to take on the financial risk if they believe the quality measures associated with payment are directly related to the care they provide and their decisions (Dreyer & Maddox, 2023). Some providers may also be reluctant to serve high-need or complex patients in a capitated model of payment due to the additional risk of the patient needing high-cost care for which they may not be adequately reimbursed (Bravo-Taylor, 2022).

Episodic or Bundled Payment Model

The **episodic or bundled payment** model focuses on specific conditions (e.g., a hip replacement) over the continuum of care for a period of time (e.g., 90 days) or episode of care, including all acute and post-acute care needs. Most episodic payment models through CMS include a 90-day episode of care, in which the provider or healthcare system is responsible for the total patient care cost (Knickman & Elbel, 2019). The initial or anchor provider or setting receives a lump-sum payment based on the health condition and expected care costs for the entire episode of care. This encourages interprofessional collaboration and care coordination across the continuum of care and decreases fragmented care.

For example, a person may be admitted to a hospital for a congestive heart failure (CHF) exacerbation. After stabilization at the hospital, they may need subacute rehabilitation (SAR) for a period of time to return to baseline mobility and activities of daily living levels. When discharged from the SAR facility, the therapy team may recommend that the patient receive home health services for continued therapies and skilled nursing services related to disease management. The initial provider (the hospital) in this episode of care would receive the lump-sum payment and then be accountable for covering the costs of the SAR and home health services throughout the 90-day episode of care and also be responsible for working with all providers to ensure coordinated care. This can be a financially risky model. Suppose the patient falls during ambulation at the hospital while recovering from their CHF exacerbation. The patient fractures their hip. Now the hospital may also be responsible for covering the costs of hip fracture repair, recovery, and rehabilitation.

This payment model may be based on a prospective or **retrospective payment** model. In prospective payment, the provider is paid a lump sum at a predetermined rate of usual costs for the condition over the episode of care. In the retrospective payment model, the provider is paid in a fee-for-service model, but costs are tracked. If costs exceed the usual and customary costs for the health condition, the third-party payer may reduce the payment (NEJM Catalyst, 2018). Episodic or bundled payment models are used by **Medicare** and **Medicaid** as well as other commercial third-party payers.

Mixed results have been found in cost savings and quality outcomes with the model. Maddox et al. (2018) found through an examination of five common conditions covered by bundled payments, that there were no significant changes in Medicare payments, length of stay, emergency department use, or readmissions (p. 269). Agarwal et al. (2020) found that cost savings depended upon the medical condition and the complexity of patient needs. However, the Tennessee Medicaid program introduced bundled payment programs and found that "costs were reduced by more than $11.1 million after the first year—a 3.4% drop in perinatal costs, an 8.8% drop in the costs of asthma exacerbation, and a 6.7% drop in the costs of total joint replacements" (TennCare, 2016, para. 4).

Bundled Payments for Care Improvement Advanced (BPCI Advanced)

The original bundled payments program initiated by the Center for Medicare and Medicaid Services (CMS) has transitioned to the BPCI Advanced payment model. The goal is to improve

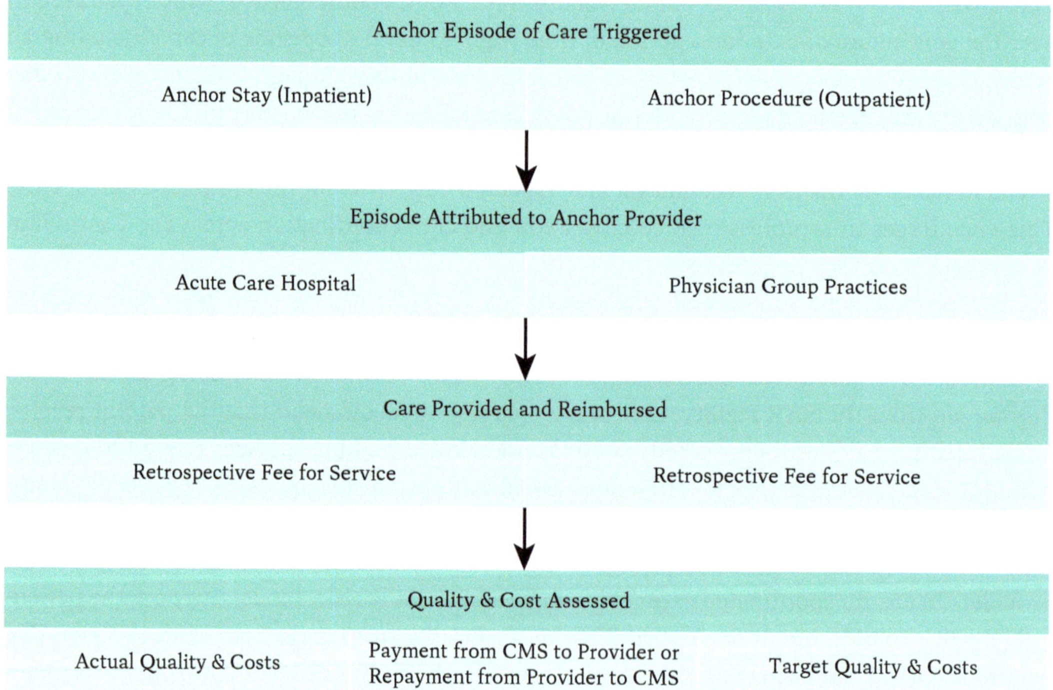

FIGURE 8.4 BPCI Advanced Payment Model

quality and reduce costs by utilizing care coordination, financial accountability, and engagement for the healthcare provider and patient. BPCI Advanced focuses on specific clinical service lines rather than individual conditions, such as cardiac care and procedures, neurological care (e.g., stroke), spinal procedures, gastrointestinal surgery and care (e.g., major bowel procedures, inflammatory bowel disease), orthopedics, and medical care (e.g., sepsis, pneumonia; CMS, 2022, October).

The BPCI Advanced model is in its third cohort of voluntary participants. BPCI Advanced uses a retrospective payment model based on target prices that are reviewed semiannually. The BPCI Advanced model provides a lump-sum payment to the initial provider who triggers the anchor stay or procedure that begins the 90-day episode of care. The payment provided is expected to cover the "bundle" costs of inpatient and outpatient hospital services, laboratory services, durable medical equipment (DME), inpatient readmissions, physician services, medications, skilled nursing facility services, inpatient rehabilitation, long-term care hospital services, home health, and hospice services. BPCI Advanced overlaps with other CMS value-based healthcare payment models, such as ACOs and shared savings programs (CMS, 2022, October). See Figure 8.4 for a flowchart of the BPCI Advanced Payment model.

Quality Measures and Value-Based Healthcare Payment Models

Quality measurement is a crucial component of all value-based healthcare payment models. Quality healthcare has several definitions, each with a slightly different focus. Nevertheless, most definitions follow the Institute of Medicine's (IOM) core elements for a 21st-century healthcare system: safety, effectiveness, person-centeredness, timely, efficient, and equitable (Busse et al., 2019; IOM, 2001). Quality in healthcare can be viewed from a systems level, which translates into organizational outcomes and performance. However, system-level outcomes depend on microlevel services and patient care delivery, translating into quality measurements and benchmarks used to calculate reimbursement rates in value-based healthcare payment models (Shi & Singh, 2019). The IOM defines quality as

> the degree to which health services for individuals and populations increase the likelihood of desired health outcomes and are consistent with current professional knowledge. (McGlynn, 1997, p. 8)

This definition ties the systems-level view into daily healthcare and nursing practices that support safe, effective, efficient, timely, equitable, and person-centered care.

Revisiting the Donabedian model of health care quality, which identifies outcomes, processes, and structural elements of quality, provides an additional framework for selecting quality measures for reimbursement purposes. A quality measure of outcomes may be the number of hospital-acquired infections or readmissions within 30 days of discharge from acute care. Process aspects may point to quality measures such as patient satisfaction or medication errors. Structural quality components might include staffing levels, patient ratios, or the number of nurses certified in care coordination or case management (Shi & Singh, 2019).

Unfortunately, an excess of quality measures has been developed with the movement to define and measure quality in healthcare delivery. Often, Medicare, Medicaid, and private third-party payers may require different clinical quality measures in collected and reported data for reimbursement purposes. This has caused confusion for providers and health systems, a burden in collecting and reporting quality measure data, and resulted in varying approaches to selecting clinical care as a quality measure (Jacobs et al., 2023).

Due to this proliferation of quality measure sets, CMS has developed a National Quality Strategy that seeks to provide direction for how providers and organizations are viewed through the lens of quality healthcare. The CMS National Quality Strategy has eight goals. The goals include (a) outcomes across the continuum of care, (b) alignment and coordination across settings, (c) equity and whole-person care, (d) patient engagement and partnership in their care, (e) safety evidenced by zero preventable harm, (f) resiliency in the healthcare system evidenced by responsiveness and quality improvement, (g) interoperability with healthcare informatics and technologies, and (h) scientific advancement used to transform healthcare (CMS, 2023, April).

CMS has introduced the building block or "universal foundation" approach to quality measures development to meet these National Quality Strategy goals. Initially, measures for the adult and pediatric population will be developed, leveraging evidence-based interventions and dashboards that inform performance and quality improvement needs. This will be achieved by promoting standardized quality metrics for value-based healthcare models. One metric will be data collection and integration of equity into quality measurements to meet the needs of underserved populations through social determinants of health (SDOH) data and equity-specific quality measures, such as screening all patients for SDOH. Increasing the use of patient-reported quality and safety measures to target quality improvement and patient engagement and reduce harm will also be a metric. Another key identified metric is ensuring support for healthcare workers and systems to reduce burnout and workforce shortages, and lastly, the metric of requiring the transition of all quality measurement data to be digitally collected for timely availability and data-driven policy development (CMS, 2023, April).

As CMS develops the universal foundation approach to clinical quality measures, the agency will focus on the following criteria when selecting a quality measure. The measure should have the following features:

- be of high national impact
- can be benchmarked nationally and globally
- be applicable to multiple populations and settings
- be appropriate for stratification to identify disparities and gaps
- have scientific acceptability
- be feasible and become digital or computable
- not have any unintended consequences (CMS, 2023d, September, para. 2)

Through implementing the universal foundation approach to quality measure development, meaningful metrics and benchmarks will be created, provider burden will be decreased, and equity in healthcare will be advanced through additional collection of equity-based quality measure data. As the quality measure collection and storage transitions to a solely digital format, data mining and identifying gaps or areas of quality improvement will be streamlined. The goal will be to have a universal foundation of quality measures that span the healthcare journey from conception to the end of life and across the continuum of care and settings, including prevention and quality mental health screenings and services. Measures focusing on care coordination after hospitalization, screenings, and follow-up services will also be included (Jacobs et al., 2023). See Table 8.1 for Preliminary Adult Universal Foundation Measures.

TABLE 8.1 Preliminary Adult Universal Foundation Measures

Domain	Measure Identification Number and Name
Wellness and prevention	139: Colorectal cancer screening 93: Breast cancer screening 26: Adult immunization status
Chronic conditions	167: Controlling high blood pressure 204: Hemoglobin A1c poor control (>9%)
Behavioral health	672: Screening for depression and follow-up plan 394: Initiation and engagement of substance use disorder treatment
Seamless care coordination	561 or 44: Plan all-cause readmissions or all-cause hospital readmissions
Person-centered care	158 (varies by program): Consumer Assessment of Healthcare Providers and Systems overall rating measures (CAHPS®)
Equity	Identification number undetermined: Screening for social drivers of health

Source: Jayne Josephsen, "Preliminary Adult Universal Foundation Measures," *Aligning Quality Measures Across CMS - the Universal Foundation*, Centers for Medicare & Medicaid Services, 2024.

Coding Considerations

As discussed, although the United States does not have a centrally funded healthcare system, CMS often leads the way for how third-party payers determine reimbursement and payment for healthcare services. This is done by introducing demonstration projects sponsored by CMS, such as the various value-based healthcare models and billing and coding guidelines, **diagnostic related groups** (DRGs), **ambulatory payment classifications** (APC), and **case mix indexes** (CMI) The nurse care coordinator must understand each of these items and how they affect resource management and care delivery to assist patients in navigating the healthcare payer system, making informed decisions regarding their care, and supporting organizational financial viability.

Diagnostic-Related Groups (DRG) and Ambulatory Payment Classifications (APC)

When a patient receives healthcare, the service is documented through a diagnosis or procedure code. Various coding formats are used, depending on whether the procedure or service is inpatient or outpatient, whether it is used by a physician, the facility in which it is used, etc. (e.g., CPT®, HCPCS, ICD-10 codes). These codes direct the assignment of the DRG (for inpatient care) or the APC (for outpatient care), which directs the providers' reimbursement and payment for the healthcare service. The DRG and APC codes represent the diagnosis of the patient and any comorbidities, complications, or co-occurring conditions.

For example, suppose a patient was admitted to an acute care hospital for a kidney infection and had a comorbidity of diabetes. In that case, they may be assigned a DRG code representing "Kidney or Urinary Tract Infection with Major Complications or Comorbidities." However, if the patient was admitted for a kidney infection without any identified comorbidities or complications, they may be given a DRG code that represents a "Kidney or Urinary Tract Infection without Major Complications or Comorbidities" (Cleverley & Cleverley, 2018, p. 26). The second DRG without complications or comorbidities would be reimbursed at a lower rate, and the DRG with identified complications or comorbidities would be reimbursed at a higher rate. Several billing code formats are utilized, and the nurse care coordinator will need to understand how they are used in their organization or practice to provide education and address patients' questions. The various types of billing codes and how they are linked to identified health conditions or procedures point to the importance of the nurse assessing and documenting patient health history, conditions, and changes in condition to ensure appropriate financial reimbursement.

Case Mix Index (CMI)

The case mix index (CMI) is used in conjunction with the DRG code to determine facility reimbursement rates for Medicare and Medicaid beneficiaries. The DRG is based on the diagnosis and procedure codes assigned to the patient for healthcare services. The CMI is the average of all the relative weights of the DRGs in a population of patients, for example, in an acute care hospital over a certain period. The relative weight is a number assigned to the DRG by CMS that represents the resource use connected to the DRG (Prescott, 2018). CMI equals the sum of all the facilities' DRG relative weights (RW) divided by the number of cases or patients discharged for that period of time (ACDIS, 2022). The CMI is affected by the patient population and their prognosis, diagnosis, severity of illness, complexity of treatment, and intensity of resources needed. The CMI is used in conjunction with the DRG to determine the average cost of care to treat the condition and the appropriate **length of stay** (LOS) for that condition (Dejelo, 2019). Higher CMIs translate into a higher reimbursement rate for the facility.

The CMI assists the hospital in allocating resources and making staffing decisions to provide appropriate care and services for the patient as it reflects patient acuity levels. The DRG and CMI information can also direct the care coordinating nurse to take actions to ensure that effective resource management is in place and LOS guidelines are met, such as beginning care coordination and discharge planning at admission, providing person-centered and relationship-centered care involving the patient and interprofessional team to ensure a safe and

CMI Formula and Example Calculation

CMI Formula: $\sum$ *DRG RWs* ÷ η *cases* = *CMI*

DRG Code	Condition	Relative Weight (RW)	Number of Discharges	Total Relative Weight (RW)
189	PULMONARY EDEMA & RESPIRATORY FAILURE	1.3542	10	13.542
541	OSTEOMYELITIS	1.3708	3	4.1124
869	OTHER INFECTIOUS & PARASITIC DISEASES DIAGNOSES	1.7834	8	14.2672
			Total cases discharged = 21	Total DRG RWs = 31.9216

CMI Formula: 31.9216 ÷ 21 = 1.52

(CMS, n.d., Final Version 22 file)

effective transition to the next level of care within the LOS guidelines available, pacing the case, and accessing community resources as needed to meet patient needs and preferences of care (Dejelo, 2019).

Third-Party Payers/Commercial Insurers

Several types of third-party payers/commercial insurers provide reimbursement for healthcare received by their members or beneficiaries. The nurse care coordinator must know what kind of insurance the patient has, as each type of insurance has specific guidelines related to coverage. In care coordination practice, the nurse may engage and communicate with the insurance provider to preauthorize care, or to recognize what benefits the patient may be eligible for. Common types of third-party payers/commercial insurers that patients may utilize to provide payment for their healthcare include Medicare, Medicaid, private commercial insurance, and self-funded insurance programs.

Medicare

Medicare is a key insurance provider, covering those 65 years of age or older or those with a disability such as end-stage renal disease (ESRD). In 2020, over 62.6 million people, or approximately 18% of the United States population, were enrolled in Medicare. The vast majority were eligible for Medicare due to age, with about 8 million receiving Medicare due to a disability. In 2020, the Medicare program spent approximately $926 billion on healthcare costs (Vankar, 2023). Medicare is a large third-party payer, and due to the number of beneficiaries and money spent in the program, CMS continually looks for innovative programs and ways to add value and quality to healthcare while managing costs and resource use. Medicare is divided into four parts: A, B, C, and D. Medicare supplementary coverage plans are referred to as **Medigap plans**. Each part has different covered items and premiums, copayments, and deductibles. Medicare is not free and does not cover all costs, as some people may think. Even if a patient has Medicare, they may have significant financial concerns about meeting copayments and deductible requirements.

Medicare Part A

Part A is designed to be the insurance that reimburses for hospital stays, skilled nursing facility care, hospice services, and some outpatient home health care. Part A does not have a premium or an amount that the patient must pay for the healthcare insurance if the patient has worked and paid Medicare taxes for at least 10 years or if they are eligible through their spouse paying enough Medicare taxes. It is essential for the care coordinating nurse to know whether the patient has Medicare Part A, as some patients may not have paid enough Medicare taxes and therefore do not have insurance coverage for their inpatient or hospice care. If a patient is not eligible for Part A without a premium, they may have the option to pay the premium and gain Part A coverage. The 2024 premium for Part A coverage for those not eligible for the premium-free version is between $278 and $505 a month, depending on income (Medicare.gov, n.d.a).

Part A has deductibles, with the 2024 deductible set at $1,632 for each benefit period. The benefit period begins from the day the patient is admitted to the hospital and ends when they have not received any inpatient care for 60 consecutive days. There may be more than one benefit period in a year depending on the patient's health condition and needs, meaning they may have to meet the deductible more than once a year. There are also copayments with Part A, which vary on where patients receive care and how many days they receive services (Medicare.gov, n.d.a). The cost of the copayment goes up as the days progress. For example, if the patient were hospitalized for 63 days, they would not have copayments for the first 60 days of the benefit period. However, they would need to meet their deductible of $1,632. Then, for days 61, 62, and 63, they would have a copayment of $408 for each day or $1,224 in copayment costs in addition to the $1,623 in deductible costs, totaling $2,847 in costs for that hospitalization.

If they went to a skilled nursing facility for SAR, they would have up to 20 days of rehabilitation with no copayments. However, each day following they would have a $204 per day copayment (Medicare.gov, n.d.a). This can be expensive for patients, and many facilities will direct the plan of care to meet the patient's healthcare needs or rehabilitation needs to fall within the benefit period so the patient does not have copayments. Additionally, some patients may prefer to receive care via home health services, which is covered 100% with Part A, or a patient may pursue outpatient services to avoid deductibles and copayments, depending on where they fall in the benefit period.

Medicare Part B

Medicare Part B is designed to meet outpatient healthcare needs, outpatient hospital services, physician services, home healthcare services, durable medical equipment needs, and other care not covered by Part A. Medicare Part B has premiums, deductibles, and copayments. For

2024, the monthly premium for Medicare Part B is $174.70, with an annual deductible of $240. The monthly premium amount is increased based on adjusted gross income calculations, with increases beginning with beneficiaries reporting an adjusted gross income greater than $103,000 individually or $206,000 jointly. Copayments usually run 20% of the Medicare-approved amount for the service or item received, but there may also be zero copay for items such as labs or home health services (CMS, 2023, October). Some patients may not have Part B Medicare due to the premiums. It is essential for the care coordinating nurse to ascertain if the patient has Part B when developing the plan of care and making referrals or follow-up appointments.

Medicare Part C

Medicare Part C is often referred to as a Medicare Advantage plan, where private or commercial insurance plans administer Medicare contracts and manage beneficiaries' care. These plans usually follow a health maintenance organization (HMO) or preferred provider organization (PPO) model. There are several models of HMO, and sometimes, they are referred to as managed care plans. The HMO model focuses on wellness and preventative care. They may offer additional services such as gym memberships or weight loss support to promote health maintenance. The HMO model usually uses the PCP as a gatekeeper for referrals, and the beneficiary usually needs to receive care from providers in the HMO network. The PPO model in Medicare Advantage plans is based upon discounted negotiated reimbursement rates for services within a network of providers. The PPO model may offer more flexibility to beneficiaries, as they may choose to see out-of-network providers at a higher copayment cost. The PPO model often does not use the PCP as a gatekeeper, so the beneficiary can see specialists without a referral (Shi & Singh, 2019).

Medicare Advantage plans have grown in popularity, with approximately 30 million beneficiaries enrolled in one during 2023, or about 50% of the Medicare beneficiary population. There are several choices of Medicare Advantage plans, with an average of 43 plans for the average Medicare beneficiary to choose from (Ochieng et al., 2023). When a person elects for a Medicare Advantage plan (Part C), they "sign over" their Medicare benefit to the plan. This means they no longer have Part A, Part B, or Part D. Medicare pays the Medicare Advantage plan a set per member per month (PMPM) amount, plus an additional amount for prescription medication coverage, and the Medicare Advantage plan manages the beneficiary's care (HHS, n.d.a).

There are premiums for Part C, with the beneficiary having to pay the Part A and Part B premiums if they are not eligible for the free Part A. Most Medicare Advantage plans do not require additional premiums, but some may. There are still deductibles and copayments, but these are often less than Part A and B, and most plans have an annual out of pocket limit, which Medicare Part A and B do not (AARP, 2023.). The most notable benefit to a Medicare Advantage plan is the lower costs when considering out-of-pocket limits and copayments, and many of these plans may also include dental, hearing, and vision care, which is not included in Medicare Part A and B (AARP, 2023.).

However, this can also be an issue in care coordination and care transitions. Due to the low costs, some Medicare Advantage plans may have lower reimbursement rates for services provided than regular Medicare or other third-party payers, causing some providers, home health agencies, or other organizations to refuse Medicare Advantage insurance or to take only a limited number of patients with that insurance. These plans may also have more requirements for pre-authorization of care and referral restrictions, making transitions in care challenging. It is essential that the care coordinating nurse know the type of Medicare Advantage plan the patient has and if there are gaps in accepting providers and facilities in their area or specific items needed for pre-authorization of services and referrals.

Medicare Part D

Medicare Part D helps cover the cost of prescription medication. Part D is optional; some patients may opt out of carrying Part D coverage, meaning they do not have prescription medication insurance coverage and pay for all medications out of pocket. To enroll in Part D, the beneficiary must also be enrolled in Part A or Part B. Medicare approves several third-party prescription medication plans, and the beneficiary will need to choose from those offered in their geographic area. If a beneficiary has enrolled in a Medicare Advantage plan or Part C, they are not eligible for Part D, as the Part C plan includes prescription medication coverage. All Medicare Part D plans have their own formulary or list of medications they cover, which the beneficiary will want to review to ensure their current medications will be covered or determine if they can change medications. Like most prescription medication plans, there are usually tiers or levels of coverage in the formulary to identify which medications may have a different cost (Medicare.gov, n.d.b).

Premiums, deductibles, and copayments vary by the plan. For 2023, CMS has projected the average monthly premium for a Part D plan to be $31.50 (CMS, 2022, July). For 2024, the deductible for all Medicare-approved Part D plans cannot exceed $545 per year, but many plans have no deductible. For the year 2024, once the beneficiary has $5,030 in prescription costs, they can pay no more than 25% of the cost of the prescription until their out-of-pocket expenses are met, which cannot exceed $8,000 annually. The beneficiary may have to pay more, depending on their adjusted gross income. For example, in 2024, if the beneficiary had an adjusted gross income of $103,000 individually or $206,000 filing jointly, they would pay an additional $12.90 plus the monthly plan premium (Medicare.gov, n.d.b).

Medicare Part D has a "donut hole," or coverage gap, that has slowly decreased since 2020. The "donut hole" is when there is a temporary limit on what the plan will cover for medications. In 2024, the beneficiary enters the "donut hole" when they have met $5,030 in prescription medication costs and continues in the "donut hole" until they reach their out-of-pocket maximum. Once the beneficiary meets the annual $5,030 amount and enters the "donut hole," they begin paying 25% of the cost of their prescription medications, which most times is an increase in cost from the copayments they were paying prior. Before 2020, beneficiaries paid 100% of the cost of their prescription medications once they entered the "donut hole" until they met their annual out-of-pocket maximum. Once the beneficiary meets their annual out-of-pocket maximum, they enter a catastrophic coverage level (Bihari, 2023). In 2024, there are no other out-of-pocket expenses once the beneficiary enters catastrophic coverage (Medicare.gov, n.d.b). Beginning in 2025, Medicare will offer beneficiaries the option of paying for out-of-pocket prescription costs in monthly installments and out-of-pocket costs will be capped at $2000. These changes will address some problems the "donut hole" presents (Medicare.gov, n.d.c).

A "Donut Hole" Example

In 2024, Ruth enrolled in a Medicare-approved Part D prescription medication plan. The deductible for the plan is $545 for the year. The amount of prescription costs Ruth will need to incur before she enters the "donut hole," including deductibles and copayments, is $5,030. After she meets this amount, Ruth will pay 25% of the cost of her medications until she reaches her total out-of-pocket expenses, a maximum of $8,000 for the year.

Ruth met the $5,030 amount in medication costs (total cost of medications, not only copayments and deductibles) and has entered the "donut hole." She is now responsible for 25% of the cost of her medications until she reaches her maximum out-of-pocket amount of $8,000. Ruth will need an additional $2,970 in medication costs before she can exit the "donut hole" and reach the catastrophic coverage level.

Ruth's total estimated expenses for the year will be $545 (deductible) + $2,450 (medication costs before the "donut hole") + $1,325 (medication costs after she enters the "donut hole") = $4,320 + her monthly Medicare Part D premiums of $31.50 a month. Ruth's total annual costs for Part D = premium costs $378 (31.50 x 12) + 4,320 = $4,698. In this scenario, Ruth never exits the "donut hole" in the year.

Medicare Supplemental Insurance or Medigap Coverage

Medigap coverage is additional insurance bought from a private insurance company and can assist with covering the costs of Medicare, such as deductibles, copayments, etc. Beneficiaries can only purchase Medigap coverage if they have Part A and B Medicare. Medigap coverage only has a one-time enrollment, for which there is no risk of denial. This is during the first month they start Medicare Part B, and they must also be 65 or older. If the beneficiary does not purchase a Medigap policy at that time, they take the risk of having higher premiums or being denied coverage. Medigap policy providers must follow all state and federal guidelines and laws regarding insurance (Medicare.gov, n.d.d).

Medigap policies are signified by a letter; A-D, F, G, and K-N. Each policy has differing monthly premiums ranging from approximately $50 to over $400 monthly. The policies vary in deductibles, copayments, and benefits, with some offering no deductibles or copayments. With Medigap coverage, Medicare pays its share of the covered healthcare costs, and then the Medigap policy pays a portion. The beneficiary is responsible for any costs that are left. If the beneficiary is enrolled in a Medicare Advantage plan or Part C, they are not eligible for a Medigap policy. Prescription drug coverage is not included in Medigap plans, and the beneficiary will need to enroll in Medicare Part D (Medicare.gov, n.d.d).

Navigating Medicare plans can confuse patients as there are many parts, each with a different focus, requirements, and premiums. The nurse care coordinator must have knowledge of what types of Medicare the patient holds if they have Medicare and where they are in their benefit period if inpatient. They must also assess for financial strains or concerns the patient is experiencing concerning deductibles and copayments, as these may affect the patient's choice of care and services or affect the ability of the patient to adhere to the plan of care and recommendations. If the patient has a Part C plan, the care coordinating nurse must ensure an understanding of authorization guidelines and which providers the insurance provider is contracted with. See Table 8.2 for an example of the types of premiums and deductibles experienced by those with Medicare. When reviewing the table, remember that many beneficiaries may not purchase a Medigap plan or choose a Medigap or Part C plan with higher or lower premiums than the example. Others may also have the additional cost of a Part A premium or increased premium costs in Part B or D due to income.

TABLE 8.2 Medicare Premiums and Deductibles Example

Type of Medicare Coverage	Example Premium	Example Annual Deductible	Total Annual Costs	Medicare and Medigap Coverage Total Annual Costs	Medicare Part C Coverage Total Annual Costs
Part A	$0/Annual	$1,632/per episode	$1,632 @ 1 episode	$1,632 @ 1 episode	N/A
Part B	$174.70/Month $2,096.40/Annual	$240	$2,336.40	$2,336.40	N/A
Part C	Part A Premium of $0/Annual Plus Part B Premium of $2,096.40/ Annual Plus Part C Premium Average of $91.95/Month $1,103.40/Annual	Varies	$3,199.80 plus deductible	N/A	$3,199.80 plus deductible
Part D	Average Premium $31.50/Month $378/Annual	$545	$923	$923	N/A
Medigap Policy	Average Premium $175/Month $2,100/ Annual	Varies	$2,100 plus deductible	$2,100 plus deductible	N/A
Total Annual Costs				$6,982 plus deductible of Medigap policy	$3,199.80 plus deductible of Part C plan

Medicaid

Medicaid is a health insurance program for those who meet low-income guidelines or have been diagnosed with certain disabilities, such as legal blindness. Medicaid covers children, pregnant women, and adults who meet federal poverty limits. Medicaid is managed and delivered by states, with state and federal financing. This means that Medicaid in one state may have different guidelines or policies regarding who qualifies for Medicaid, how the program is administered, and reimbursement rates and systems (Knickman & Elbel, 2019). The Affordable Care Act Medicaid expansion program aimed to cover all adults with incomes up to 138% of the federal poverty level, or $20,120 for an individual in 2023. The expansion program offered states enhanced federal matching rates to expand Medicaid in their state. However, states can opt out of accepting these enhanced funds for their Medicaid programs. As of 2023, 10 states are not participating in the federal expansion Medicaid program. These are Wyoming, Kansas, Texas, Wisconsin, Tennessee, Mississippi, Alabama, Georgia, South Carolina, and Florida (KFF, 2023).

Unlike Medicare, Medicaid covers only those who fall into income guidelines. Each state determines the income and other eligibility criteria. Medicaid covers all healthcare services under the Medicaid program and often offers services that Medicare does not cover, such as custodial care in a nursing home and personal care services. Usually, there is a low copayment or no copayment and no deductible in Medicaid programs (HHS, n.d.b.). As of July 2023, approximately 91.5 million people were enrolled in Medicaid programs in the United States, with just over 7 million enrolled in the Children's Health Insurance Program (CHIP), which provides health coverage to children in families who do not qualify for Medicaid. In some states, CHIP also covers pregnant women (HealthCare.gov, n.d; Medicaid.gov, n.d.).

Medicaid programs often utilize value-based payment models, such as shared savings and capitated payment programs. These programs usually link reimbursement rates with the organization or provider meeting identified clinical quality measures such as immunization rates in children or screenings for depression at every primary care visit. They may also utilize a PMPM model, where the primary care provider is offered a flat monthly rate to provide care for Medicaid beneficiaries in that clinic's practice.

The care coordinating nurse will have several considerations when working with a patient covered by Medicaid. Often, Medicaid offers lower reimbursement rates so that fewer providers may accept Medicaid, or the patient may need to be placed on waiting lists for services like nursing home care, as the facility may only have a few beds dedicated to patients with Medicaid (Shi & Singh, 2019). Another care coordination consideration is whether the patient is dual eligible, meaning they have both Medicare and Medicaid.

Dual-eligible beneficiaries generally meet poverty or low-income guidelines put forth by the state Medicaid program and are also enrolled in Medicare. There is a partnership between Medicare and Medicaid for the dually eligible, sharing the costs and covering premiums, copayments, and deductibles at differing rates depending on the beneficiary's situation and income (CMS, 2022, February). There were 12.5 million dual-eligible beneficiaries in 2020. Dual-eligible beneficiaries have lower incomes and tend to be in poorer health with more extensive healthcare needs, some having serious physical or mental health conditions (Pena et al., 2023). It is important for the care coordinating nurse to understand this so that assessment, plan of care development, and targeted interventions can be delivered and developed in a person-centered and relevant manner that addresses the patient's global healthcare needs.

Third-Party Commercial Insurance

Approximately half of the United States population receive health insurance through commercial insurance plans, either employer, association, or union-sponsored or purchased privately (Choudhury, 2023). Commercial insurance as we know it has evolved over the years, beginning in the 1930s to pay for the costs of medical care. The model initially sought coverage of rare events or catastrophic accidents and has evolved into insurance models that provide coverage for preventative care, predictable health issues, and unforeseen healthcare needs. A pioneer in commercial insurance was the nonprofit Blue Cross and Blue Shield plan, which established a contract with a hospital in Texas to provide care for a group of teachers. This prompted the fee-for-service model, with Blue Cross enrollees receiving hospital admission at a 50% higher rate than the rest of the nation by the late 1930s. This also led to specialization and medical technology development, as well as the hospital setting serving as the center of care. About a decade later, for-profit commercial insurance plans were introduced, which began the practice of charging higher insurance premiums for those who were less healthy or had a pattern of frequent insurance claims compared to lower premiums for those who were healthier (Young & Kroth, 2018).

Due to rising healthcare costs, by the 1970s, other insurance models were introduced, such as Managed Care, HMOs, PPOs, or a Point of Service (POS) plan, which allowed more flexibility in seeking care from out-of-network providers. These are all current models in healthcare today, and they continue to evolve to meet beneficiary, provider, and payer needs and priorities. Many organizations and providers were not satisfied with the Managed Care plans in the 1970s, feeling they were too restrictive. Due to this, by the 1990s, legislation concerning patient rights and those with provider protections was introduced. By the 2000s, various consumer-driven insurance plans, such as high-deductible plans, were beginning to be introduced (Young & Kroth, 2018).

A commercial insurance plan has key elements, including an outline of the benefits, how the plan is designed and delivered, reimbursement methods, and coverage policies. Commercial insurance plans have defined services covered with listed limitations, such as the number of visits for a specific care need, such as physical therapy, and identified out-of-pocket costs, such as copayments and deductibles (American Hospital Association, 2022, January). For example, a commercial insurance plan may have a limit of 20 mental health visits per year, copayments of $20 for primary care office visits, $40 for specialist care office visits, and an annual deductible of $1,700 per individual or $3,000 per family. The insurance plan may have lifetime benefit limits, such as a $10,000 hospice benefit. Alternatively, they may not cover a specific type of care, such as chiropractic or acupuncture. Each plan will have unique coverage and benefit features.

Commercial insurance plans have different service models, some based on an HMO, PPO, or POS model, another model, or a hybrid of models. The type of service delivery will often direct the reimbursement strategies, which may vary, including a fee for service, a capitated

PMPM payment, a bundled payment, or a shared saving payment. All commercial insurance providers must follow federal laws and guidelines, as well as those in the states where they offer insurance policies (American Hospital Association, 2022, January).

The care coordinating nurse must be aware of a critical issue when working with patients who carry commercial insurance plans for their health care coverage. Sometimes the commercial plan may have utilization review or pre-authorization practices that appear to hinder timely access to care, which may drive up healthcare costs due to longer LOS or readmissions. A poll conducted by Morning Consult found "that 84% of nurses say insurers' administrative policies delay patient care, and 80% of physicians say that burdensome insurer policies affect their ability to practice medicine, taking them away from their patients' bedside" (Pollack, 2023, para. 6). The complicated coding, billing, authorization, and denial of claims process add cost and resource use to the healthcare organization or provider. During a sample of denials from June 1–7, 2019, it was found that 13% of prior authorization denials and 18% of payment denials met coverage rules and should have been approved (American Hospital Association, 2022, November, p. 5). This leads to resubmission of claims, provider-to-insurance-company advocacy, financial stress for patients and organizations, and it can negatively affect timely access to care and services. This calls for the care coordinating nurse to pace the case and proactively communicate with the commercial insurance provider to ensure there are no delays in needed care.

Self-Funded Insurance Plans

In the late 1970s, **self-funded insurance** plans began with larger employers to decrease the costs of healthcare premiums and give more control over the benefits provided. In a self-funded plan, the employer pools premiums collected from employees into an account and then pays for medical claims out of that account, instead of utilizing a commercial insurance provider. The employer may contract a third-party administrator to manage the plan, administer the benefits, pay the medical claims, collect needed data, and coordinate care for high-risk or high-cost patients. This type of insurance plan can offer the employer various tax benefits, decreased administrative costs, and flexibility in benefit offerings and costs (Young & Kroth, 2018). For the care coordinating nurse, a self-funded plan works like a commercial insurance plan. The nurse will need to understand the benefits available, review and authorization processes, and out-of-pocket expenses the patient may incur when managing care across the continuum.

Uninsured

Those who do not have health insurance impact the financing strategies of providers and organizations, affecting the ability of care to be delivered and quality measures and outcomes. Approximately 7.7% of United States residents are uninsured according to the Office of the Assistant Secretary for Planning and Evaluation (ASPE, 2023, para. 1). Many of the uninsured are working adults or have at least one working adult in their family but are financially ineligible for programs like Medicaid or financial assistance to purchase insurance through the marketplace. Some may not have access to insurance coverage through their employer, or they may be undocumented emigrants, so they are not eligible for public health insurance programs.

An analysis of the 2021 National Health Interview Survey found that approximately 20% of nonelderly uninsured adults identified that they did not have insurance because the process to apply was confusing or too complicated, and 64% of uninsured adults indicated that they were uninsured because of cost (Tolbert et al., 2022).

This population of patients may pay for their medical care out of pocket, access funds from organizations that offer financial assistance to the uninsured, seek care from sliding-scale payment clinics in their community, or not seek regular care due to the costs. Those uninsured present challenges to the coordination of care due to the inability to create connections and

Taylor's Story: Medical Costs and Follow-Up Care

Deductibles, copayments, and lack of health insurance can lead a patient not to follow care plan recommendations or receive follow-up care for health conditions. Sometimes a patient may collaboratively develop a care plan with the interprofessional team and agree to plan recommendations and follow-up care, only to not follow through with the appointments or care suggested due to the costs. Below is an example of one such situation, which identifies the essential need of the care coordinator to assess for and address social and economic barriers to care.

Taylor has commercial health insurance through her employer but only has income 9 months out of the year, as her employer closes during the winter. Taylor works as a server in a local restaurant to supplement her income throughout the year and cover the three months without income from her primary employer. Recently, Taylor had a skiing accident in which she experienced 3 small fractures in her hand, wrist, and elbow. She went to the local urgent care clinic, which gave her a sling and soft cast and referred her to an orthopedist. Taylor went to the specialist appointment. The orthopedist instructed Taylor to continue to wear the soft cast and sling and not to work as a server for 6 weeks. Taylor was to return in 2 weeks for a follow-up x-ray and examination to ensure the fractures were healing correctly. Taylor then received her copayment bill from the urgent care clinic for $536.72 and a copayment bill for the orthopedic specialist appointment for $94 ($40 for the visit and $54 for the x-ray).

Taylor is a single parent of two children and has no foreseeable income for the 6 weeks. She has rent due and needs money for food, utilities, laundromat use, and transportation costs. Taylor received care from two different healthcare organizations. The urgent care organization agreed to work with her on a payment plan for the $536.72. The orthopedic organization is demanding immediate payment for her $94 bill, or interest will be added to her bill. Taylor decides she will not go to any follow-up appointments or have any more x-rays as she has no way to pay for them.

It is now 12 weeks since her injury, and she is having continued pain and difficulty performing her server work. Taylor called the orthopedist, but they could not get her in for another 4 weeks. They suggested she go to the emergency room. Taylor does not do this either, as she is still paying her urgent care bill. She decides to live with the pain, see how it goes, and hope it will get better without having to seek any more healthcare.

continuity in care delivery from providers and organizations that may not be reimbursed for the care delivered. Many providers and organizations will not accept patients without insurance or require payment before providing care. Uninsured patients likely will not have a PCP to follow them, coordinate continued referrals, sign needed orders for care, or adjust medications (Balasubramanian et al., 2021).

Even if the care coordinating nurse can make a needed referral or organize admission to a facility that will deliver needed care, the patient may refuse due to concern about being unable to pay for care. Many uninsured patients are less likely to receive preventive care or care for significant health conditions and chronic conditions, leading the patient to seek care through the emergency department at a local hospital after first allowing a condition to progress significantly, to be unable to get in to see a PCP, or not to receive any systematic follow-up in care.

The care coordinator must address barriers for uninsured patients who may be experiencing significant social and economic barriers to care. Sometimes an uninsured patient may not fill a prescription or go to follow-up appointments due to concern over medical debt or inability to pay. Engagement with the organizational leadership concerning awareness of the uninsured status of the patient, effective communication across the interprofessional team, connection with community resources, and assistance with accessing financial support programs such as Medicaid, veteran's benefits, or other funding sources are required (Balasubramanian et al., 2021). This calls for significant advocacy, facilitation of transitions in care, flexibility concerning needed care plan modifications, and education so that the patient and those involved in their care are clear about any needed follow-up items or actions, as well as who to contact with questions or for assistance and the expected financial or reimbursement outcomes.

Healthcare Financing and Value-Based Current Events

Due to the complicated healthcare financing system and the increasing healthcare costs, several pieces of legislation, CMS demonstration projects, and final rules have been introduced to protect patients and advance healthcare accessibility, quality, and equity. As the health system advances in the transformation to value-based healthcare delivery, more legislation, policies, and programs will continue to be developed and implemented. Nurses must be aware of current initiatives, be a voice for patients, and be involved in constructing a health system that delivers quality, safe, accessible, and equitable care. A few recent events that address issues of costs, financing, and innovative healthcare delivery methods are the No Surprises Act, the Hospital-at-Home Program, and the introduction of rural emergency hospitals.

The No Surprises Act

The No Surprises Act legislation was passed to protect patients from receiving "surprise" medical bills related to care from out-of-network providers, such as air ambulance services or care from an in-network facility provided by an out-of-network provider. If the patient had received care from an out-of-network provider, they may have charged more than the negotiated rate that an in-network provider would have charged. In this case, the out-of-network provider may have billed the patient the difference between what the insurance company reimbursed and what was charged. The No Surprises Act protects patients who, through no choice of their own, received care from an out-of-network provider (e.g., an emergency room provider or an anesthesiologist). In this case, the patient is only responsible for the in-network costs (CMS, 2022, January). If the patient understands the provider is out of network and chooses to receive care from that provider, then a notice of the provider being out of network, as well as an estimate of the charges, must be provided in advance, and the patient needs to consent to the out-of-network care and increased costs (Luhby, 2021).

Additionally, the No Surprises Act offers a dispute resolution process for disputes between insurance plans and providers and those who are uninsured and receive a bill significantly larger than the original good faith estimate. The dispute resolution process considers several factors, including in-network rates, quality and outcomes, patient acuity, CMI, good faith efforts, etc. There is some criticism of this process and controversy about who is responsible for covering the remainder of the cost of care, between the in-network and out-of-network rates or the additional costs above a good faith estimate (Luhby, 2021).

Hospital-at-Home Program

Another innovative value-based approach introduced by the CMS during the COVID-19 pandemic is the Hospital-at-Home program. This demonstration project allows patients needing acute-level hospital care to receive it at home instead of the hospital, if appropriate. Most Hospital-at-home programs focus on medium-acuity patients who are stable. Each Hospital-at-Home program may have a different approach to care provision, such as offering the service out of the emergency department, admitting eligible patients to their home rather than to a hospital bed, using specialist clinics as the admission point, or focusing on specific patient populations, such as post-surgical monitoring in the home. This assists with costs and resource use. Some programs have focused on geographic areas such as rural and frontier areas, where admission to the hospital can have multiple challenges, including transportation or places for the family to stay during an inpatient admission, thus increasing accessibility to care. The Hospital-at-Home program utilizes health information technologies, such as video-based provider visits and continuous remote patient monitoring, in conjunction with needed in-person visits to provide continuous support and care (American Hospital Association, 2020).

Studies have shown that the Hospital-at-Home program can offer quality and appropriate care at a lower cost, an average of 25% less. Kaiser Permanente found that readmission rates and 7-day returns to the emergency department decreased with the Hospital-at-Home implementation and comparable LOS compared to brick-and-mortar hospital admission (Donlan, 2023). The Veterans Affairs and health systems, with their own insurance plans, have navigated the model and created healthcare reimbursement and financing strategies for this model of care; however, many commercial insurance providers do not cover the Hospital-at-Home service (American Hospital Association, 2020).

Hospital-at-Home

"Hospital-at-home care programs are at the forefront of improving acute care to save money and time while improving patient satisfaction. Due to the COVID-19 pandemic and the explosion of programs across the country, payment options are improving and implementation is streamlining" (Eisley & Mcilvena, 2022, "The Bottom Line").

Rural Emergency Hospitals (REHs)

Many areas of the United States are considered rural. In these areas, they may have critical access hospitals (CAHs), which are small hospitals that primarily operate in rural areas and meet specific guidelines, such as providing 24/7 emergency care and having 25 inpatient beds or less (Shi & Singh, 2019). Medicare has historically paid CAHs for services on a cost-based reimbursement model (CBR), which typically equaled 101% of the cost of the inpatient, outpatient, or post-acute care swing bed services (MacKinney et al., 2023; MedPac, 2021). CBR is not based on the type or number of services given but rather on the service's total cost. This leads to a zero-profit model, which can most often lead to a lack of financial viability, and the CAH usually operates at a loss (MacKinney et al., 2023). CAHs are more likely to serve patients primarily receiving Medicare or Medicaid or those who are uninsured, experiencing an estimated $4.6 billion in losses from unreimbursed or uncompensated care in 2020 (American Hospital Association, 2022, September, p. 6). Additionally, with the advent and implementation of value-based payment models, which often rely on a specific volume of patients to meet quality metrics and do not address the operational costs of being ready to provide emergency care 24 hours a day, the CAHs more frequently experience dire financial losses. Many are opting to close, with a reported 106 CAHs completely closing since 2005 (UNC, 2014).

CAHs fill a significant need in the healthcare system, providing healthcare to rural and underserved populations who may be unable to travel to urban areas for healthcare. However, the financial viability of the CAH is in question as it relates to new payment models and issues such as staffing and the number of patients served. CMS has created a final rule that went into effect in 2023 to allow some CAHs to change to rural emergency hospitals (REHs) to support healthcare delivery in these underserved areas, promote health equity, and support the Quintuple Aim. If a CAH converts to an REH, it can still provide emergency service, observation care, and outpatient medical services that do not exceed an average LOS of over 24 hours per patient. Inpatient services can only be provided as part of SAR or other post-acute care services (CMS.gov, 2023). CAHs can apply to be REH beginning in 2023 and start receiving payments from Medicare. CMS will cover outpatient services in REHs and add an additional 5% payment per service, and they will not charge the beneficiary copay for this extra 5% payment. CMS will also pay the REH a monthly payment to the facility. However, inpatient beds are not allowed in the REH model, and any extended post-acute services, like SAR, need to be licensed separately and will not be eligible for the 5% payment per service (CMS.gov, 2022). "The new REH designation aims to maintain access to emergency services, observation care, and additional medical and outpatient services in rural areas" (NCSL, 2023, para. 3).

CHAPTER SUMMARY

Healthcare financing and payment models can be complicated for patients, providers, and nurses to navigate. Value-based healthcare payment models have been introduced to move the healthcare system from a fee-for-service model to one based on better outcomes and management of healthcare costs. Nurses must understand healthcare financing, the value-based payment models used by their organizations, and which insurance provider the patient has in order to provide adequate patient education and advocacy, promote good outcomes, and manage resources and costs.

Value-based healthcare is measured by the patient outcomes versus the cost to receive that outcome, aligning person-centered care approaches with the goal of better health outcomes and reduced healthcare costs. Value-based healthcare supports the Quintuple Aim, the seven rights of care coordination, and an organizational culture of quality care delivery. There are several value-based payment models, such as the ACO, shared savings programs, hospital value-based purchasing programs, and capitated and episodic or bundled payment models. All value-based healthcare payment models utilize quality measurement data or benchmarking to direct reimbursement rates. Many quality measure sets have been developed, often with different third-party payers using divergent sets. This has caused confusion and redundancy in data collection for providers and organizations to obtain reimbursement for healthcare services rendered. There are also many coding considerations when examining healthcare financing and payment models, such as diagnostic-related groups (DRG), ambulatory payment classifications (APC), and case mix indexes (CMI). The care coordinating nurse must understand each of these items and how they affect resource and cost management.

The nurse will need to engage and communicate with the third-party payer to obtain pre-authorization of care, understand which providers are contracted with the payer, and determine what benefits the patient may be eligible for. Some common types of third-party payers/insurers are Medicare, Medicaid, private commercial insurance, and self-funded insurance programs. Many people may be uninsured, pay for medical care out of pocket, access organizations offering financial assistance, or not seek regular healthcare due to the costs. As each plan and situation has unique requirements, guidelines, authorization processes, and reimbursement strategies, the care coordinating nurse must know what funding source the patient has in order to provide the most appropriate advocacy and education, support informed decision-making, and promote positive health outcomes.

Value-based payment models and legislation are constantly evolving to address the need for the healthcare system to provide safe, effective, person-centered, timely, efficient, and equitable care that provides good outcomes while managing resources and costs. The No Surprises Act, the Hospital-at-Home program, and the REH are examples of this. Nurses will continue to see value-based payment models and legislation advance, with CMS likely leading the effort through innovative demonstration projects and working to identify ways to create value in healthcare. Table 8.3 shows that by 2025, it is expected that between 38.4% and 53.5% of healthcare financing and funding will be provided by Medicare and Medicaid, depending on the service. This points to the great need for nurses to understand healthcare funding sources, as the reimbursement policies and guidelines of Medicare and Medicaid may direct much of the care authorized for patients and inform the types of quality measures data collected, as well as set benchmark measures that nurses, providers, and the healthcare system will be required to meet for reimbursement purposes.

TABLE 8.3 Projected Funding Sources Year 2025

Funding Source	Hospital	Physicians	Prescription Medications	Nursing Home Care
Year	2025	2025	2025	2025
Private Insurance	35.6%	39.3%	39.7%	9.1%
Out-of-pocket Payments	3%	7.7%	12.4%	27.8%
Medicare	27%	25.1%	35%	28%
Medicaid	18.6%	13.3%	9.6%	25.5%
Medicare/ Medicaid Total	45.6%	38.4%	44.6%	53.5%

(Cleverley & Cleverley, 2018, p. 35)

CHAPTER 8 GLOSSARY

Accountable Care Organization (ACO): A group of providers or organizations that take responsibility and accountability for the cost of healthcare for a population of patients they serve.

Ambulatory Payment Classifications (APC): A coding system for outpatient healthcare services that direct reimbursement amounts.

Capitated Payment: A reimbursement model that offers fixed payments, often in a per member per month (PMPM) style, in which the healthcare organization or provider receives a set amount in advance for each patient served, incentivizing cost and resource management.

Case Mix Index (CMI): A formula used in conjunction with DRG codes to determine reimbursement rates for beneficiaries with Medicare or Medicaid.

Critical Access Hospitals (CAHs): A hospital usually located in a rural area that offers 24/7 emergency care and, most times, has 25 or fewer inpatient beds. The CAH may also use inpatient beds as "swing beds" for longer-term inpatient rehabilitative services. It typically serves underserved populations or those who experience healthcare access and equity issues.

Diagnostic-Related Group (DRG): A coding system for inpatient healthcare services that direct reimbursement amounts.

Dual-Eligible: A person who has both Medicare and Medicaid.

Episodic Payment/Bundled Payment: A reimbursement model that focuses on a specific condition or service line over an episode of care or the entire treatment period of an illness, including all acute and post-acute care needs. The initial or anchor provider receives a lump-sum amount based on the health condition and is accountable for covering the costs of care throughout the episode of care.

Fee-for-Service: A reimbursement model in which a provider or organization is paid for each healthcare service or procedure provided, often leading to quantity or volume-based care delivery.

Healthcare Financing: How healthcare organizations and providers are reimbursed or paid for services and supplies provided.

Length of Stay (LOS): A clinical quality measure that identifies the average time between admission and discharge in an acute care setting. The LOS often points to whether efficient and quality care is delivered.

Medicaid: A health insurance program for those who meet low-income guidelines or have been diagnosed with certain disabilities. Medicaid is managed and delivered by individual states with state and federal financing.

Medicare: A federal government-based third-party payer that provides healthcare insurance coverage to those 65 years of age and older or with an identified disability. There are several parts of Medicare: parts A (inpatient care), B (outpatient care), C (Medicare Advantage plans), and D (prescription coverage).

Medigap Plan: Additional private insurance that a Medicare Part A and B beneficiary may purchase to assist with covering the costs of Medicare, such as deductibles and copayments.

Prospective Payment: A payment model that sets a predetermined reimbursement amount for a healthcare service or procedure.

Retrospective Payment: A payment model in which the provider or organization is reimbursed in a fee-for-service model, but costs are tracked, and if they exceed usual and customary costs for the health condition, the third-party payer may reduce the reimbursement amount.

Rural Emergency Hospital (REH): A hospital in a rural area that can provide emergency services, outpatient services, and observation services but cannot have inpatient beds unless provided as part of SAR or other post-acute care services.

Self-Funded Insurance: An insurance plan funded by the employer, pooling insurance premiums collected from employees into an account and then paying for medical claims out of that account. Often these plans use a third-party administrator to manage the plan and pay out the claims.

Shared Savings: A reimbursement model in which the provider or organization is incentivized to keep patients healthy and receives a third-party payer payment based on the realized cost savings.

Third-Party Payer: An organization that pays for a patient's healthcare. These may be commercial insurance companies, governmental payers, or employers who sponsor self-funded plans.

Value-Based Healthcare: A healthcare model designed to improve health outcomes and assist with cost management, viewed from the perspective that healthcare value equals the quality of care divided by the cost of care.

DISCUSSION QUESTIONS AND ACTIVITIES

Discussion Questions

1. Explain the differences between a fee-for-service model and a value-based payment model. Identify and discuss at least one way each payment model may create barriers to meeting one aspect of the Quintuple Aim.
2. Discuss why nurses must understand value-based payment and healthcare financing models to provide appropriate patient advocacy, education, and resources.
3. Explore and discuss the reasoning and evidence for integrating coordinated and continuity of care into value-based payment models.
4. Discuss the possible effect of diagnostic related groups (DRGs) and case mix index (CMI) on reimbursement, nurse staffing levels, acuity of interventions offered, and patient outcomes.
5. Discuss whether there are potential difficulties with new value-based payment models confusing the roles and differences between providers and payers. If so, how? If not, why not?

Activities

1. The Centers for Medicare and Medicaid Services (CMS) are developing a universal foundation approach to clinical quality measures to be paired with value-based payment models. Utilizing the seven criteria of quality measures identified in the chapter section titled "Quality Measures and Value-Based Healthcare Payment Models," create two clinical quality measures that would be appropriate for CMS to integrate into the Universal Foundation of Measures. Provide a rationale concerning why you created/chose the measure and describe how the measure contributes to value-based healthcare delivery.
2. Create a Medicare and Medicaid comparison fact sheet that you would use to provide health education to a patient and their family or support system on what each type of funding source offers in benefits and what eligibility requirements they may have.
3. Case Study

You are the care coordinator in a local emergency department (ED). A patient arrives at the ED accompanied by a man and a woman unrelated to the patient. They state that the patient has been squatting in their home, and they have tried to get him to leave, but he will not. The patient is a 67-year-old man who uses a walker to ambulate. Upon assessment, you find that the patient does not have a primary care provider (PCP), reports a history of diabetes, which he has not been treating due to being unable to purchase medications or go to a provider, and has a wound on his left lower extremity that is red and with purulent drainage. Upon review of the patient's labs, you see he has a slightly elevated white blood cell count, which indicates an infection. The ED provider believes the patient can be treated in an outpatient setting with home health nursing for medication management and disease education and physical therapy for mobility, prescribes an oral antibiotic and oral antidiabetic, orders home health, and asks you to make a referral to a PCP to follow up on diabetes management and wound healing. You want to talk to the couple that brought the patient about these recommendations and discharge plans, but they have left the building. The ED nurse assigned to the patient indicated that the couple said they would not take him back into their home as he had no right to be there, and they left about 15 minutes earlier.

You find that his only source of income is his social security check of $607 a month and that he is not eligible for the premium-free Medicare Part A, does not have Part B or D, and is uninsured. You begin to work on a Medicaid application with the patient so that he can access a skilled nursing or assisted living facility that takes Medicaid. You discuss options for temporary living arrangements with the patient. The patient states he has no family or friends, and no other options are available. You begin contacting assisted living and skilled nursing facilities, hoping that one will take the patient pending Medicaid approval. The patient has been in the ED for 4 days as he does not have an inpatient or observation-level medical need for admission purposes but is unsafe to discharge without support. You have not found a facility, a home health agency, or a primary care provider that will take the patient pending Medicaid approval and have been unable to contact any family member or friend for assistance.

1. The care coordination supervisor is now contacting you as the hospital administration is concerned about the patient's length of stay in the ED and his uninsured status. Discuss why the hospital administration may be concerned about this from a healthcare financing and a patient outcome perspective.
2. What other resources might the care coordinating nurse consider when creating a care plan for this patient?
3. A local assisted living facility has agreed to accept the patient pending Medicaid approval. To ensure continuity of care and good patient outcomes what other interventions must the care coordinating nurse implement before transferring care to the assisted living facility?
4. As you reflect upon this case study, did you find that you held any biases or assumptions concerning the situation, or were gaps in knowledge made apparent? If so, what were they?

NCLEX STYLE QUESTIONS

1. What are the primary aims of value-based payment models?

    a. Assist patients in attaining better outcomes
    b. Manage healthcare costs
    c. Patient engagement
    d. All of the above

2. You are orienting a new nurse to care coordination duties at your organization. As you begin discussing value-based payment models, you want to ensure that the new nurse understands the common payment models used. Which of the payment models listed below would you include in your education on this issue for the new nurse?

    a. Capitated payment models
    b. Shared savings payment models
    c. Episodic payment models
    d. All of the above

3. Describe the basic value-based care formula (short answer).
4. An Accountable Care Organization (ACO) assists with potential fragmentation of care through which of the following actions?

    a. Sharing information only with those organizations and providers who are part of the ACO system.
    b. Focusing on patient engagement and ensuring patients understand they are accountable for their health outcomes.
    c. Providing a microlevel approach to managing costs.
    d. Using health information technology to ensure duplicate or unnecessary services are eliminated.

5. Which of the following does the hospital value-based purchasing program (VBP) provide?

    a. A good total performance score (TPS) for all hospitals participating in the program
    b. Use of a retrospective payment model based upon the case mix index
    c. The ability to increase value in care received in psychiatric and specialty hospitals
    d. Linking payment with clinical outcomes

6. Capitated payment models may be financially risky for providers. Why is this?

   a. Complex patients may need high-cost care.

   b. Payment quality measures are always directly linked to the provider's delivered care and decisions.

   c. Coordinated care is incentivized.

   d. Insurance premiums fund the model.

7. Match the healthcare financing model to the correct description.

   Medicare Part A ______

   Is often based on an HMO or PPO model of care delivery and may be referred to as a Medicare Advantage Plan.

   Medicare Part B ______

   An optional private insurance plan that can assist in covering copayment and deductible costs.

   Medicare Part C ______

   Has a "donut hole" where the beneficiary potentially will experience a temporary limit on what the plan will cover for prescription medications.

   Medicare Part D ______

   Requires the person to work and pay Medicare taxes for at least 10 years or be eligible through their spouse for the premium-free option.

   Medigap Plan ______

   Reimburses for outpatient healthcare needs, outpatient hospital services, physician services, home healthcare services, and durable medical equipment.

8. Which of the following is not a potential problem concerning clinical quality measures?

   a. An excess of differing clinical quality measure sets

   b. Varying approaches in how a clinical quality measure is selected

   c. The implementation of the National Quality Strategy

   d. Confusion on how to collect and report quality measures

9. Which of the following can affect reimbursement rates in an acute-care hospital? (Select all that apply.)

a. CMI
b. DRG
c. APC
d. RW

10. You are the care coordinating nurse at your local hospital. You are meeting with a patient who has been admitted for potential sepsis and discussing their insurance coverage. You have found that the patient does not have Medicare Part A but does have Parts B and D. What information and education will you need to give the patient so that they understand how this will affect their cost of care?

    a. Ensure they understand that they will be solely responsible for all inpatient stay costs.
    b. It will not affect their cost of care as they have Medicare Part B and D.
    c. Recommend that they obtain a Medigap plan as soon as possible to cover any large deductibles or copayments.
    d. Explain to them that they will need a 3-day stay to qualify for a skilled nursing facility subacute rehabilitation stay post-discharge.

11. Which of the following insurance programs is funded through state and federal funds? (Select all that apply.)

    a. CHIP
    b. BPCI Advanced
    c. Medicaid
    d. Self-Funded

12. You are a nurse care coordinator who works in a low-cost community clinic. A patient who has a history of schizophrenia, uncontrolled Type 2 diabetes, and is persistently homeless presents complaining of a severe headache. Upon assessment of funding sources, you find the patient has Medicare and Medicaid. What is this referred to as it relates to healthcare financing?

    a. Dual-Enrolled
    b. Dual-Diagnosis
    c. Dual-Eligible
    d. Dual-Served

Questions 13 and 14 relate to the following scenario:

You are the care coordinating nurse in the local emergency department (ED). A 57-year-old woman arrives with a productive cough and chest and throat pain. You find that the patient does not have any health insurance.

13. As you plan your care coordination interventions, you consider that patients may not have health insurance for which of the following reasons?

    a. The patient is financially ineligible for Medicaid or financial assistance with insurance costs.

    b. The patient found that applying for insurance was too complicated.

    c. The patient is an undocumented person/emigrant.

    d. All of the above.

14. The ED provider recommends that the patient be discharged with outpatient follow-up and a prescription for an oral antibiotic. You are developing your discharge plan for the patient, and you know which of the following is the most appropriate care coordination intervention:

    a. Referral to a primary care provider who will work with an uninsured patient

    b. Planning and organizing ability to obtain prescription medications

    c. Connection with community resources and alternate funding sources

    d. All of the above

15. Which issue in healthcare insurance was the No Surprise Act passed to address?

    a. The lack of price transparency for patients

    b. The lack of complexity in billing, coding, and insurance appeals

    c. The lack of knowledge about how much it will cost to receive care from an out-of-network provider when a patient has no choice in provider

    d. The lack of good faith estimates provided by providers

REFERENCES

AARP. (2023, January 30). *What is Medicare Advantage?* https://www.aarp.org/health/medicare-qa-tool/what-is-medicare-advantage.html

Agarwal, R., Liao, J. M., Gupta, A., & Navathe, A. S. (2020). The impact of bundled payment on health care spending, utilization, and quality: A systematic review. *Health Affairs, 39*(1), 50–57. https://doi.org/10.1377/hlthaff.2019.00784

Alguire, P. C. (n.d.). *Understanding capitation*. American College of Physicians. https://www.acponline.org/about-acp/about-internal-medicine/career-paths/residency-career-counseling/resident-career-counseling-guidance-and-tips/understanding-capitation

American Hospital Association (AHA). (2020, December). *Creating value by bringing hospital care home* (issue brief). https://www.aha.org/system/files/media/file/2020/12/issue-brief-creating-value-by-bringing-hospital-care-home_0.pdf

American Hospital Association (AHA). (2022, January). *Commercial health insurance primer.* https://www.aha.org/system/files/media/file/2022/03/commercial-health-insurance-primer.pdf

American Hospital Association (AHA). (2022, September). *Rural hospital closures threaten access: Solutions to preserve care in local communities.* https://www.aha.org/system/files/media/file/2022/09/rural-hospital-closures-threaten-access-report.pdf

American Hospital Association. (2022, November). *Addressing commercial health plan challenges to ensure fair coverage for patients and providers.* https://www.aha.org/system/files/media/file/2022/10/Addressing-Commercial-Health-Plan-Challenges-to-Ensure-Fair-Coverage-for-Patients-and-Providers.pdf

American Nurses Association (ANA). (2015). *Code of ethics for nurses with interpretive statements.* American Nurses Association.

American Nurses Association (ANA). (2019). *Nursing scope and standards of practice* (4th ed.). American Nurses Association.

Association of Clinical Documentation Integrity Specialists (ACDIS). (2022, August). *Demystifying and communicating case-mix index* [white paper]. https://acdis.org/taxonomy/term/14

Balasubramanian, B. A., Higashi, R. T., Rodriguez, S. A., Sadeghi, N., Santini, N. O., & Lee, S. C. (2021). Thematic analysis of challenges of care coordination for underinsured and uninsured cancer survivors with chronic conditions. *JAMA Network Open*, *4*(8), e2119080. https://doi.org/10.1001/jamanetworkopen.2021.19080

Bihari, M. (2023, April 28). *Understanding the Medicare Part D coverage gap.* https://www.verywellhealth.com/understanding-the-medicare-part-d-donut-hole-1738872

Bravo-Taylor, E. (2022, June 2). *Four downside-risk payment models to consider.* RTI Health Advance. https://healthcare.rti.org/insights/downside-risk-payment-models-providers-should-consider

Busse, R., Panteli, D., & Quentin, W. (2019). An introduction to healthcare quality: defining and explaining its role in health systems. In R. Busse, N. Klazinga, D. Panteli, et al., (Eds.). *Improving healthcare quality in Europe: Characteristics, effectiveness and implementation of different strategies.* European Observatory on Health Systems and Policies (Health Policy Series, 53). https://www.ncbi.nlm.nih.gov/books/NBK549277/

Centers for Medicare and Medicaid Services (CMS). (n.d.). *DRG relative weights: Final version 22* (file download). https://www.cms.gov/Medicare/Medicare-Fee-for-Service-Payment/AcuteInpatientPPS/Acute-Inpatient-Files-for-Download-Items/CMS022597

Centers for Medicare and Medicaid Services (CMS). (2022, January 3). *No surprises: Understanding your rights against surprise medical bills.* https://www.cms.gov/newsroom/fact-sheets/no-surprises-understand-your-rights-against-surprise-medical-bills

Centers for Medicare and Medicaid Services (CMS). (2022, February). *Beneficiaries dually eligible for Medicare & Medicaid.* https://www.cms.gov/Outreach-and-Education/Medicare-Learning-Network-MLN/MLNProducts/Downloads/Medicare_Beneficiaries_Dual_Eligibles_At_a_Glance.pdf

Centers for Medicare and Medicaid Services (CMS). (2022, July 29). *CMS releases 2023 projected Medicare basic Part D average premium.* https://www.cms.gov/newsroom/news-alert/cms-releases-2023-projected-medicare-basic-part-d-average-premium

Centers for Medicare and Medicaid Services (CMS). (2022, October). *BPCI advanced model overview fact sheet—Model year 6 (2023).* https://www.cms.gov/priorities/innovation/innovation-models/bpci-advanced

Centers for Medicare and Medicaid Services (CMS). (2023, April). *National quality strategy (NQS).* https://www.cms.gov/files/document/cms-national-quality-strategy-handout.pdf

Centers for Medicare and Medicaid Services (CMS). (2023a, September 6). *What are the value-based programs?* https://www.cms.gov/medicare/quality/value-based-programs

Centers for Medicare and Medicaid Services (CMS). (2023b, September 6). *Hospital value-based purchasing program.* https://www.cms.gov/medicare/quality/initiatives/hospital-quality-initiative/hospital-value-based-purchasing?ref=marco.health

Centers for Medicare and Medicaid Services (CMS). (2023c, September 6). *Capitated model.* https://www.cms.gov/medicaid-chip/medicare-coordination/financial-alignment/capitated-model

Centers for Medicare and Medicaid Services (CMS). (2023d, September 6). *Aligning quality measures across CMS—the universal foundation.* https://www.cms.gov/aligning-quality-measures-across-cms-universal-foundation

Centers for Medicare and Medicaid Services (CMS). (2023, October 12). *2024 Medicare parts A & B premiums and deductibles.*https://www.cms.gov/newsroom/fact-sheets/2024-medicare-parts-b-premiums-and-deductibles

Centers for Medicare and Medicaid Services (CMS). (2023, November 2). *Shared savings program.* https://www.cms.gov/medicare/payment/fee-for-service-providers/shared-savings-program-ssp-acos

Choudhury, J. S. (2023, October 27). *The employer strikes back: The hollowing of the commercial health insurance market and its impact on payers and providers.* Healthcare Financial Management Association. https://www.hfma.org/payment-reimbursement-and-managed-care/the-employer-strikes-back-the-hollowing-of-the-commercial-health-insurance-market-and-its-impact-on-payers-and-providers/

Cleverley, W. O., & Cleverley, J. O. (2018). *Essentials of health care finance* (8th ed.). Jones & Bartlett Learning.

CMS.gov. (2022). *Rural emergency hospitals proposed rulemaking* [Fact Sheet]. https://www.cms.gov/newsroom/fact-sheets/rural-emergency-hospitals-proposed-rulemaking

CMS.gov. (2023). *Rural emergency hospitals.* https://www.cms.gov/medicare/health-safety-standards/guidance-for-laws-regulations/hospitals/rural-emergency-hospitals

Dejelo, A. (2019). *Diagnosis related groups (DRGs) and impact on hospital length of stay (LOS).* https://www.nahsehouston.org/2019/06/24/diagnosis-related-groups-drgs-and-impact-on-hospital-length-of-stay-los/

DiChiara, J. (2015, February 19). *History of value-based, accountable care models at CMS.* Xtelligent Healthcare Media. https://www.revcycleintelligence.com/news/history-of-value-based-accountable-care-models-at-cms/

Donlan, A. (2023, February 6). *Where hospital-at-home programs go next.* Home Health Care News. https://homehealthcarenews.com/2023/02/where-hospital-at-home-programs-go-next/

Dreyer, T., & Maddox, K. J. (2023, March 30). *What's the value in value-based care?* AAMC Research and Action Institute. https://www.aamcresearchinstitute.org/our-work/issue-brief/whats-value-value-based-care

Eisley, A., & Mcilvena, L. (2022, October 4). *5 health systems that are getting hospital-at-home care right.* GoodRx Health. https://www.goodrx.com/hcp/providers/hospital-at-home-care

Finkler, S. A., Calabrese, T. D., & Ward, D. M. (2019). *Accounting fundamentals for health care management* (3rd ed.). Jones & Bartlett Learning.

HealthCare.gov. (n.d.). *Medicaid expansion & what it means for you.* https://www.healthcare.gov/medicaid-chip/medicaid-expansion-and-you/

Institute of Medicine (IOM). (2001). *Crossing the quality chasm: A new health system for the 21st century.* National Academy Press.

Itchhaporia, D. (2021). The evolution of the Quintuple Aim: Health equity, health outcomes, and the economy. *Journal of the American College of Cardiology, 78*(22), 2262–2264. https://doi.org/10.1016/j.jacc.2021.10.018

Jacobs, D. B., Schreiber, M., Seshamani, M., Tsai, D., Fowler, E., & Fleisher, L. A. (2023). Aligning quality measures across CMS—The universal foundation. *New England Journal of Medicine, 388*(9), 776–779. https://www.nejm.org/doi/10.1056/NEJMp2215539

KFF. (2023, October 4). *Status of state Medicaid expansion decisions: Interactive map.* https://www.kff.org/medicaid/issue-brief/status-of-state-medicaid-expansion-decisions-interactive-map/

Knickman, J. R., & Elbel, B. (Eds.). (2019). *Jonas & Kovner's healthcare delivery in the United States* (12th ed.). Springer Publishing Company.

Lewis, C., Horstman, C., Blumenthal, D., & Abrams, M. K. (2023, February 7). *Value-based care: What it is, and why it is needed* (explainer). The Commonwealth Fund. https://doi.org/10.26099/fw31-3463

Luhby, T. (2021, December 28). Patients won't have to fear as many surprise medical bills come January. *CNN.* https://www.cnn.com/2021/12/28/politics/no-surprises-act-2022/index.html

MacKinney, C., Mueller, K., Ferdinand, A., Knudson, A., Lundblad, J., & McBride, T. (2023). Modernizing payment to critical access hospitals: A proposal for the next iteration of the Flex Program. *Journal of Rural Health, 39,* 716–718. https://doi.org/10.1111/jrh.12750

Maddox, K. E., Orav, J., Xheng, J., & Epstein, A. M. (2018). Evaluation of Medicare's bundled payments initiative for medical conditions. *The New England Journal of Medicine, 379*(3), 260–269. https://www.nejm.org/doi/full/10.1056/nejmsa1801569

McGlynn, E. A. (1997). Six challenges in measuring the quality of health care. *Health Affairs (Project Hope), 16*(3), 7–21. https://doi.org/10.1377/hlthaff.16.3.7

Medicaid.gov. (n.d.). *Children's Health Insurance Program (CHIP).* https://www.medicaid.gov/chip/index.html

Medicare.gov. (n.d.a). *What does Medicare cost?* https://www.medicare.gov/basics/get-started-with-medicare/medicare-basics/what-does-medicare-cost#:~:text=Costs%20for%20Part%20A%20(Hospital%20Insurance)&text=If%20you%20don%27t%20qualify,worked%20and%20paid%20Medicare%20taxes.

Medicare.gov. (n.d.b). *Drug coverage Part D.* https://www.medicare.gov/drug-coverage-part-d

Medicare.gov. (n.d.c). *Costs in the coverage gap.* https://www.medicare.gov/drug-coverage-part-d/costs-for-medicare-drug-coverage/costs-in-the-coverage-gap

Medicare.gov. (n.d.d). *What's Medicare supplement insurance (Medigap)?* https://www.medicare.gov/health-drug-plans/medigap

MedPac. (2021). *Critical access hospitals payment system.* https://www.medpac.gov/wp-content/uploads/2021/11/medpac_payment_basics_21_cah_final_sec.pdf

National Conference of State Legislators (NCSL). (2023). *Rural emergency hospitals.* https://www.ncsl.org/health/rural-emergency-hospitals

NEJM Catalyst. (2017). *What is value-based healthcare?* https://catalyst.nejm.org/doi/full/10.1056/CAT.17.0558

NEJM Catalyst. (2018). *What are bundled payments?* https://catalyst.nejm.org/doi/full/10.1056/CAT.18.0247

Ochieng, N., Binniek, J. F., & Freed, M. (2023, August 9). *Medicare Advantage in 2023: Enrollment update and key trends.* https://www.kff.org/medicare/issue-brief/medicare-advantage-in-2023-enrollment-update-and-key-trends/

Office of the Assistant Secretary for Planning and Evaluation. (2023, August 3). *National uninsured rate reaches an all-time low in early 2023.* https://aspe.hhs.gov/reports/national-uninsured-rate-reaches-all-time-low-early-2023

Pena, M. T., Mohamed, M., Burns, A., Biniek, J. F., Ochieng, N., & Chidambaram, P. (2023, January 31). *A profile of Medicare–Medicaid enrollees (dual eligibles).* https://www.kff.org/medicare/issue-brief/a-profile-of-medicare-medicaid-enrollees-dual-eligibles/

Pollack, R. (2023, July 14). *Let's end commercial insurer barriers that reduce access to care.* American Hospital Association. https://www.aha.org/news/perspective/2023-07-14-lets-end-commercial-insurer-barriers-reduce-access-care

Prescott, L. L. (Ed.). (2018). Q & A: Understanding case mix index. *CDI Strategies, 12*(14). https://acdis.org/articles/qa-understanding-case-mix-index

Shi, L., & Singh, D. (2019). *Essentials of the U.S. health care system* (5th ed.). Jones & Barlett Learning.

Teisberg, E., Wallace, S., & O'Hara, S. (2020). Defining and implementing value-based health care: A Strategic Framework. *Academic Medicine: Journal of the Association of American Medical Colleges, 95*(5), 682–685. https://doi.org/10.1097/ACM.0000000000003122

TennCare. (2016, October 15). *TennCare's new approach to payment shows savings.* https://www.tn.gov/tenncare/news/2016/10/5/tenncare-s-new-approach-to-payment-shows-savings.html

Tolbert, J., Drake, P., & Damico, A. (2022, December 19). *Key facts about the uninsured population.* https://www.kff.org/uninsured/issue-brief/key-facts-about-the-uninsured-population/

Tretina, K. (2021, April 21). *What are accountable care organizations?* Medicareguide.com. https://medicareguide.com/accountable-care-organizations-299579

U.S. Department of Health and Human Services (HHS). (n.d.a) *What is Medicare Part C?* https://www.hhs.gov/answers/medicare-and-medicaid/what-is-medicare-part-c/index.html

U.S. Department of Health and Human Services (HHS). (n.d.b). *What's the difference between Medicare and Medicaid?* https://www.hhs.gov/answers/medicare-and-medicaid/what-is-the-difference-between-medicare-medicaid/index.html

U.S. Department of Health and Human Services (HHS). (2023, August 2). *Medicare shared savings program saves Medicare more than $1.8 billion in 2022 and continues to deliver high-quality care.* https://www.hhs.gov/about/news/2023/08/24/medicare-shared-savings-program-saves-medicare-more-1-8-billion-2022-continues-deliver-high-quality-care.html

University of North Carolina at Chapel Hill (UNC). (2014). *Rural hospital closures.* https://www.shepscenter.unc.edu/programs-projects/rural-health/rural-hospital-closures/

Vankar, P. (2023, September 1). *Medicare—statistics & facts.* https://www.statista.com/topics/1167/medicare/#topicOverview

Young, K. M., & Kroth, P. J. (2018). *Sultz & Young's health care USA: Understanding its organization and delivery* (9th ed.). Jones & Bartlett Learning.

Credits

Fig. 8.1a: Copyright © by Microsoft.

Fig. 8.2: Source: https://www.cms.gov/medicare/quality/value-based-programs.

CHAPTER 9

Health Technology

Health Information Technology, Informatics, and Digital Health

LEARNING OBJECTIVES

1. Examine health information technology, informatics, and digital health.
2. Apply health technology-related regulations to care coordination practice.
3. Explore challenges to the integration and application of health technologies.
4. Outline health technology-supported coordination and continuity of care practices.

KEY TERMS

- big data
- data
- data integration
- data integrity
- data security
- digital health
- digital inclusivity
- disruptive technologies
- Health Information Exchange (HIE)
- health information technology (HIT)
- Health Information Technology for Economic and Clinical Health (HITECH) Act
- Health Insurance Portability and Accountability Act (HIPAA)
- informatics
- interoperability
- Meaningful Use
- technological knowing

Introduction

The Institute of Medicine (IOM) identified that "constraints on exploiting the revolution in information technology" (2001, p. 25) were a key underlying reason for the lack of quality healthcare delivery in the United States. Since the IOM report, there has been a continuous influx of innovative and, at times, disruptive technologies into the healthcare system. These **disruptive technologies** are innovative but have significantly altered workflows, structures, processes, and how healthcare is delivered. This has, at times, caused confusion and required significant changes in the system and the structure of healthcare delivery (Twin, 2023). Though sometimes disruptive to the status quo, innovative technologies can ultimately positively impact upstream and downstream healthcare outcomes and support value in healthcare by enhancing quality, safety, and care coordination. This has led to somewhat of a disconnect between the healthcare system's ability to integrate promising and innovative technologies into the system's infrastructure and simultaneously address barriers to effective technology integration. Yet, technology assimilation into clinical practice and today's healthcare system is critical to providing quality, cohesive, and coordinated care across the continuum (Dixon et al., 2018).

Additionally, the variety of terms used to reference technology use in healthcare has contributed to a healthcare workforce that may not have a shared understanding of the how, why, and what of technology in supporting quality, safe, efficient, and effective care. For example, a nurse may refer to the electronic health record (EHR) system as health information technology (HIT), informatics, or digital health. It is essential to understand each of these technology components, how they contribute to quality healthcare, and the nurse's role in using and implementing these technologies for successful care coordination.

Several regulations have also directed the integration and use of HIT and informatics in the healthcare system. Three critical regulations regarding HIT are the Health Information Technology for Economic and Clinical Health (HITECH) Act, the Health Insurance Portability and Accountability Act (HIPAA), and Meaningful Use. Knowledge of these regulatory requirements is essential to meeting coordination and continuity of care standards, as specific regulatory requirements pair with care coordination practices, such as the privacy and security concerns from HITECH and HIPAA that accompany the Meaningful Use requirement for electronic transfer of patient discharge summaries across settings to provide for continuity of care. Violating these regulations can mean fines or decreased reimbursement rates for the healthcare organization, affecting resource and cost management, which is a key goal of care coordination.

The care coordinating nurse needs to be cognizant of the pillars to data management concerning the integration of HIT, informatics, and digital health in the healthcare system, and proactively address potential issues to continuity and coordination of care. These data management pillars include data security, integrity, and integration. Through a cohesive understanding of the regulatory requirements, data management pillars, and the role of HIT, informatics, and digital health in delivering quality healthcare, the nurse can support efficient and effective care coordination practice and person-centered care.

Health Information Technology (HIT)

Health information technology (HIT) is the "hardware, software, and systems that comprise the input, transmission, use, extraction, and analysis of information ..." (Jen et al., 2023, para. 1). Examples of HIT might include the EHR computerized physician order entry (CPOE), or collecting information electronically to identify overcrowding scores in real time to proactively address emergency room overcrowding (Jen et al., 2023). The foundation for HIT development is the belief that using HIT can improve accountability, outcomes, and efficient healthcare delivery, while decreasing healthcare costs (Jen et al., 2023).

The HIT system has a focused scope and function in healthcare. It includes hardware and software that manages inputting, searching, organizing, managing, and extracting of health data in an electronic environment. **Data** is a collection of discrete facts or statistics that communicates information that can be aggregated, retrieved, and used in the transfer and analysis of quality or other measures or material. This database function of HIT dramatically increases safety, quality, and coordinated care and is critical for value-based payment structures that rely on extraction of accurate quality measures data (Sherifi et al., 2021). The use of HIT increases accountability through various avenues, such as retrieving quality data, improving medication safety with CPOE, ensuring that orders are appropriate through red flag alerts, and generating preventative care or appointment reminders for a large patient population. Notably, the healthcare HIT database enables cross-setting electronic communication and transfer of pertinent patient information, leading to successful care transitions.

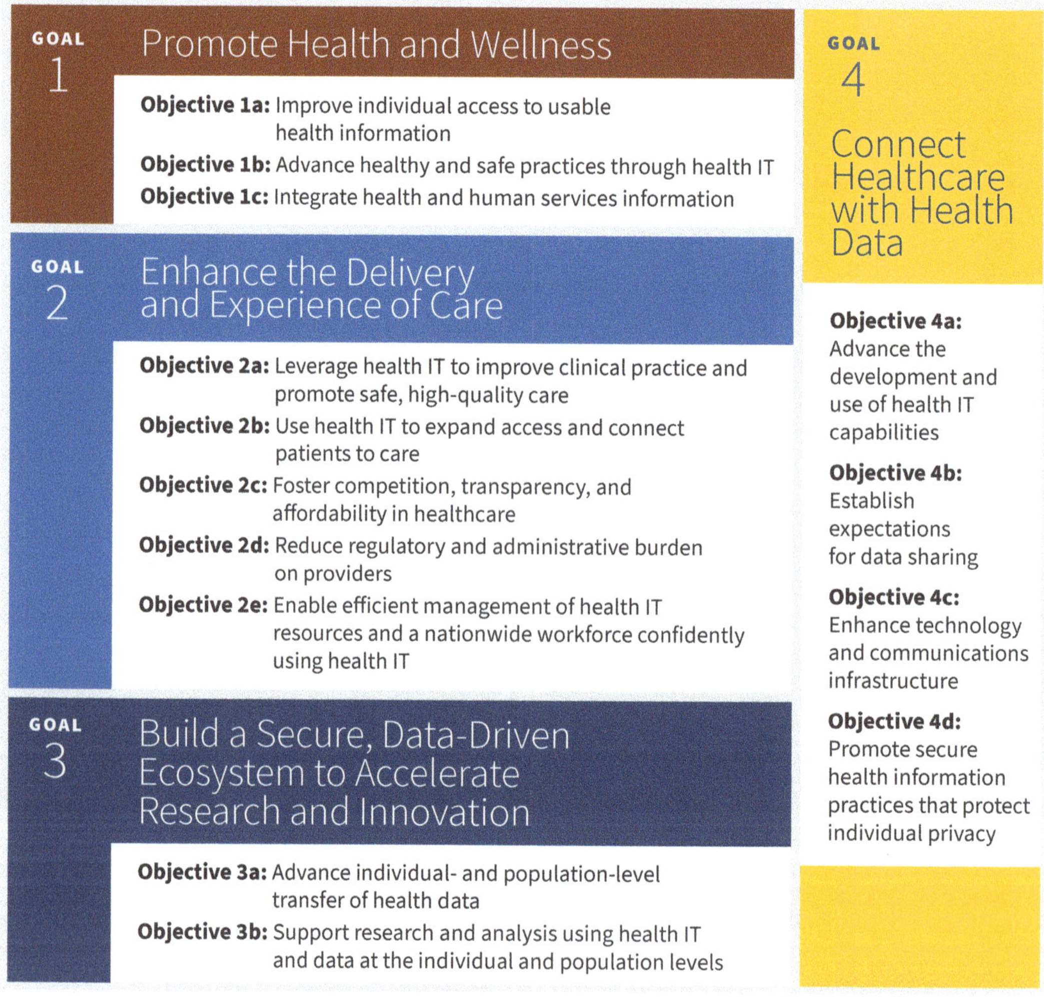

FIGURE 9.1 Strategic Plan Framework

Standards for HIT have been developed and outlined by the Office of the National Coordinator for Health Information Technology (ONC). The ONC was legislatively mandated in the Health Information Technology for Economic and Clinical Health (HITECH) Act of 2009 to advance HIT capabilities and establish data-sharing expectations. The ONC is also responsible for supporting "the adoption and promotion of HIT and a nationwide standards-based health information exchange" (HIE; HealthIT.gov, 2022, *About ONC*). The ONC has developed a federal strategic plan for using HIT, which includes goals to promote health and wellness, enhance the delivery and experience of care, build a secure, data-driven environment to accelerate research and innovation, and connect healthcare with health data (ONC, 2020).

See Figure 9.1 for a visual of the Federal HIT Strategic Plan. It is evident from the ONC goals and the structure and function of HIT that it has broad impact. The data generated and retrieved from the HIT systems often directs healthcare reimbursement based upon quality measures, such as LOS guidelines or all-cause readmission within 30 days. This data is also used to direct continuous quality improvement strategies and policy development on an organizational or national level (Sheikh et al., 2021).

Informatics

Informatics has been described as the data-driven "logic of healthcare" and the "rational study of how we think about patients and how treatments are defined, selected, and evolved" (Sherifi et al., 2021, p. 5). The American Nurses Association (2014) defines nursing informatics as the integration of "nursing science with multiple information and analytical sciences to identify, define, manage and communicate data, information, knowledge and wisdom in nursing practice" (para. 1). The AACN *Essentials* identifies that information technology is combined with informatics to "provide care, gather data, form information to drive decision-making, and support professionals as they expand knowledge and wisdom for practice" (2021, p. 46). The American Medical Informatics Association states that informatics concerns data collection, analysis, and application to care decisions to improve outcomes, lower costs, and increase safe and quality healthcare services (AMIA, 2024, para. 1–2).

These definitions show that informatics builds upon the foundation of HIT. Informatics is more than inputting data into an EHR and more than being able to navigate a computer. Informatics is the ability to use technology to access and process information and then critically

Wisdom in Nursing

Wisdom in nursing is using knowledge and information appropriately to solve problems. "Wisdom guides the nurse in recognizing the situation at hand, based on the nurse's expertise, patient's and family's values, and patient's healthcare knowledge" (Hebda et al., 2019, p. 24). Wisdom is an iterative process where nursing knowledge is applied to clinical judgment, and actions implemented are evaluated through reflective practice, initiating learning and professional development (Hebda et al., 2019).

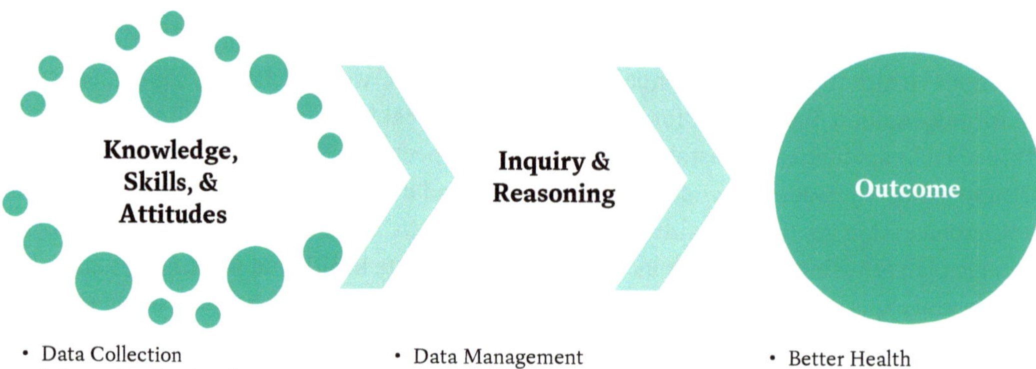

FIGURE 9.2 Nursing Informatics Process

synthesize and apply that information to direct evidence-based decision-making and deliver quality and coordinated healthcare, improving patient outcomes. It involves both practical computer/technology navigation skills and cognitive, perceptive, and analysis abilities, utilizing a person-centered perspective, leading to individualized person-centered care decisions. See Figure 9.2 for a visual of the nursing informatics process.

Digital Health

Digital health describes how technology, such as HIT, converges with healthcare delivery to improve outcomes and service for patients and providers (Bernstein, n.d.; Steckelman, 2019). It is a global concept encompassing a person's health and the healthcare system, changing the interface between health, the healthcare system, and technology. Digital health includes the use of "digital, mobile, and wireless Internet-connected technologies to work with health data (e.g., electronic patient records), health information (e.g., health online and social media sites), and health services (e.g., telehealth)" (The University of Melbourne, 2023, para. 1). It is the overarching construct of how HIT and informatics can be used to create a culture of digital health delivery systems that transform the healthcare system into one with the patient and patient interface as a focal point (Mesko, 2018). Digital health is part of a cultural transformation that includes disruptive technologies that provide digital and objective data accessible to patients and their support systems, leading to equalizing the doctor–patient relationship by including shared decision-making and the "democratization of care" (Mesko, 2018, p. 431).

The change driver of consumerism and the explosion of health technologies have provided opportunities for the patient to be the driver of their care, shifting the culture of healthcare to a system of partnership, involving the patient at the center with a variety of other professions, services, and resources supporting the patient as the driver of their health. This is the opposite of the traditional hierarchical patient-provider dyad where the provider acts as the director of the healthcare experience and the patient, in an unengaged and inactivated fashion, complies or does not comply with health provider directives.

We can view digital health in the sense of technology in healthcare as the node or sensor of the healthcare system. A combination of technologies that support a culture of patient-provider partnership through patient engagement and activation, including detecting changes, monitoring events, sending and receiving information, and connecting all aspects of the healthcare system with the patient at the center. Digital health combines all technologies to improve the patient-provider interface and communication, enhancing wellness, health, and quality of life (Bernstein, n.d.).

The digital health concept and structure support consumer-focused and person-centered care and activated and engaged roles for the individual patient in their healthcare. Aspects of digital health, such as the patient portal, have been shown to improve health awareness and medication adherence and increase preventative care (Dixon et al., 2018). Digital health can also benefit patient outcomes and experiences by leveraging artificial intelligence (AI) to construct predictive modeling through data mining and analysis to inform population health-level interventions on an organizational, local, or national level (Ronquillo et al., 2023). Advantages of integrating digital health into healthcare delivery include supporting person-centered and individualized care for patients, increasing accessibility to care, improving quality of care, and managing resource use and costs.

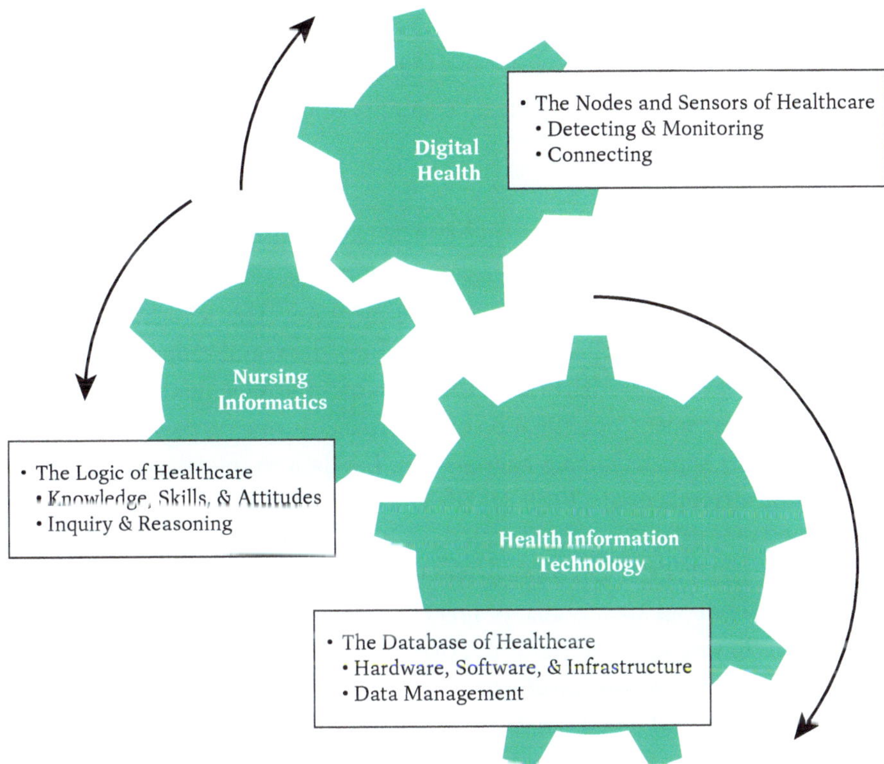

FIGURE 9.3 The Symbiosis of HIT, Informatics, and Digital Health

When considering HIT, informatics, and digital health, we see the connection between the three; this technology-based healthcare system supports a symbiotic relationship. The foundation of HIT supports nurse-directed informatics applications and digital health technology, and informatics and digital health maximize the benefits of HIT in healthcare. Nurses must engage in the logic of informatics and understand how data collection, storage, and retrieval drive and inform their nursing practice and decision-making (Sweeney, 2017). The connection, communication, and monitoring technologies provided by digital health support the overall transformation of the healthcare system and the promotion of health and wellness (Benis et al., 2022). The essential interface of HIT, informatics, and digital health strengthens safe, quality, and coordinated care and healthcare transformation to value-based care delivery. See Figure 9.3 for a visual of the symbiotic relationship.

Regulatory Considerations

The future of healthcare involves optimizing technologies and increasing the ability to transfer information among providers (Sherifi et al., 2021). The evolution of HIT has contributed to the ability to transition to value-based payment models, the transformation to an interprofessional and across-the-continuum approach to care, population health-based interventions advancement, and the enhancement of patient engagement and self-management of health. These advances have also required the development and implementation of regulations concerning information technology use in healthcare. A few notable healthcare regulations affecting information technology use include the Health Information Technology for Economic and Clinical Health (HITECH) Act, the Health Insurance Portability and Accountability Act (HIPAA), and Meaningful Use.

Health Information Technology for Economic and Clinical Health (HITECH) Act

The Health Information Technology for Economic and Clinical Health (HITECH) Act was enacted in 2009 as part of the American Recovery and Reinvestment Act. This legislation provides incentives for EHR use, provides guidelines for the use of EHR data, and supports the development of **Health Information Exchanges** (HIE) with the goals of improving quality, safe, and efficient healthcare, patient engagement, coordination of care, and ensuring privacy and security of data. Additionally, HITECH supports using aggregate or big data to inform quality improvement and policy decisions (Hebda et al., 2019). HITECH allows providers to receive incentivized or enhanced payments for using "certified" EHRs and demonstrating that the EHR is being used in a "meaningful" way. HITECH was a key driver to the implementation of EHRs in healthcare. Before HITECH, only about 10% to 20% of hospitals were using an EHR system, while now almost all hospitals have an EHR system, and over 90% of ambulatory care clinics are using a certified EHR (D'Amore, 2019, *The Good*).

HITECH has had mixed results in meeting its goals of quality, safety, and efficiency of healthcare and coordination of care through Meaningful Use and transmission of data. In the Office of National Compliance (ONC) 2016 report to Congress, it was shown "that 84 percent of academic studies examining health IT functionalities required under the Medicare and Medicaid EHR Incentive Programs had a positive or mixed positive effect on quality, safety, and efficiency of care" (p. 8), supporting the integration of the EHR for meeting HITECH goals. Unfortunately, the United States Government Accountability Office (2023) found that many providers and systems still rely on mail or traditional fax to send or receive patient health information, especially in small or rural hospitals or clinics. This finding is supported by Hsiao et al. (2015), who found that many providers use fax or written documents to exchange patient information, even if they have an EHR system.

Additionally, by incentivizing the EHR and HIT, HITECH supported the development and expansion of HIEs (Alder, n.d.a). An HIE supports the coordinated exchange of patient healthcare data and information electronically across organizations, communities, or systems (NPPES, 2016). This differs from the EHR, which is utilized more on a system or organizational level. The HIE allows for the exchange of essential patient data among different patient information systems. Depending on the system and point-to-point contacts, the HIE can work on a local, regional, state, or national level. The HIE electronic system facilitates the exchange of patient information across providers, organizations, and systems, regardless of where the patient has received care.

For example, the Nationwide Health Information Network (NHIN) provides standards and policies to facilitate the secure exchange of protected health information (PHI) on the Internet. PHI is any individually identifiable data, including demographics, past, present, or future health conditions, information concerning care received, information about payment for care, and anything that can reasonably identify the patient. The NHIN became operational in 2023 under the Trusted Exchange Framework and Common Agreement℠ (TEFCA). The following agencies are the first to be officially designated as Qualified Health Information Networks™ (QHINs™): Epic Nexus, Health Gorilla, KONZA, and MedAllies. It is hoped that many more agencies will participate in QHINs™, resulting in patients having increased access to their health records and providers, systems, and payers being able to enhance the security of electronic records exchange (HHS, 2023).

Health Information Exchanges (HIEs)

HIEs are often funded through membership and transaction fees, where stakeholders such as payers, providers, agencies, hospitals, or clinics pay a membership fee to support the operational costs of the HIE. There may also be transaction fees for specific services offered by a regional or state HIE system. These services could include technical assistance or the amount of HIE use over the month. There may also be a program fee for purchasing and/or implementing the HIE system (Hebda et al., 2019). This can cause barriers to HIE acceptance and implementation. For example, a home health agency may opt not to pay the membership, organization, and program fees for a statewide HIE system access, due to not seeing the value in the costs or believing the costs are prohibitive for their agency.

Health Insurance Portability and Accountability Act (HIPAA)

Part of the HITECH Act addressed privacy and security concerns related to the electronic transmission of health information, strengthening enforcement of the **Health Insurance Portability and Accountability Act (HIPAA)** rules and enhancing fines (HHS, 2021). The HIPAA Act, passed in 1996, requires healthcare organizations and providers to use a variety of privacy protections and safeguards for patient records and identifiable information that is in oral, written, or electronic form (Kelly et al., 2018). HIPAA legislation provides guidelines for the sharing or transmitting of patient information, ensuring that privacy and security protections are in place. HIPAA rules outline these guidelines and enforce procedures for fines or other consequences for rule violations.

HIPAA concerns how patient information is shared through the use of standardized terms and the secure transfer of that data. HIPAA requires that organizations have physical, technical, and administrative processes to protect patient information. This is known as the security rule. HIPAA also requires that organizations not share patient health information without their knowledge or permission, the privacy rule. Organizations must also have processes in place to notify patients if their personal information has been breached within 60 days of the incident and to comply with patients' requests for medical records. These are known as the breach and omnibus rules. Lastly, an enforcement rule outlines standards and procedures for processing complaints and enforcing the rules (HHS, 2021; Secureframe, n.d.). Not following any of the rules is considered a HIPAA violation, which can be as simple as not turning your computer screen off when you step away or looking at a patient health record when you do not have permission or an authorized need. To support the standardization of terms used, HIPAA also includes rules related to the use of transaction and code sets, such as ICD-10 or CPT® codes, and unique identifiers, such as identifiers for a health plan or a unique patient identifier (HIPAA 101, 2024).

HIPAA violations for 2023 had a minimum fine of $137 per violation to a maximum of approximately $69,000 per fine for a Level 1 or a lack of knowledge violation. A Level 1 violation is one in which the violation was unknown and due diligence was exercised. The maximum violation is Level 4, a violation of gross negligence or one in which the HIPAA rules were willfully not followed and were not corrected within 30 days. The fines for a Level 4 violation for 2023 were a minimum fine of approximately $69,000 to a maximum of roughly $2,000,000 per instance and/or jail time (Alder, n.d.b, Table 1). See Figure 9.4 for the levels of HIPAA violations. Fines for HIPAA violations not only put the healthcare organization at risk but also neglect provision 3.1 of the nursing code of ethics, which identifies the need to protect the patient's rights to privacy and confidentiality (ANA, 2015, p. 9).

HIPAA applies to healthcare organizations, payers, health plans, and any business associates that perform services on behalf of one of those entities. For example, a health insurance plan may contract with an agency to provide care management and coordination for their beneficiaries with chronic health conditions; although the contracted agency is not part of the health insurance plan, they still need to follow HIPAA privacy rules. However, HIPAA also identifies when a care coordinator may disclose patient health information, such as to the

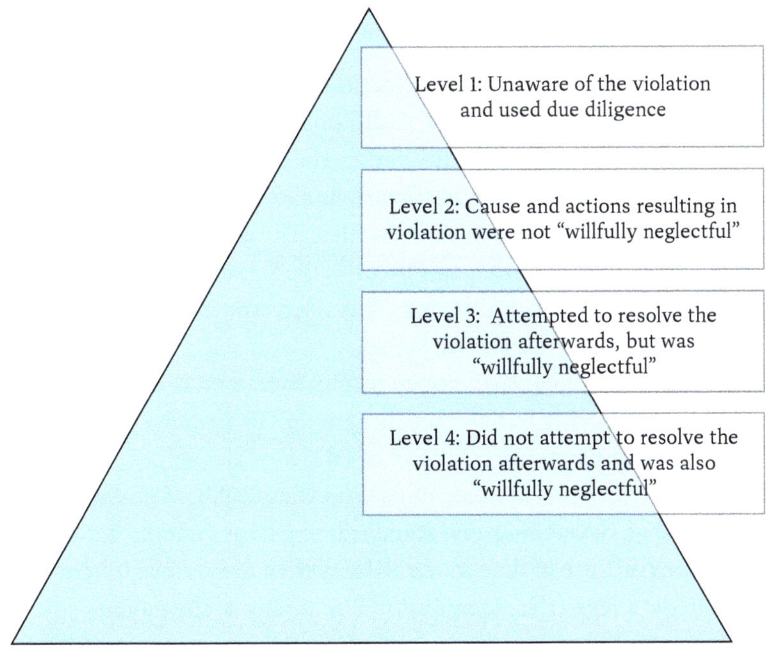

FIGURE 9.4 Levels of HIPAA Violations

patient themselves, for the purposes of treatment, payment, or healthcare operations, or when conducting care coordination, including care planning.

Specifically, HIPPA privacy rules (HHS, 2003) identify that treatment "is the provision, coordination, or management of health care and related services ..." (p. 5). Healthcare operations are defined as "quality assessment and improvement activities, including case management and care coordination ..." (p. 5). So, in these cases, HIPAA rules identify that obtaining patient consent to share their PHI for treatment, payment, or healthcare operations is optional. This does not exclude the care coordinating nurse from ensuring that PHI transmitted arrives to the correct person or organization and only for those purposes outlined in HIPAA rules. The nurse must make "reasonable efforts to use, disclose, and request only the minimum amount of protected health information needed to accomplish the intended purpose ..." (p. 10). The healthcare provider or organization must have policies and procedures and provide training to their workforce to prevent violations of HIPAA, as well as safeguarding data to prevent intentional or unintentional transmission of PHI that violates the HIPAA privacy rule.

It is evident that proactively addressing HIPAA when using HIT is essential in healthcare. Nurses transmitting patient information in care coordination duties must be cognizant of and follow organizational policies and procedures concerning patient information to ensure HIPAA rules are not violated. HIT, informatics, and digital health support the need for timely transfer and sharing of patient information, guiding better decision-making and problem-solving, decreasing costs and resource use, and increasing patient engagement. However, their use must be thoughtfully approached and precautions taken to ensure the patient remains at the center of care and their rights are respected.

Meaningful Use

The healthcare system and HIT support the collection of vast amounts of data. Yet, this data often comes from various sources, and there is difficulty with sharing the data, sometimes making it more of a siloed collection of "stuff" rather than contributing to quality healthcare delivery (Hebda et al., 2019). This data can be in various forms, such as an EHR, emails, shared documents, or Word, PowerPoint, and multimedia files. The data must be used meaningfully for quality and coordinated care, but this can be difficult if there is no outline or framework for how the data should best be used and stored. This need contributed to the development of **Meaningful Use** in 2009 as part of the HITECH Act.

The HITECH Act provided incentive money to providers and organizations to transition to EHR systems. Due to this, poorly but quickly designed EHR systems that catered to organizational desires or skepticism concerning the use of HIT were developed, rather than systems that contributed to the seamless coordination of care (Settles, 2015). Meaningful Use legislation provided standards for using, developing, and standardizing EHR systems. It tied EHR incentive payments to the "meaningful" use of data in the EHR system to improve outcomes, coordinate care, and participate in data registries. Meaningful Use is part of the payment system through the Centers for Medicare and Medicaid Services (CMS) EHR incentive payment programs and requires the organization or provider to demonstrate use of the EHR meaningfully through data capture and sharing, clinical processes, and improving outcomes (HealthIT.gov, 2013).

By 2011, Stage 1 of Meaningful Use was implemented, and incentive payments were made for data capture and sharing use of the EHR (Anumula & Sanelli, 2012; Settles, 2015). In 2012, Stage 2 was implemented, and incentive payments were made to expand Stage 1 to include increased expectations for health information exchange, e-prescribing, and electronic transmission of patient care summaries (Anumula & Sanelli, 2012). In 2016, Stage 3 was implemented, focusing on improving outcomes through the expanded transmission of information across settings, coordination of care, public and clinical data registry reporting, and reporting protection of patient information factors (American Academy of Pediatrics, 2021; CMS, 2024).

One goal of Meaningful Use is to encourage using Certified Electronic Health Record Technology (CEHRT), which promotes interoperability and data exchange. For an organization or provider to be identified as a "meaningful user" and avoid payment penalties, they must show that their EHR system meets CEHRT requirements using the most current standards (CMS, 2024). For 2023, this included meeting the 2015 Edition Cures Update, which has a broad application to the abilities of the CEHRT system and how it is used for patient, clinician, hospital, and CEHRT developer purposes. For example, the key goal of the ONC certification of EHR technologies is to "support clinician engagement in clinical practice, improvement in care coordination activities using health IT—including participation in CMS programs" (HealthIT.gov, 2023, Figure 1). This means that developers of CEHRT products must create products that meet all standards to fulfill this overarching goal, and providers and organizations must have and use tools in the CEHRT system to engage in clinical practice, care coordination, and quality improvement. See Figure 9.5 for a descriptive figure concerning Certified Health IT.

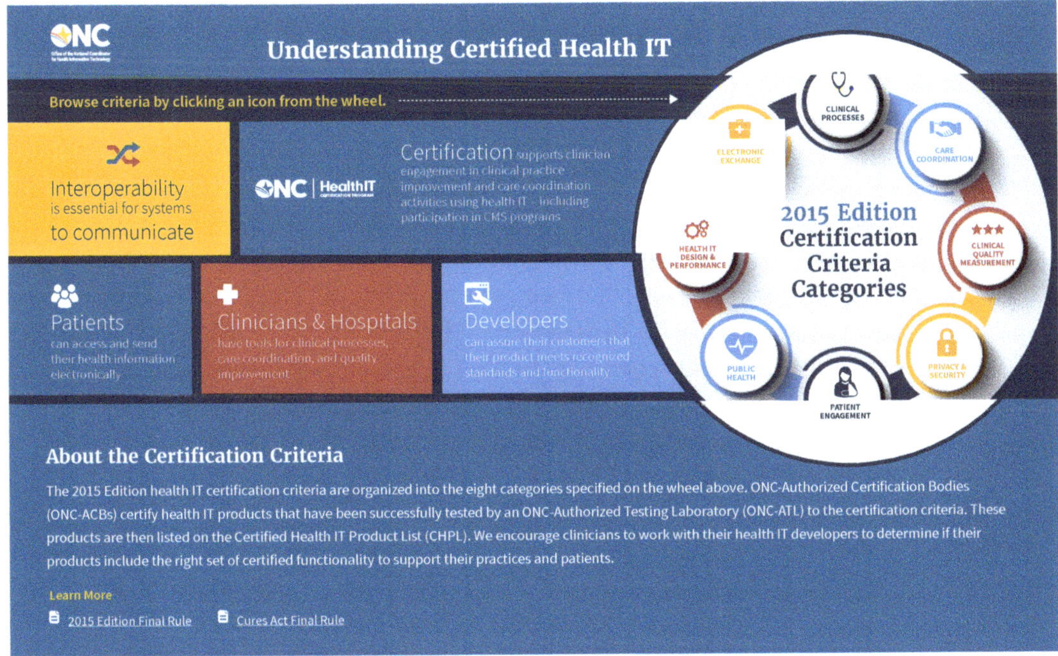

FIGURE 9.5 Understanding Certified Health IT

Considering the certification area of care coordination, some particular areas of the CEHRT are essential for the care coordination nurse to understand and support person-centered care. The first is that the CEHRT must support good transitions of care by being able to create and receive discharge, care, and referral summaries that assist the receiving provider or facility in having the needed information to provide safe and quality care (ONC, n.d.). Secondly, the CEHRT must have clinical information reconciliation and incorporation (CIRI) abilities where a patient's information can be incorporated into the CEHRT from external sources, such as pharmacies or specialist providers (ONC, n.d.). In this way, patient information can be imported into the health record and reconciled to current treatments, medications, and conditions, decreasing the possibility of duplication and poor outcomes. The third area under care coordination is e-prescribing, where prescriptions are entered and sent electronically and stored in the patient's health record for convenient review at follow-up appointments or when transitioning to another setting (ONC, n.d.). This assists with patient and provider satisfaction as well as decreased medication errors. The CEHRT must also have an integrated care plan feature that allows for structured documentation of patient identified goals, assessment data, interventions offered, etc., that supports shared care plan development and person-centered care (ONC, n.d.).

The following care coordination certification areas focus on information transfer, a critical aspect of the CEHRT. Data export functionality is required to export patient information to payers, providers, or other third parties that may use a different CEHRT system (ONC, n.d.). As interoperability is an issue with HIT, this is a function that care coordinating nurses may use extensively, and they must understand the policies and procedures of their organization to ensure that data export follows HIPAA rules. This data export may include a summary of care that the CEHRT generates. It will contain PHI, so it must include a security-tagged care summary, identifying that PHI is included and the data's disclosure restrictions when sent or received (ONC, n.d.). Additionally, the CEHRT must support the export of the entirety of electronic health information related to a specific patient per their request or when the organization changes to a different CEHRT system and needs to export or import the entire patient population electronic health information to the new system (ONC, n.d.).

Meaningful Use is a comprehensive set of regulations that provide the foundation of how to use the EHR to provide patient-centered care that meets HIPAA rules and contributes to the continuing transformation of healthcare to a value-based system. This requires the nurse to understand that each time the EHR is used, it should contribute to "meaningful" patient experiences, quality and safe care delivery, provider and organizational needs, and care coordination across the continuum. Suppose barriers are found to Meaningful Use in care coordination practice. In that case, the nurse must advocate for the discipline and patient experience, reporting issues and suggesting EHR use or documentation improvements. As nurses spend significant amounts of time interfacing with the EHR system, their voice is essential to ensure that future regulations, EHR designs, and organizational policies and procedures support seamless care coordination and value-based nursing care.

Data Management Considerations

Data security is one critical consideration for the care coordinating nurse who is managing data for export to other providers, such as in the transition of care or when they are adding to the patient record assessment or care plan data. When inputting or transmitting electronic data, security is attained through authentication, authorization, and encryption, protecting the data from being altered or falsified. Data is authenticated through processes that confirm the origin and validity of the data, such as in email messages, faxing PHI, or sharing information via internal EHR messaging systems. For example, many email messages received outside of a healthcare organization may have a header or flag indicating that the message is from an external source and one should be cautious with the message.

Much of data authorization can be performed from database management or built-in EHR processes, in which only authorized users can access the email or EHR messaging systems through assigned logins and secure passwords and limiting access to data to only people who have a role in the patient's care (Chin, 2022). In this way, only those who have permission and a need to document, retrieve, and send data, review orders, etc., concerning a patient are given authorization and the ability to perform these actions in the EHR system. The nurse must follow the procedures set in place, not sharing logins and passwords or attempting to access or send data that is not relevant to the care coordination process.

Data encryption is the encoding of the data so that only those authorized can receive and view the data (Puranik, 2020). Encryption is used when data is pulled from the secure EHR system and stored or transferred, such as in an email. HIPAA requires data encryption so that authorized users only access the data, which is securely stored and transmitted. Additionally, data encryption enhances data integrity, as the encryption process can often detect changes to data content (Lau, 2023). The nurse must follow organizational procedures and processes

Data Security and Ransomware

Healthcare data and patient health information are increasingly coming under cyberattack, resulting in the data being held ransom. For example, a hacker was paid a $17,000 Bitcoin ransom for returning HIT access to the Hollywood Presbyterian Hospital after the hacker used malware to infect and lock down the hospital's computer systems, preventing the hospital from being able to use their EHR and other technologies (Winton, 2016).

concerning data encryption and protect patient privacy by not moving secure PHI to nonsecure places, such as USB drives or personal email accounts.

Data integrity means that the data is accurate, complete, and maintained through using standardized terms, reconciling data, and ensuring data is up-to-date. This is a need in healthcare, as the data that the provider, nurses, and others in the interprofessional team access are used to make decisions concerning patient care. Inconsistencies, inaccuracies, or missing data can lead to impaired decision-making and poor patient outcomes (Stearns, n.d.). If the care coordinating nurse fails to ensure that proper coding or standardized terms are used for conditions or interventions, this can affect appeals and claims for the healthcare service, causing additional resource use in processing denials or appeals of claims. Further, the nurse must ensure that data inputted is complete, connects to the patient's diagnoses or conditions, and is relevant, using standardized terms (Stearns, n.d.).

The interprofessional team will review documentation to guide clinical decision-making. If a vague or unstandardized term is used, this may affect how the interprofessional team interprets the data and negatively affect the clinical pathways or decisions made. Furthermore, the care coordinating nurse must make every effort to ensure the data in the EHR or other technology is the most up-to-date; older data needs to be identified or archived if appropriate with organizational policies and procedures (Stearns, n.d.). Lastly, if there are contradictions in the patient record, the nurse needs to document additional context as to why there may be a contradiction when reconciling patient data to assist with quality, safe, and coordinated care delivery.

A common error in data integrity is using synonyms or alternate nonnormative or unstandardized terms in documenting patient information. For example, if a nurse performed a depression screening using the PHQ-9 screening tool and then documented "depression screening conducted" or "screening P9 performed" rather than the designated organizational EHR standardized documentation "PHQ-9 completed," when the data is pulled for quality measure reporting, it will look as though this patient did not have a PHQ-9 screening as it will not register as that in the EHR. For data to be retrievable and aggregated for quality measure benchmarking and continuous quality improvement initiatives, standardized terms and language must be used when inputting data into the EHR (Hebda et al., 2019). If unstandardized terms and language are used, there is potential for loss of critical data, which may cause repetitive screenings or delayed treatment for a positive screening, leading to poor patient outcomes.

Data integration refers to the ability to merge data from different electronic sources. This may occur when a patient is transitioning to a new provider and the past provider exports the

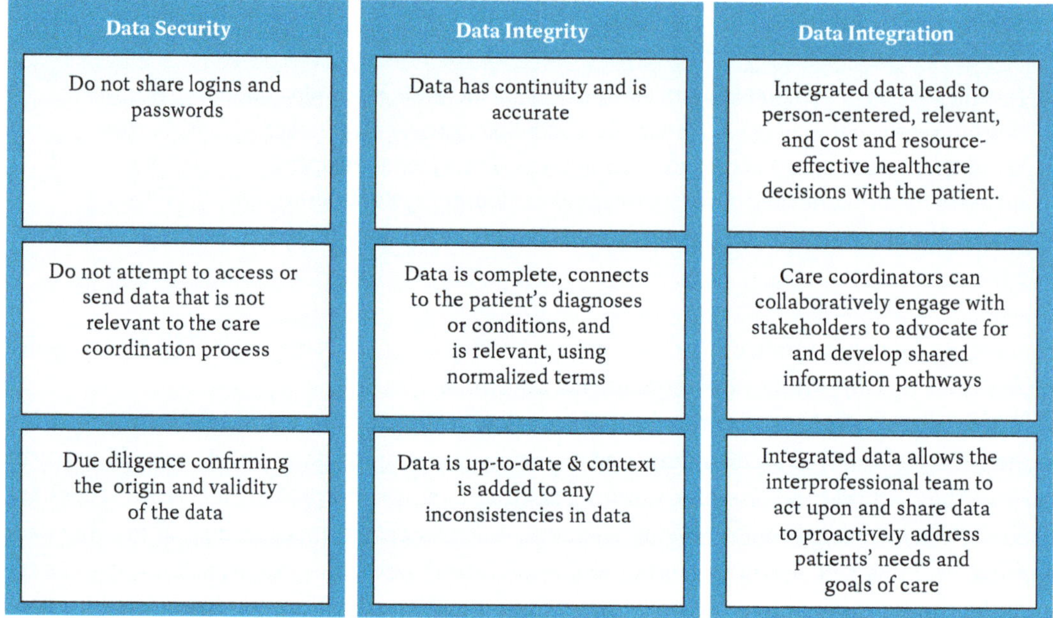

FIGURE 9.6 Data Management Pillars and Care Coordination

patient data to the new provider's office through a secure EHR system. Then the new provider can integrate that patient data into their records. Alternatively, this may occur when an organization moves from one EHR system to another and needs to export all its patient data into the new system.

In care coordination, we can think of this need for data integration as a way to dismantle silos in care. As patient data becomes more integrated, available at all points of care, up-to-date, and accurate, the need for extensive care coordination efforts may decrease (Poku et al., 2019). If data is integrated, each provider can access needed patient information to make person-centered, relevant, and cost-effective and resource-effective healthcare decisions with the patient. For data integration to move beyond just the CEHRT guidelines, nurse care coordinators will need to engage collaboratively with the interprofessional team, payers, community resources, healthcare organizations, and patients to advocate for and develop shared information pathways or processes that are appropriate for their patient population and community so that all stakeholders in the patient's care can "effectively share and act upon information" (Poku et al., 2019, p. 1907). In this way, data integration can be improved, decreasing unnecessary resource use, proactively addressing patients' needs and goals of care, and improving outcomes. See Figure 9.6 for a visual of the application of data management pillars to care coordination practice.

Trade-Offs and Considerations

Technology in healthcare delivery can address many quality and safety of care issues, as well as support coordinated and person-centered care. Yet, several areas need further development or support to integrate technology use, such as HIT, informatics, and digital health. One is the continuing development of solutions to user interface issues that support using technologies for person-centered and coordinated care. Furthermore, although technology can address many issues concerning health equity and accessibility, it also can create barriers to those with lower digital health literacy, those who lack access to technological tools, or those who have sensory, functional, or cognitive impairments, resulting in a lack of digital inclusivity (Fulmer et al., 2021). Lastly, education is needed concerning current regulations such as HIPAA to address privacy and ethical concerns providers may have, as well as infrastructure and interoperability needs on a systems level rather than in a siloed HIT system.

User Interface Considerations

The use of technology in healthcare is often viewed as impersonal or is met with distrust by patients and providers alike. These perceptions may be reinforced by time spent training on use of HIT or digital health applications, disruption to workflows and processes, and design issues that may feel they are clicking through several windows or having to input redundant information. Most of these issues can be resolved with education, time to learn how to use the tools, and organizational support (Vehko et al., 2019). However, two prevalent concerns related to HIT integration into healthcare are based more on the nurse's perceptions and attitudes. These include alert fatigue and the nurse–patient relationship.

Alert Fatigue

The goal is to prevent errors and improve safe and quality care delivery with the support of health technologies, yet without sufficient consideration of user interface or workflow processes, this may not occur. The concept of alarm fatigue is not new. It happens when equipment alarms, such as a cardiac monitor, bring attention to a potential safety issue or change in a patient's condition. This concept also translates to the use of HIT in the form of alert fatigue, where red flag warnings or other alerts are flashed or sent but ignored. When there are many alerts, they may slow or interrupt the workflow or documentation or desensitize the nurse to the alert. This may encourage the view that the alerts are not relevant or important and increase a tendency to ignore the alerts (Jen, 2023).

Research has shown that many alerts may be false or repetitive. If a nurse experiences several false or repetitive alerts, they may develop the perspective that alerts are not that important, and they may only give them a cursory look rather than critically thinking through the alert and whether some action is required. For example, in one study, it was identified that approximately 25% of drug alerts and about 33% of clinical reminders received by a primary care provider (PCP) were repeated alerts, and after the first alert reminder, alert acceptance by the PCP dropped significantly, indicating that many subsequent alert reminders were ignored (Ancker et al., 2017). Nurses need to understand that alerts are key data points that affect their clinical decision-making; ignoring an alert is a decision, but one that can lead to poor patient outcomes and a lack of safe and quality care delivery (Hebda et al., 2019). Nurses are key in promoting quality and safe care delivery and must act accordingly to address alert fatigue (Kelly et al., 2018).

Alert Fatigue Example

A HIT medication alert system in the EHR and CPOE sent an alert to a provider and pharmacist that an order was a 3,800% overdose of a medication. The provider and pharmacist saw the alert but ignored it because they had experienced receiving enormous amounts of prescription alerts, which had primarily been false alarms. They began the habit of only giving the alerts a quick look over and moving on with their work. They had alert fatigue. The patient was given an overdose of medication and went into seizures, which ultimately had significant health consequences, although the patient survived (Wachter, 2015).

Nurse–Patient Relationship

Nurses and patients may feel that the use of HIT, such as charting at the bedside, diminishes the ability to develop caring and trusting relationships. Yet technology has been integrated into nursing care for quite some time in the form of cardiac monitors, vital sign machines, etc. These types of technology are tools for quality and safe nursing care delivery. HIT is the same; it is a tool that can be used to enhance the delivery of nursing care, decrease error potentials, and increase person-centered care. Nurses must understand and communicate to the patients the importance of technology as a tool for enhanced safe and quality care, communication, and data collection so that the healthcare interprofessional team can provide person-centered care. Suppose the nurse does not understand the purpose and function of HIT or does not educate the patient concerning the value and application of HIT. In that case, negative perspectives of HIT use may be reinforced and indirectly contribute to a view of a healthcare system that is not person-centered (Grys, 2022).

HIT is a valuable tool in the nursing "toolbelt" that can build relationships if used effectively and appropriately, allowing the nurse to know more about their patients. However, if the nurse moves their focus to the technology itself rather than how it can assist patient care, it can build a barrier to the nurse–patient relationship (Krel et al., 2022). This concept has more to do with the nurse's perception of technology use and nursing behaviors than the technology itself. Nurses must be competent in **technological knowing** by viewing the patient as a whole person and effectively using technologies to provide holistic care and support patient activation and self-management of health (Krel et al., 2022). Nurses can enhance and support other ways of understanding and knowing patients through the competent use and combination of technology with person-centered nursing practice. The use of HIT does not mean that a caring relationship cannot be developed or supported. Rather, through technological knowing, nurses have another way of understanding their patients "through the competent use of technologies" (Locsin, 2017, p. 163).

By integrating data available in HIT systems into nursing practice, nurses can obtain an enhanced view of the patient as a dynamic and multidimensional being that changes over time and may have unpredictable behaviors or outcomes (Locsin, 2017). Technology and person-centered care can coexist with competent and dynamic engagement of the patient and technology interface. The use of technology does not replace a caring and person-centered approach. It augments nursing and care coordination practice through enhanced communication abilities, error prevention tools, and whole-person data-driven clinical decision-making and informatics.

Ethical, Equity, and Accessibility Considerations

Part of technological knowing is retaining a humanity perspective when using HIT and other technologies for healthcare. There is an ethical obligation to apply technologies individually to patient care delivery, rather than indiscriminately using them without a person-centered approach and perspective. One such ethical issue is that of **digital inclusivity**. On a broad level, digital inclusivity ensures that all individuals have access to and can use information and communication technology, including access to the Internet and Internet-equipped devices, and addresses barriers to technology use. Necessary activities for digital inclusivity include affordable Internet access, Internet devices that meet the user's needs, digital literacy training, technical support, and applications and content that enable users to be engaged and activated in self-management of health (NDIA, n.d.).

The extensive and integral use of technology in healthcare delivery can potentially exclude specific populations from receiving technology-based care, contributing to health inequities and lack of accessibility to care (Sheikh et al., 2021). For example, those who may have visual or hearing disabilities or those who have lower digital literacy levels may be at risk for exclusion from digital healthcare delivery and support. Adaptive interfaces may be needed for those with differing abilities, allowing the applications or devices to alter layouts or features, such as text-to-speech or alternate light modes, so that they may access and utilize health technologies effectively. Digital inclusion requires intentional strategies to reduce and eliminate barriers to the use of technology (NDIA, n.d.).

Digital inclusion can be considered a social determinant of health because if patients cannot access or use technological healthcare services such as telemedicine or their patient portal, they may be disadvantaged in health outcomes (CTN, 2023). Additionally, if they do not have access to digital literacy education, they may have reduced access to health information, which can affect their healthcare decision-making and self-management of health. Furthermore, if they cannot access Internet-capable devices or the Internet, they may be unable to use mobile health applications, track health or fitness goals, or utilize remote patient monitoring devices for things like their blood pressure or oxygen saturation. This requires the nurse to thoroughly assess patient needs, resources, and digital literacy so that support can be provided to the patient. This also means that nurses must advocate for patient needs and policy and process development or reforms prioritizing digital inclusion strategies and interventions on an organizational, community, and national level. "By providing equal access to digital technologies, we can close healthcare disparities, empower patients, and improve health outcomes for all" (CTN, 2023, para. 5). See Figure 9.7 for a visual of aspects of digital inclusivity in healthcare.

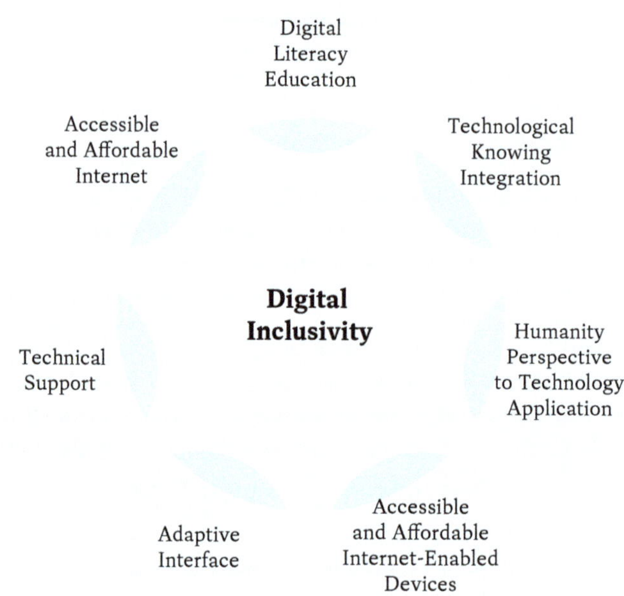

FIGURE 9.7 Digital Inclusivity in Healthcare

Privacy and Infrastructure Considerations

Several challenges become apparent when considering the need to protect patient privacy and the security of their PHI while enhancing continuity and coordination of care. As part of the value-based healthcare transformation, there is a need to collect multiple types and large amounts of data to ensure that quality care is being delivered. Data security is not only an issue for individual EHR systems used on an organizational level, but also concerns where the data is stored. In addition, providers and organizations may be reluctant to share their patients' PHI due to the desire not to violate HIPAA rules. Lastly, a significant consideration in implementing HIT, HIEs, and other technologies is infrastructure and the interoperability of systems. These security and connection issues can cause challenges to the seamless coordination of care and the import and export of PHI.

Big Data Sets

An HIT-specific issue is one involving big data or large data sets. For example, quality measure data sets are collected for reimbursement purposes. They are analyzed by the CMS and other stakeholders, such as payers or national organizations, to inform improvements to the coordination of care practices (Hebda et al., 2019). **Big data** are large sets of data that support digital healthcare delivery and quality healthcare delivery through analysis, identifying data patterns, facilitating predictive modeling, and informing population- or system-level interventions and improvements that support quality healthcare delivery and outcomes. Frequently, this data is stored in a cloud-based system, as the amount of data collected is often too large for any one facility to store or manage. Cloud-based systems deliver computing services, such as data storage, networking, analytics, etc., over the Internet or the cloud (HHS Cybersecurity Program, 2021). These systems must follow the Omnibus Final Rule, requiring that business associates/contractors are HIPAA compliant and will be held accountable for meeting these requirements. Yet cloud-based systems are still vulnerable to security breaches and either loss or movement of data from one storage location to another or ransomware attacks.

Provider Patient Privacy Concerns

Due to HIPAA, some healthcare providers or organizations are unwilling or hesitant to share data with other organizations/providers because they feel they may violate patient privacy and security rules. "Confusion about the Health Insurance Portability and Accountability Act (HIPAA) often prevents physicians from sharing electronic protected health information without a patient's authorization" (Parks, 2016, para. 1). The HIPAA rules are designed to protect PHI from misuse. Still, the rules also identify that PHI can be accessed, used, and shared without the patient's permission for healthcare delivery purposes. There are some guidelines to this, including that both the sender and receiver of the PHI must have a relationship with the patient, only what PHI is needed is disclosed, and the PHI shared must relate to the patient–provider relationship (HHS, 2022). Unfortunately, confusion about the HIPAA rules and fear of fines or litigation have created barriers to the efficient and timely data sharing for care coordination and transition management purposes.

Further education for healthcare providers and nurses concerning HIPAA rules and the need for data-sharing is essential for care coordination and value-based reimbursement processes. Value-based care relies on coordination across the continuum of care and easy access to essential PHI and data. If patient information is incomplete, not shared, or inaccessible, coordinated care may not be possible (ASPE, n.d.). Prompt patient data sharing is needed to ensure that LOS guidelines are met and that the patient receives timely follow-up care. This will decrease healthcare costs and increase positive patient outcomes.

Infrastructure Considerations

Implementation of an EHR can be costly and cost-prohibitive for some providers or organizations. It is not just the purchase of the technology; the cost also includes hardware, software, Internet expansion, added information technology support staff, and staff training. All these costs are just to support the initial integration of the EHR. This does not include the costs of revising workflows or updating policies or procedures (Jen, 2023). It has been estimated that the upfront and yearly expenses for EHR implementation for a five-person practice are approximately $162,000 in the first year and $85,000 a year in maintenance costs (Palabindala et al., 2016, p. 3). These high costs require all stakeholders to collaborate and develop strategies, regulations, and infrastructure supporting EHR adoption.

Interoperability is another infrastructure issue that has affected the ability to share data amongst different systems and providers. Interoperability is the ability of the EHR to securely exchange and receive electronic health information with other EHR systems, allowing for data access and use. There are many aspects of interoperability, including organizational processes and procedures, standardized terms, standardized data exchange formats and guidelines, and the actual technical interoperability to securely export and import data between EHR systems

(Knickman & Elbel, 2019). Inconsistency in standardized data formats and guidelines is one of the primary barriers to interoperability in healthcare (Ali, 2022). Even if two EHR systems could securely export and import data, if the data is formatted differently, it may not be able to be integrated into the other EHR system. The variety of formats and guidelines, workarounds, and organizational EHR adaptations may signify one of the most significant obstacles to quality care coordination: siloed care delivery.

For interoperability to be attained, all stakeholders will need to collaborate concerning standards, formats, processes, and regulations, and data will need to be viewed as the *basis* of coordinated care delivery, not as a commodity or strategic resource in a siloed and fragmented healthcare system (Riesman, 2017). "The future of EHR and its ability to be an important tool in care coordination and team-based care will depend on the action taken by the EHR vendor industry and the federal government to ensure interoperability is a major focus" (Reisman, 2017, p. 575).

CHAPTER SUMMARY

Care coordination and continuity of care depend on data and data sharing. Technology in care coordination is essential as it improves the quality of care through all disciplines having access to the same EHR or patient record. It improves patient satisfaction as the patient has to repeat themselves less often when their PHI is on a localized record that the entire health team can access. It also assists in controlling costs by minimizing duplications of care. Furthermore, using a variety of technology-based healthcare delivery systems provides timely and proactive care, potentially decreasing readmissions and emergency room use.

Communication is a critical aspect of HIT integration into care coordination practice. Communication with the patient can occur through a patient interface or with other providers and organizations involved in the patient's care delivery and payment. Communication is essential to facilitate transitions in care and securely exchange patient information so that the receiving provider or facility can deliver quality and safe patient care. Communication of patient goals, priorities, and needs for care can be facilitated with HIT by developing person-centered care plans and documenting assessment data in the EHR system so the interprofessional team can engage in coordinated care planning and care delivery.

Moreover, communication via HIT can support follow-up, monitoring, and self-management of health through integrated clinical pathways, alert and reminder systems, and health education resources (AHRQ, 2014). Technology in care coordination practice assists in standardizing assessment, data quality, creating person-centered care plans and pathways, and real-time data accessibility that can support interprofessional collaboration (Iorfino et al., 2021). Standards of nursing practice also support using standardized classification systems, technology, decision support tools, and data to effectively communicate diagnoses, issues, or patient problems (ANA, 2021).

HIT, informatics, and digital health tools are essential to promote quality, safe, and coordinated care. Health technologies will continue to evolve and address patient and population-level health needs, focusing on supporting patient activation, engagement, and self-management of health (Ronquillo et al., 2023). Yet there are barriers and other considerations to the use of

EHRs and Care Coordination

"EHRs bring a meaningful medium to enhance continuity of care, care coordination, access to information, and satisfaction for both patient and provider, while decreasing costs" (Hebda et al., 2019, p. 12).

technology in healthcare, and the nurse must ensure that equitable access and digital inclusivity of technology is supported, as well as patients obtaining the advocacy and education needed to use healthcare technology to improve and manage their health (ANA, 2021).

HIT use in care coordination facilitates person-centered care by supporting seamless care transitions and essential PHI exchange, communication, and handoffs. HIT also allows the care coordinating nurse to access evidence-based clinical pathways and decision trees for proactive care planning and leverage alert systems to ensure that gaps in care or potential barriers to positive outcomes are addressed timely and efficiently (Haas et al., 2014). Furthermore, care coordination efforts supported by HIT can facilitate patients' utilization of patient portals, monitor their health and care needs, schedule appointments, and proactively communicate with and amongst multiple providers (Chen et al., 2022).

In addition, HIT-supported care coordination promotes one of the main goals of care coordination—managing costs and resources. The EHR system can monitor the LOS and safety events, capturing clinical quality measure data and alerting the care coordinating nurse to areas that may need to be dealt with. HIT can also assist the care coordinating nurse in risk stratifying patients to determine which ones may need more urgent care coordination intervention or to identify specific patient populations with direct care coordination efforts, such as those with chronic health conditions or those with high care costs or frequent visits (Haas et al., 2014).

HIT-supported data collection can also support the achievement of the Quintuple Aim through the ability to utilize and manage data for intentional and actionable care coordination interventions, policy and process development, and patient advocacy (Campbell, 2023). Care coordination supported by HIT enhances the understanding of and interventions provided to address SDOH, such as digital inclusivity. These HIT-enhanced abilities may offer new challenges to integration and use in the healthcare system. Still, they also provide ample opportunities to support health equity, clinician well-being, patient satisfaction, positive outcomes, cost, and resource use, and overall healthcare transformation.

CHAPTER 9 GLOSSARY

Big Data: Large sets of data that are analyzed, identifying data patterns, facilitating predictive modeling, and informing population- or system-level interventions and improvements that support quality healthcare delivery and outcomes.

Data: A collection of discrete facts or statistics that communicates information that can be aggregated, retrieved, and used in the transfer and analysis of quality or other measures or material.

Data Integration: The ability to merge data from different electronic sources.

Data Integrity: Data that is accurate, complete, and maintained through using standardized terms, reconciling data, and ensuring data is up-to-date.

Data Security: When inputting or transmitting electronic data, security is attained through the use of authentication, authorization, and encryption, protecting the data from being altered or falsified.

Digital Health: A combination of technologies that support a culture of patient–provider partnership through patient engagement and activation, detecting changes, monitoring events, sending and receiving information, and connecting all aspects of the healthcare system with the patient at the center.

Digital Inclusivity: Ensuring that all individuals have access to and can use information and communication technology, including access to Internet and Internet-equipped devices, and addressing barriers to technology use.

Disruptive Technologies: Innovative technology that significantly alters workflows, structures, or processes and the way healthcare is delivered.

Health Information Exchange (HIE): An electronic system that facilitates the exchange of patient information across providers, organizations, and systems, regardless of where the patient has received care.

Health Information Technology (HIT): A system, including hardware and software, that manages the inputting, searching, organizing, managing, and extracting of health data in an electronic environment.

Health Information Technology for Economic and Clinical Health (HITECH) Act: Legislation that provides incentives for EHR use, provides guidelines for the use of EHR data, and supports the development of Health Information Exchanges (HIE), with the goals of improving quality, safe, and efficient healthcare, engaging patients, coordinating care, and ensuring privacy and security of data.

Health Insurance Portability and Accountability Act (HIPAA): Legislation that provides guidelines for the sharing or transmitting of patient information, ensuring that privacy and security protections are in place. HIPAA rules outline these guidelines and enforce procedures for fines or other consequences for rule violations.

Informatics: Using practical technology skills and cognitive, perceptive, and analytic abilities to access, process, critically synthesize, and apply electronic information to direct evidence-based decision-making and deliver quality, person-centered, and coordinated healthcare.

Interoperability: The ability of an EHR to securely exchange and receive electronic health information with other EHR systems, allowing for access and use of the data.

Meaningful Use: Legislation that provides standards for the use, development, and standardization of EHR systems and ties EHR incentive payments to the "meaningful" use of data available in the EHR system to improve outcomes, coordinate care, and participate in data registries.

Technological Knowing: The competent use and combining of technology with person-centered nursing practice, enhancing and supporting other ways of understanding and knowing patients.

DISCUSSION QUESTIONS AND ACTIVITIES

Discussion Questions

1. Choose health information technology (HIT), informatics, or digital health and describe how the technology can support quality and safe nursing care delivery. Then identify one barrier to its implementation and integration into nursing practice.
2. Discuss how health information technology (HIT) can improve patient outcomes, reduce healthcare costs, and improve care coordination.
3. Identify and discuss how digital health contributes to equalizing the provider–patient relationship and explain how this benefits healthcare delivery.
4. Explain how digital inclusion can be considered a social determinant of health and discuss how the nurse can promote it in their nursing practice.
5. Discuss the issue of alert fatigue, identifying what it is, how it can affect effective nursing informatics, and how nurses can address the issue in their practice.

Activities

1. Choose one of the following regulations regarding health technology: HITECH, HIPAA, or Meaningful Use. Write a short essay summarizing the regulation's main points, goals, and how the regulation can affect care coordination practices. Identify one aspect of the regulation that you believe could be improved or revised to enhance implementation in the healthcare system.
2. In a small group, create a definition of health technology-supported care coordination. Then give examples of how the care coordinating nurse might apply health technology-supported care coordination to each nursing process step (ADOPIE).
3. Case Study

   An 85-year-old woman arrives in the emergency room on a Sunday night from a long-term care facility where she has resided for the last 2 years. The patient is nonresponsive after experiencing a fall, and the examination and testing show that the patient had a berry aneurysm that ruptured. Because of her age, health history, and length of time since the aneurysm ruptured, the patient is not a candidate for surgical intervention. The neurologist on duty is recommending supportive and comfort care, as the prognosis is grave, with death imminent.

The family has arrived, and the care coordinating nurse enters the room to determine if the patient has an advanced healthcare directive. The family indicates that the patient did complete an advanced directive last year with her primary care provider, but they do not know what is included in the advanced directive. Unfortunately, the patient was brought to a local hospital that was not in the primary care provider's health system. The care coordinating nurse attempts to access the advanced directive through the state Health Information Exchange (HIE) but can only access data that indicates the patient has an advanced directive, not the actual document. The care coordinating nurse calls the hospital associated with the patient's primary care provider records department to request that the advanced directive be sent to the emergency room provider for review. The records department indicates they will need to look for it, but they are short staffed, so it will be 1 to 2 hours.

While the care coordinating nurse awaits this information, the family begins to want the patient admitted to the intensive care unit (ICU) for all possible care, including surgery if needed. The emergency department provider is reluctant and discusses the grave prognosis with the family members. The family becomes quite upset, expressing their dissatisfaction with the care the patient has received, and demands that the patient be admitted to the ICU and emergent surgery be given immediately.

The advanced directive finally arrives by fax, and the care coordinating nurse is notified of this by the unit clerk. The advanced directive states that the patient wants no heroic measures and to be on comfort measures if the condition is likely nonreversible. The care coordinating nurse shares this information with the family and discusses how the advanced directive applies to the patient's condition. The family agrees to follow the patient's wishes. The patient is admitted to the medical floor for end-of-life comfort measures and supportive care.

1. What health technologies could have been used to improve communication between the two healthcare systems/hospitals and the family? What barriers to communication existed?
2. How would having the patient's up-to-date advanced directive available improve the emergency room providers' and neurologists' ability to admit patients promptly and appropriately and assist with person-centered and relationship-centered care?
3. How would having a Health Information Exchange (HIE) with complete and accessible information ensure that the patient's advanced directive care goals would be followed?

NCLEX STYLE QUESTIONS

1. Which of the following allows healthcare information to be shared electronically across systems, organizations, and communities?

    a. Meaningful Use

    b. Business Associate Agreement

    c. Health Information Exchange

    d. Informatics

2. What is the nurse care coordinator assessing when determining the ability of the patient to access the Internet, Internet-enabled devices, and barriers to technology use?

    a. Health literacy

    b. Digital Inclusivity

    c. Digital health

    d. Health equity

3. What is the name for practical technology skills and cognitive, perceptive, and analytic abilities to access, process, critically synthesize, and apply electronic information to direct evidence-based decision-making and deliver quality, person-centered, and coordinated healthcare?

    a. Interoperability

    b. Critical thinking

    c. Informatics

    d. Health information technology

4. Which of the following is an outcome of the nursing informatics process?

    a. Information retrieval

    b. Interprofessional practice

    c. Decreased resource use and costs

    d. Navigation of health information technology

5. Digital health is a combination of technologies that support which of the following: (Select all that apply.)

    a. The provider-patient hierarchy

    b. Connecting aspects of the healthcare system

    c. Health awareness

    d. Emergent care

6. What type of relationship do health information technology, nursing informatics, and digital health have?

    a. Adversarial

    b. Interprofessional

    c. Person-centered

    d. Symbiotic

7. This regulation has the goals of quality, safe, and efficient healthcare and coordination of care through the meaningful use and transmission of data.

    a. HIPAA

    b. Meaningful Use

    c. CEHRT

    d. HITECH

8. The Nationwide Health Information Network (NHIN) provides standards and policies concerning which of the following?

    a. The secure exchange of personal health information on the Internet

    b. Meaningful use of EHR systems

    c. The exchange of personal health information across settings

    d. Fines and procedures for HIPAA violations

9. You are orienting a new nurse concerning HIPAA policies and procedures in your unit. You know the nurse understands your teaching when they say which of the following?

    a. HIPAA violations occur only when nurses knowingly violate the HIPAA rules.

    b. If there is a ransomware attack and the health information is ultimately returned, the healthcare organization does not need to notify the patient according to HIPAA.

    c. It is not a HIPAA violation if I try to access a patient record for a patient not assigned to me if I know the patient.

    d. HIPPA concerns the sharing or transmission of patient information and violations can put the organization at risk.

10. HIPPA allows the care coordinating nurse to share patient information without patient permission under which of the following circumstances?

    a. The information is being shared for healthcare operations or payment purposes.

    b. Only the minimum amount of health information needed is shared.

    c. The sender and receiver of the health information must have a relationship with the patient.

    d. All of the above.

11. Data security is essential when inputting or transmitting electronic data. Which of the following are ways that data security can be attained?

    a. Certification, Endorsement, and Encryption

    b. Accommodation, Authorization, and Encoding

    c. Authentication, Authorization, and Encryption

    d. Authentication, Permission, and Encoding

12. The ability of health information technology (HIT) to securely exchange and receive electronic health information with other HIT systems is referred to as which of the following?

    a. Integration

    b. Integrity

    c. Interoperability

    d. Infrastructure

The following three questions relate to the following scenario.

Fiona Garth is a 52-year-old woman who has been diagnosed with Stage 4 breast cancer and has been admitted to the unit for surgical removal of a metastatic lung tumor. Fiona has been previously identified as having low health literacy and has been reluctant to discuss her diagnosis and condition with her family or her assigned nurses. She frequently expresses how the hospital is impersonal and full of beeping computers.

13. You are the assigned nurse for Fiona, have just completed your initial assessment for the shift, and are about to begin documenting the assessment in the bedside computer EHR system. Which of the following would you say to Fiona before starting your documentation?

    a. Fiona, I will step over here to the computer and chart. I will only be a few minutes.

    b. Fiona, I will be documenting on this computer for a few minutes. This will allow your care team to access the information they need to provide safe and quality care.

    c. Fiona, I need to chart on the bedside computer for a few minutes. It takes my attention to ensure I don't miss an area, so please don't interrupt me.

    d. Fiona, do you need anything else? If not, I will finish this charting and see you after lunchtime.

14. As you finish your assessment documentation, you notice a new note from the social worker has been entered. You pull it up and review it, discovering that Fiona has asked the social worker about hospice care services, but she does not want her family to know as they want her to "keep fighting." She expressed to the social worked that she is exhausted and does not like going to the hospital or the doctor anymore. You decide to gently explore how Fiona is feeling and her thoughts concerning her scheduled surgery so you can offer support and resources if needed. This is an example of what?

    a. Technological competence

    b. Technological innovation

    c. Technological informatics

    d. Technological knowing

15. As you discussed the situation and upcoming surgery with Fiona, she said she has just been doing what the doctor and her family want as everyone talks so fast. She does not ever understand what anybody says to her when they are explaining things to her about her breast cancer, so she does not say anything. But a friend at church had mentioned hospice to her, and it sounded like something she might want. Fiona explains that she has tried to look up more information about hospice and what it is, but she only has a

small cellular phone. She can never see words on the screen due to having significant vision problems, and she cannot afford to pay for Internet in her home or to purchase a computer. What Fiona is describing represents which of the following?

a. Reduced access to health information

b. Lack of adaptive technologies

c. Inability to use information and communication technologies

d. All of the above

REFERENCES

Agency for Healthcare Research and Quality (AHRQ). (2014). *Chapter 3. Care coordination measurement framework.* Author. https://www.ahrq.gov/ncepcr/care/coordination/atlas/chapter3.html

Alder, S. (n.d.a). What is the HITECH Act? *The HIPAA Journal.* https://www.hipaajournal.com/what-is-the-hitech-act/

Alder, S. (n.d.b). HIPAA violation fines. *The HIPAA Journal.* https://www.hipaajournal.com/hipaa-violation-fines/

Ali, N. (2022). EHR interoperability challenges and solutions. *EHR in Practice.* https://www.ehrinpractice.com/ehr-interoperability-challenges-solutions.html

American Academy of Pediatrics. (2021). *Meaningful Use overview.* https://www.aap.org/en/practice-management/health-information-technology/meaningful-use-overview/

American Association of Colleges of Nursing (AACN). (2021). *The Essentials: Core competencies for professional nursing education.* https://www.aacnnursing.org/Portals/0/PDFs/Publications/Essentials-2021.pdf

American Medical Informatics Association (AMIA). (2024). *Why informatics?* https://amia.org/about-amia/why-informatics

American Nurses Association (ANA). (2014). *Nursing informatics: Scope and standards of Practice* (2nd ed.) (For Historical Reference Only). https://www.nursingworld.org/nurses-books/nursing-informatics-scope-and-standards-of-practice-2nd-ed/

American Nurses Association (ANA). (2015). *Code of ethics for nurses: With interpretive statements.* Author.

American Nurses Association. (2021). *Nursing: Scope and standards of practice* (4th ed.). American Nurses Association.

Ancker, J. S., Edwards, A., Nosal, S., Hauser, D., Mauer, E., Kaushal, R., & the HITEC Investigators (2017). Effects of workload, work complexity, and repeated alerts on alert fatigue in a clinical decision support system. *BMC Medical Informatics and Decision Making, 17*(1), 36. https://doi.org/10.1186/s12911-017-0430-8

Anumula, N., & Sanelli, P. C. (2012). Meaningful Use. *AJNR. American Journal of Neuroradiology, 33*(8), 1455–1457. https://doi.org/10.3174/ajnr.A3247

Assistant Secretary for Planning and Evaluation (ASPE). (n.d.). *Supporting value-based care transformation through interoperability and care coordination.* https://aspe.hhs.gov/sites/default/files/2021-07/value-based-care.pdf

Benis, A., Grosjean, J., Billey, K., Montanha, G., Dornauer, V., Crişan-Vida, M., Hackl, W. O., Stoicu-Tivadar, L., & Darmoni, S. J. (2022) Medical informatics and digital health multilingual ontology (MIMO): A tool to improve international collaborations. *International Journal of Medical Informatics, 167*, 104860. https://doi.org/10.1016/j.ijmedinf.2022.104860

Bernstein, C. (n.d.). Digital health (digital healthcare). *TechTarget Health IT.* https://www.techtarget.com/searchhealthit/definition/digital-health-digital-healthcare

Campbell, M. (2023). *Achieving the Quintuple Aim through data-driven transformation.* https://www.linkedin.com/pulse/achieving-quintuple-aim-through-data-driven-transformation-t3gzc/

Centers for Medicare and Medicaid Services (CMS). (2024). *2023 program requirements.* https://www.cms.gov/medicare/regulations-guidance/promoting-interoperability-programs/2023-program-requirements

Chen, J., Buchongo, P., Spencer, M. R. T., & Reynolds, C. F. (2022). An HIT-supported care coordination framework for reducing structural racism and discrimination for patients with ADRD. *The American Journal of Geriatric Psychiatry, 30*(11), 1171–1179. https://doi.org/10.1016/j.jagp.2022.04.010.

Chin, K. (2022). Authenticity vs. non-repudiation. *UpGuard*. https://www.upguard.com/blog/authenticity-vs-non-repudiation

Community Tech Network (CTN). (2023). *Why digital inclusion matters for healthcare*. https://communitytechnetwork.org/blog/why-digital-inclusion-matters-for-healthcare/

D'Amore, J. (2019). 10 years since HITECH: The good, the bad and the ugly. *Healthcare IT Today*. https://www.healthcareittoday.com/2019/12/19/10-years-since-hitech-the-good-the-bad-and-the-ugly/

Dixon, B. E., Embi, P. J., & Haggstrom, D. A. (2018). Information technologies that facilitate care coordination: Provider and patient perspectives. *Translational Behavioral Medicine, 8*(3), 522–525. https://doi.org/10.1093/tbm/ibx086

Fulmer, T., Reuben, D. B., Auerbach, J., Fick, D. M., Galambos, C., & Joshnson, K. S. (2021). Actualizing better health and health care for older adults. *Health Affairs, 40*(2). https://www.healthaffairs.org/doi/full/10.1377/hlthaff.2020.01470

Grys, C. A. (2022). Digital health: The next evolution of healthcare delivery. *Nursing, 52*(10), 40–43. https://doi.org/10.1097/01.NURSE.0000872464.40584.87

HealthIT.gov. (2013). *Meaningful Use*. https://www.healthit.gov/faq/what-meaningful-use

HealthIT.gov. (2022). *About ONC*. https://www.healthit.gov/topic/about-onc

HealthIT.gov. (2023). *2015 edition*. https://www.healthit.gov/topic/certification-ehrs/2015-edition

Hebda, T., Hunter, K., & Czar, P. (2019). *Handbook of informatics for nurses and healthcare professionals* (6th ed.). Pearson.

HHS Cybersecurity Program. (2021). Threats in healthcare cloud computing [PowerPoint Slides]. https://www.hhs.gov/sites/default/files/threats-in-healthcare-cloud-computing.pdf

HIPAA 101. (2024). *HIPAA rules & standards*. http://www.hipaa-101.com/hipaa-rules.htm

Hsiao, C. J., King, J., Hing, E., & Simon, A. E. (2015). The role of health information technology in care coordination in the United States. *Medical care, 53*(2), 184–190. https://doi.org/10.1097/MLR.0000000000000276

Iorfino, F., Piper, S. E., Prodan, A., LaMonica, H. M., Davenport, T. A., Lee, G. Y., Capon, W., Scott, E. M., Occhipinti, J. A., & Hickie, I. B. (2021). Using digital technologies to facilitate care coordination between youth mental health services: A guide for implementation. *Frontiers in Health Services, 1*, 745456. https://doi.org/10.3389/frhs.2021.745456

Institute of Medicine (IOM). (2001). *Crossing the quality chasm: A new health system for the 21st century*. National Academy Press.

Jen, M. Y., Kerndt, C. C., & Korvek, S. J. (2023). Health information technology. In *StatPearls*. StatPearls Publishing. https://pubmed.ncbi.nlm.nih.gov/29262233/

Kelly, P., Vottero, B. A., & Christie-McAuliffe, C. A. (Eds.). (2018). *Introduction to quality and safety education for nurses: Core competencies for nursing leadership and management* (2nd ed.). Springer Publishing Company.

Knickman, J. R., & Elbel, B. (Eds.) (2019). *Jonas & Kovner's health care delivery in the United States* (12th ed.). Springer Publishing Company.

Krel, C., Vrbnjak, D., Bevc, S., Štiglic, G., & Pajnkihar, M. (2022). Technological competency as caring in nursing: A description, analysis and evaluation of the theory. *Slovenian Journal of Public Health, 61*(2). 115–123. https://doi.org/10.2478/sjph-2022-0016

Lau, V. (2023). HIPAA encryption: Requirements, best practices & software. *Kiteworks*. https://www.kiteworks.com/hipaa-compliance/hipaa-encryption/

Locsin, R. C. (2017). The co-existence of technology and caring in the theory of technological competency as caring in nursing. *The Journal of Medical Investigation, 64*(1.2), 160–164. https://doi.org/10.2152/jmi.64.160

Mesko, B. (2018). Health IT and digital health: The future of health technology is diverse. *Journal of Clinical and Translational Research, 3*(Suppl 3), 431–434. https://www.ncbi.nlm.nih.gov/pmc/articles/PMC6412600/

National Plan and Provider Enumeration System (NPPES). (2016). Health information exchange (HIE) page. *CMS*. https://nppes.cms.hhs.gov/webhelp/nppeshelp/HEALTH%20INFORMATION%20EXCHANGE.html

NDIA. (n.d.). *The words behind our work: The source for definitions of digital inclusion terms*. https://www.digitalinclusion.org/definitions/

Office of the National Coordinator for Health Information Technology (ONC). (n.d.). *Understanding certified health IT* [Infographic]. https://www.healthit.gov/sites/default/files/page/2020-12/ONC_Policy_Infographic_2020_508.pdf

Office of the National Coordinator of Health Information Technology (ONC). (2016). 2016 report to Congress on health IT progress: Examining the HITECH era the future of health IT. *HealthIT.gov.* https://www.healthit.gov/sites/default/files/2016_report_to_congress_on_healthit_progress.pdf

Office of the National Coordinator of Health Information Technology (ONC). (2020). 2020–2025 Federal Health IT Strategic Plan. *HealthIT.gov.* https://www.healthit.gov/sites/default/files/page/2020-10/Federal%20Health%20IT%20Strategic%20Plan_2020_2025.pdf

Palabindala, V., Pamarthy, A., & Jonnalagadda, N. R. (2016). Adoption of electronic health records and barriers. *Journal of Community Hospital Internal Medicine Perspectives,* 6(5), 32643. https://doi.org/10.3402/jchimp.v6.32643

Parks, T. (2016). *Sharing health data: HIPAA may allow more freedom than you think.* https://www.ama-assn.org/practice-management/hipaa/sharing-health-data-hipaa-may-allow-more-freedom-you-think

Poku, M. K., Kagan, C. M., & Yehia, B. (2019). Moving from care coordination to care integration. *Journal of General Internal Medicine, 34*(9), 1906–1909. https://doi.org/10.1007/s11606-019-05029-z

Puranik, M. (2020). Why encryption is essential in healthcare cybersecurity strategies. *Health IT Answers.* https://www.healthitanswers.net/why-encryption-is-essential-in-healthcare-cybersecurity-strategies/

Reisman M. (2017). EHRs: The challenge of making electronic data usable and interoperable. *P & T: A Peer-Reviewed Journal for Formulary Management, 42*(9), 572–575. https://www.ncbi.nlm.nih.gov/pmc/articles/PMC5565131/

Ronquillo, Y., Meyers, A., & Korvek, S. J. (2023). Digital Health. In *StatPearls.* StatPearls Publishing. https://pubmed.ncbi.nlm.nih.gov/29262125/

Secureframe. (n.d.). *HIPAA violations: Examples, penalties + 5 cases to learn from.* https://secureframe.com/hub/hipaa/violations

Settles, C. (2015). A history of Meaningful Use. *Technology advice.* https://technologyadvice.com/blog/healthcare/history-of-meaningful-use-2015/

Sheikh, A., Anderson, M., Albala, S., Casadei, B., Franklin, B. D., Richards, M., Taylor, D., Tibble, H., & Mossialos, E. (2021). Health information technology and digital innovation for national learning health and care systems. *The Lancet. Digital health, 3*(6), e383–e396. https://doi.org/10.1016/S2589-7500(21)00005-4

Sherifi, D., Ndanga, M., Hunt. T. J., & Srinivasan, S. (2021). The symbiotic relationship between health information management and health informatics: Opportunities for growth and collaboration. *Perspectives in Health Information Management, 18*(4), 1c. https://www.ncbi.nlm.nih.gov/pmc/articles/PMC8649705/

Stearns, M. (n.d.). *Data integrity fundamentals.* https://michaelstearns.net/data-integrity-fundamentals/

Steckelman, E. (2019). *Why differentiate digital health from health tech?* https://assets.ctfassets.net/srtasg51sesp/3cYTNM2OZqxaX267Ueo8Pt/3f1d70318672420ea0b7b49ea217241f/Evoke_POV_-_Health_Tech_vs_Digital_Health_-_Eric_Steckelman_-_July_2019.pdf

Sweeney, J. (Feb, 2017). Healthcare informatics. *Online Journal of Nursing Informatics* (OJNI), *21*(1). https://www.himss.org/resources/healthcare-informatics

Twin, A. (2023). *Disruptive innovation: Meaning and examples.* https://www.investopedia.com/terms/d/disruptive-innovation.asp

United States Department of Health & Human Services (HHS). (2003). *Summary of the HIPAA Privacy Rule: HIPAA compliance assistance.* https://www.hhs.gov/sites/default/files/privacysummary.pdf

United States Department of Health and Human Services (HHS). (2021). *HIPAA for professionals.* https://www.hhs.gov/hipaa/for-professionals/index.html

United States Department of Health and Human Services (HHS). (2022). *Your rights under HIPAA.* https://www.hhs.gov/hipaa/for-individuals/guidance-materials-for-consumers/index.html

United States Department of Health and Human Services (HHS). (2023). *HHS marks major milestone for nationwide health data exchange.* https://www.hhs.gov/about/news/2023/12/12/hhs-marks-major-milestone-nationwide-health-data-exchange.html

United States Government Accountability Office. (2023). *Electronic health information exchange: Use has increased but is lower for small and rural providers (report to congressional requestors).* https://www.gao.gov/assets/gao-23-105540.pdf

University of Melbourne. (2023). *Health informatics and digital health.* https://unimelb.libguides.com/healthinformatics

Vehko, T., Hyppönen, H., Puttonen, S., Kujala, S., Ketola, E., Tuukkanen, J., Aalto, A. M., & Heponiemi, T. (2019). Experienced time pressure and stress: Electronic health records usability and information technology competence play a role. *BMC Medical Informatics and Decision Making, 19.* 160. https://doi.org/10.1186/s12911-019-0891-z

Wachter, R. (2015). How medical tech gave a patient a massive overdose. *Medium.* https://medium.com/backchannel/how-technology-led-a-hospital-to-give-a-patient-38-times-his-dosage-ded7b3688558

Winton, R. (2016). Hollywood hospital pays $17,000 in bitcoin to hackers: FBI investigating. *Los Angeles Times.* https://www.latimes.com/business/technology/la-me-ln-hollywood-hospital-bitcoin-20160217-story.htm

Credits

Fig. 9.1: The Office of the National Coordinator for Health Information Technology, https://www.healthit.gov/sites/default/files/page/2020-10/Federal%20Health%20IT%20Strategic%20Plan_2020_2025.pdf, 2020.

Fig. 9.5: The Office of the National Coordinator for Health Information Technology, https://www.healthit.gov/topic/certification-ehrs/2015-edition, 2015.

CHAPTER 10

The Health System, Trends, and the Future of Care Coordination

LEARNING OBJECTIVES

1. Apply health system science and thinking to the coordination of care.
2. Consider the impact of legislation and policies on the health system.
3. Assess trends in the health system and relevance to care coordination practice.
4. Examine ethical issues in care coordination practice.
5. Explore the future of care coordination, the health system, and the nurse's role.

KEY TERMS

- advocacy leadership
- artificial intelligence (AI)
- biopsychosocial model
- healthcare social influencers
- health system science
- health systems thinking
- machine learning
- nursing metaparadigm
- proactive care coordination
- reverse quackery
- well-being

Introduction

Integrating care coordination across the continuum is essential for healthcare transformation and transitioning to a value-based healthcare system that will provide better outcomes for all. This requires not only a change in how we practice nursing and deliver healthcare but also a change in perspective and a connection of the value of coordinated care to health outcomes. At the foundation of this change in perspective, values, and nursing practice is the acknowledgment that the health system contributes either positively or negatively to health outcomes. There is an essential need to understand the road map for transforming healthcare into a value-based system, understanding the complexity of that system, and taking a system-level approach to nursing practice.

Moreover, nurses must understand the impact of regulations and legislation and how these can affect care coordination practice. In the transforming health system, nurses must be a voice and leader in introducing, developing, and implementing policies, legislation, and practices that will advance health and integrate coordinated care into daily nursing practice. Nurses will need to gain a health system viewpoint and an awareness of current trends and events that impact people's health, as well as identify ways to support patients in self-determination and self-management of their health. The healthcare culture is changing, with coordinated and person-centered care as the focal point. While applying their nursing knowledge to health conditions, nurses will also be asked to embrace the multidimensionality of health and well-being and expand their scope of reference. Nurses will influence the future construct of care coordination practice and healthcare transformation by understanding health system science and thinking, legislative issues, health system trends, and current ethical concerns.

Health System Science

The definition of **health system science** is "a foundational platform and framework for the study and understanding of how care is delivered, how health professionals work together to deliver that care, and how the health system can improve patient care and health care delivery" (AMA, 2023, para. 1). This concept of a systematic study of the healthcare system is foundational for the development of evidence-based practice, policies, and theoretical approaches concerning health. A common theoretical view of health in nursing is the nursing metaparadigm, which looks at health as part of a system of factors of health. The **nursing metaparadigm** is defined by four aspects of health: (a) the person—e.g., physical body and spiritual dimension, (b) environment—e.g., internal and external factors, (c) health—e.g., healing and harmony, and (d) nursing—e.g., caring, holistic approach (Nikfarid et al., 2018). There are also other systems of health models, such as the **biopsychosocial model**, which connects biological (e.g., age, gender), psychological (e.g., beliefs, emotional health), and sociological (e.g., social support, socioeconomics) factors to health (Johnson et al., 2020). Whatever type of system-level view of health is taken, today's healthcare system is part of the factors influencing health.

The Institute of Medicine (IOM, 2001) initialized this concept and recognition of the health system influencing health by creating a systems-level framework to support healthcare delivery improvement through health systems science and thinking. This framework included 10 rules for healthcare redesign. Rule one is based on a continuing healing relationship with the patient where the patient can receive care in a variety of formats (e.g., telehealth, face-to-face visits) from a responsive healthcare system that offers care at all times—for instance 24-hour availability (IOM, 2001, p. 61). We have seen changes in access points of care and responsiveness, yet these remain system-level issues, especially in areas with provider shortages and rural or frontier areas.

Rule two calls for care based on individualized patient needs and values. This is the crux of person-centered care and appeals to the healthcare system for adaptability and flexibility to meet and provide for individualized needs and preferences (IOM, 2001, p. 61). Personalized care coordination and relationship-centered care can meet this need through comprehensive assessment, resource connections, and customized care delivery.

Rule three supports rule two and changes the provider–patient dynamic, calling for the patient to be the source of control for their healthcare (IOM, 2001, p. 61). Care coordinating nurses are vital to this rule through assessing health and digital literacy and providing appropriate education and materials so that the patient can engage in informed and shared decision-making and action regarding their health.

Rule four calls for information exchange, a critical aspect of health information technologies and care coordination (IOM, 2001, p. 62). This rule directs that information should be available to healthcare organizations, clinicians, and patients so that crucial information can be shared amongst patients, providers, and settings.

Rule five points directly to the need for health system science, identifying that healthcare should be grounded in evidence-based practice and provided consistently among settings and providers (IOM, 2001, p. 62). Quality improvement processes and systematic evaluation of outcomes are essential to identify best practices and inform system-level healthcare delivery redesigns needed to provide quality care across the continuum.

Rules six and seven requires system-level accountability for safety in care delivery, transparency concerning the quality and safety of care delivered, and patient satisfaction (IOM, 2001, p. 62). We have seen aspects of this rule implemented through the Hospital Consumer Assessment of Healthcare Providers and Systems (HCAHPS®) survey, as well as the Center for Medicare and Medicaid Services (CMS) star ratings, clinical quality benchmarks data collection, and reimbursement rate decreases or lack of reimbursement for hospital-acquired infections or "never events" such as wrong-site surgeries.

Rules eight and nine seek to transition the healthcare system from a reactive to a proactive system that anticipates patient needs and aims to decrease waste through ineffective use of resources or patient time (IOM, 2001, p. 62). Lastly, rule 10 directs the healthcare system to cooperate, not to be siloed, to use interprofessional practice, and to communicate and exchange information with others (IOM, 2001, p. 62).

Care coordination practices actively seek to implement all these IOM rules through person-centered, holistic care. The care coordinating nurse addresses system-level healthcare delivery issues by supporting patient autonomy, utilizing shared decision-making, exchanging appropriate and timely essential information, communicating effectively, and using evidence-based practice guidelines and quality measures to inform care coordination practice. Care coordination practice is proactively assessing for and planning to meet patient needs safely and transparently based on interprofessional practice and contributing to the science of healthcare delivery through systems-level coordination across the care continuum.

The IOM rules for a 21st century health system were created over 20 years ago, and the health system continues to struggle to meet these guidelines and transform. The push for coordinated care across the system has prompted the healthcare system's advancement in this transformation process, transitioning from a disease-oriented approach to a holistic one, considering the myriad of factors influencing health and health outcomes. The health system's future is "a group of interfacing, interrelated, or interdependent components that form a complex and unified whole" (Johnson et al., 2020, p. 3) that will meet patient needs across settings and factors influencing health. This will require that all parts of the health system dismantle

Coordinated Care and Health System Questions

Nurses are responsible for a comprehensive assessment of the patient and their support or family system to ensure that all potential barriers to the care transition or discharge back into the community setting can be addressed proactively. Nurses may neglect assessment of the health system itself as they may not be familiar with assessment questions, which point to problematic areas that must be addressed. Some common questions nurses can ask to assess their patients concerning their experience and needs with the health system are the following:

1. "Do you ever have trouble getting the care you need?" (Fraser et al., 2018, p. 291). This question will identify if there are issues such as transportation, lack of a primary care provider, etc.
2. "Do you have trouble paying for medical care?" (Fraser et al., 2018, p. 291). This question can identify if there are financial issues related to copayments, deductibles, or insurance plans that do not cover specific aspects of needed healthcare.
3. "If you see multiple providers, do you know if they communicate regarding your care?" (Fraser et al., 2018, p. 291). This question can identify providers that may not be known and whether the patient knows how to communicate with them and how they communicate with each other, distinguishing possible communication barriers that may need to be addressed.

siloed aspects of care, embrace the view of healthcare as an integrated service that offers interprofessional team care, and endeavor to understand the person, not just the disease process.

Within the nursing discipline, there will be a need for a diversity of thought and a commitment to engaging with and supporting others to bring their voice to decision-making and information-generating processes. There will also need to be continued emphasis on relationship-building in the healthcare setting amongst all workers, clinicians, and nonclinicians, dismantling hierarchies and silos of care. Nurses at all levels and in all settings must embrace their role in leading the advancement of the discipline and the health system, developing better ways to do the work of healthcare (Johnson et al., 2020). Through these actions, nurses can contribute to advancing the complex health system by changing the how, what, where, and why of healthcare delivery to meet whole-person-centered needs and offer coordinated, proactive, and responsive healthcare.

Health Systems Thinking

Health system transformation will necessitate nurses to engage in **health systems thinking** processes. Nurses may be very familiar with critical thinking but should become more familiar with the need to think on a systems level about healthcare delivery. Health systems thinking is a proactive process applied to the health system that looks for patterns and relationships in problem areas, engages stakeholders, and implements systematic problem-solving approaches to health system needs, rather than one-off siloed solutions. Health systems thinking supports the World Health Organization's (WHO) definition of health: "Health is a state of complete physical, mental and social well-being and not merely the absence of disease or infirmity" (WHO, 2024, para. 1). This will require the healthcare system to move to a coordinated framework to utilize resources effectively and integrate processes for good outcomes (Shi & Singh, 2019).

The healthcare system will need to incorporate and infuse coordinated care values, methods, and actions into all system structures across the continuum of care. Health system science and thinking can inform the future of healthcare by examining the multiple elements that influence how healthcare is delivered, as well as multidimensional health factors: social, biological, socioeconomic, cultural, etc. To think broadly about the health system and integrate care coordination across the continuum of care, initiatives for system reform can be developed and implemented to meet the holistic needs of patients, populations, communities, and the nation. See Figure 10.1 for a visual of the interrelated elements of Health and the Health System.

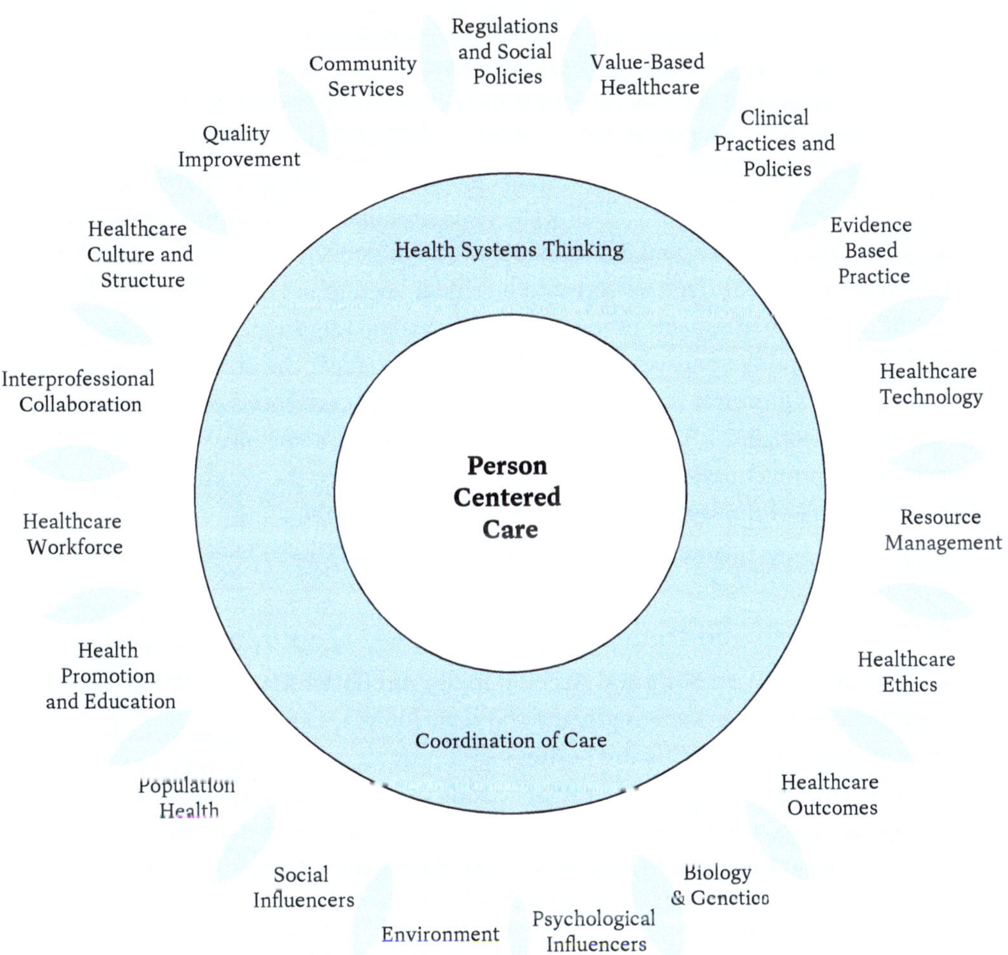

FIGURE 10.1 Interrelated Elements of Health and the Health System

Legislative Trends and Issues

Several legislative issues are at the forefront of the health system's transformation. Some challenges that significantly affect the need for coordination of care are the growth and impact of chronic or longer-term health conditions and the intersection of physical health, mental health, and social conditions, such as housing insecurity. The health system was primarily developed to address acute care needs with short, intermittent, but intensive periods of care. The growth in the number of people with chronic or longer-term conditions has shown that the current health system is ill-designed to meet the needs of those who need regular, less intensive, but more holistic and proactive healthcare. For example, approximately 60% of adults in the United States have at least one chronic health condition. Chronic and mental health conditions have been attributed to 90% of healthcare costs, along with economic costs through loss of productivity (Hoffman, 2022, para. 4–5). Additionally, the prominent fee-for-service reimbursement model in which the health system was designed does not support the critical need for care coordination among these patient populations (Mason et al., 2021).

Further, the increase in the number of people with chronic conditions has influenced the cost of private insurance, with the cost of an employer-sponsored health insurance plan increasing by 87% since the year 2000 (Hoffman, 2022, para. 7). This has exacerbated the number of those who are uninsured, with some finding the costs prohibitive. Currently, approximately 8% of people are uninsured, and about 36% of people receive publicly funded insurance (Peter G. Peterson Foundation, 2023). This has created a critical need to set appropriate national-level legislation for regulation of aspects of the healthcare system, requirements and funding for the Medicare and Medicaid systems, and national initiatives to meet the holistic needs of populations, advancing the Quintuple Aim and the central tenets of care coordination practice (Peter G. Peterson Foundation, 2023; Tikkanen et al., 2020) Moreover, some pieces of legislation have been developed to protect patients and their rights and enhance the coordination of care. Yet unanticipated effects of the legislation can sometimes hinder the ability to provide seamless care coordination. Let's consider three legislative examples.

Example One: Health Information Portability and Accountability Act (HIPAA)

The Health Information Portability and Accountability Act (HIPAA) is legislation that has had several unanticipated effects, such as privacy and security issues creating a reluctance to share patient information among healthcare settings and providers. This becomes a more significant issue if the healthcare setting or provider needs to collaborate and coordinate care with non-healthcare settings or services. Even though HIPAA allows for the secure transmission of patient health information for healthcare operations, treatment, payment, or care coordination, it also signifies that this information should be limited to only what information is necessary for the immediate issue or transition of care and only transmitted securely. Yet many people with chronic or longer-term conditions, as well as those with mental health or significant social factors influencing their health, also receive services outside the health system, such as meal services and housing assistance, or funding from charity programs. Many of these community programs are not required to follow HIPAA and do not have secure information transmission systems, which can cause increased reluctance for healthcare organizations to share pertinent patient information with these community resources (Qin, 2020).

In this case, HIPAA has created a scope that is too exclusive and specific to healthcare organizations or those identified as business partners with healthcare organizations for the capacity of care coordination to encompass the holistic needs of patients. This requires HIPAA-covered organizations to either implement some business agreement with social service agencies or obtain permission from the patient to contact and coordinate care with these organizations (Qin, 2020). These workarounds can be costly to implement and time-consuming, delaying critical information exchange to meet patient needs and coordinate care in a timely fashion. This has prompted the call for some modification and updating of HIPAA to either create a "care coordination associate" or to expand exceptions to the minimum necessary information principle to allow sharing of patient health information to provide holistic and person-centered care coordination (Qin, 2020).

Example Two: Connecting Care Coordination to Behavioral Health and Social Conditions

Meeting patient needs, including social conditions that affect overall health and health outcomes, is essential to successful holistic and person-centered care coordination. "Health care services contribute only 10% to 20% of the variance in health outcomes. Seventy percent of the variation can be explained by the patients' social conditions, including housing, physical environment, social circumstances, education level, and economic stability" (Mason et al., 2021, p. 316). A legislative example of meeting patients' holistic care coordination needs is House Bill 773, introduced as the Homelessness and Behavioral Health Care Coordination Act of 2023. H. R. 773 has been introduced to address one specific aspect of social conditions—homelessness (H.R. 773, 2023–2024). This bill acknowledges that homelessness is sometimes the result of behavioral health conditions, defined as mental health and/or substance use disorders. Due to this, H.R. 773 calls for person-centered, coordinated care to be integrated into health services for this population.

Additionally, H.R. 773 acknowledges that the health system needs capacity expansion to link health and homelessness services. H.R. 773 seeks to develop a grant program for organizations to build or expand their capacity to coordinate healthcare and homelessness services for people with cocurrent behavioral health issues. The capacity building includes infrastructure improvements, expansion of healthcare technology used for behavioral healthcare services, and increased connections with healthcare services (H.R. 773, 2023–2024). If approved, identified outcome measures of H.R. Bill 773 include improved participants' health, primary care provider access, and individualized care plans (H.R. 773, 2023–2024).

Example Three: Connecting Care Coordination and Cancer Outcomes

Another House bill introduced to improve care coordination is H.R. 6338. This bill concerns a potentially longer-term health condition: gynecological cancer. Approximately 35% to 50% of patients survive gynecological cancer for more than 10 years, depending on the type of cancer

(Cancer Research UK, 2021; Cancer Research UK, 2023). In addition, those with gynecological cancer often experience depression, anxiety, and impaired quality of life (Jónsdóttir et al., 2023). The H.R. 6338 bill has been introduced as the Veterans' Cancer Care Coordinator Act of 2023 to address these issues related to a potentially longer-term condition that may require coordinated care between the Veterans Affairs and community gynecological cancer specialists and/or mental health providers (H.R. 6338, 2023–2024).

H.R. 6338 seeks to establish a pilot gynecological cancer care coordination program in several Veterans Affairs centers. This care coordinator would coordinate care amongst the providers of the Veterans Affairs and community healthcare settings. Additionally, this care coordinator would facilitate authorizations for community care for veterans who screen positive for military sexual trauma, depression, intimate partner violence, or post-traumatic stress disorder, regularly contacting these veterans and providing a comprehensive needs assessment (H.R. 6338, 2023–2024). Key aspects of this bill include documentation of specific information in the patient's electronic health record (EHR) and outcome measures related to cancer-related mortality, remission, mental health diagnosis, patient satisfaction, safety, and timeliness of care (H.R. 6338, 2023–2024).

The Role of the Nurse in Advancing Care Coordination in Legislation

These national bills and recommendations for current legislative reform identify that care coordination is a critical aspect of offering person-centered and holistic care that can meet multiple needs, including social conditions of health, socioeconomic barriers, or other aspects of health that can contribute to poor health outcomes. With this introduced legislation, we can see that the nation's leaders and organizations are looking for ways to improve the integration of coordinated and person-centered care into healthcare transformation. However, there are difficulties in the process, including the fact that multiple stakeholders and levels of government are often involved in creating and implementing legislation and funding, all with competing priorities. Secondly, there is a notable lack of patient and nursing voices in legislative decisions. Furthermore, many legislators, lobbyists, community stakeholders, etc., do not have the expert knowledge base or health systems-level view concerning the impact of proposed legislation. This is why nurses must engage in advocacy leadership to proactively address barriers to seamless care coordination on an organizational, local, state, and national level and work to create a healthcare system that recognizes and addresses the multifaceted nature of person-centered care and the health system (Porter-O'Grady & Malloch, 2018, p. 463). Through proactive **advocacy leadership**, nurses can support health system transformation, dismantle barriers to quality healthcare delivery, and promote all participants in the health system to achieve their full potential.

Furthermore, nurses can bring an ethical lens to legislation development, ensuring that the created legislation is responsive and meets ethical standards of person-centered care practices. For example, cost and resource management are significant needs and priorities in healthcare legislation. Yet, there is also a need to ensure that those receiving or seeking healthcare are treated with respect and that their needs and priorities of care are considered. Additionally,

Patient-Centered Research

The Patient-Centered Outcomes Research Institute (PCORI) is an organization that focuses on empowering patients through research that results in actionable health information and helps inform better health decisions. Several PCORI-funded research projects focus on care coordination and patient-centered outcomes and provide evidence to inform practice and policy decisions that can reduce adverse health outcomes, especially for those with chronic illnesses that can result from a fragmented healthcare system (Cook, 2023).

any unintended consequences of implementing the legislation should be examined (Davis et al., 2010). These could be unintended consequences such as decreased healthcare access, lack of integrated coordination of care across health and social service settings, or excessive costs or regulatory requirements that are prohibitive for some organizations or providers. The President's Commission (1983) identified that

> If the nation concludes that too much is being spent on healthcare, it is appropriate to eliminate expenditures that are wasteful or that do not produce benefit comparable to those that would flow from alternate uses of these funds. But measures designed to contain healthcare costs that exacerbate existing inequities or impede the achievement of equity are unacceptable from a moral standpoint. (President's Commission for the Study of Ethical Problems in Medicine and Biomedical and Behavioral Research, 1983, p. 31)

This statement from 40 years ago points to the need for nurses to be actively involved in developing ethically based healthcare legislation concerning coordination of care and healthcare transformation.

Ethical Health Policy

"In clarifying policy options from an ethical perspective, one must consider the impact of deductibles and coinsurance on the poor, who may be discouraged by them from seeking medical care until their medical conditions are far advanced or they are forced to seek care in an emergency room" (Davis, et al., 2010, p. 158).

Health System Trends and Issues

Several trends and issues are occurring in the health system that will affect how healthcare is delivered and the role of the nurse and care coordination in healthcare transformation. Many current societal conditions and events are acting as influencers and drivers of change in the health system, such as the current healthcare workforce shortage, lack of accessible and equitable care, and the increasing influence of things like social media influencers on health behaviors. Nurses must be cognizant of these drivers of health system change and proactively engage in professional development if needed, as well as advocacy for patients and the discipline of nursing. Some trends and considerations on the horizon are positive, such as the focus on well-being and proactive care coordination. However, other trends—including the culture of the health system and the integration and use of technology in healthcare delivery—will need nurses to have a leading voice in the changes to ensure that these trends retain a person-centered care focus and contribute positively to the transition of value-based healthcare.

Well-Being

With workforce shortages and a renewed interest in prevention and wellness in healthcare, the **well-being** of the healthcare workforce and patients will be a continued focus. Health system changes will be required to address issues such as the healthcare environment, resources available, and education and training needs to ensure well-being is supported for the healthcare workforce and patients (GE Healthcare, 2023). "Well-being" is often used interchangeably with "wellness" or "health." Yet, well-being is a multidimensional construct of wellness and health that includes physical, mental, social, and spiritual aspects that are interrelated and interdependent. Well-being relates to the quality of these aspects on an individual level and includes both objective aspects (e.g., illness) and subjective aspects (e.g., how someone feels; Lomas & VanderWeele, 2022). Well-being is often viewed as a linear event in the form of a ladder or pyramid, with well-being attained when the top is reached. Yet, these approaches do not adequately integrate the multidimensionality of well-being, the human condition, and influencers of well-being.

If we compare the health system to an orchestra, a person's well-being is like an instrument, and the health system desires the person to play harmoniously and to its full potential. We can easily see how the physical, mental, and social aspects of well-being are integrated. Physical well-being may be how the instrument is designed and cared for. Are there genetic factors, social conditions, or determinants influencing health? Is there stress, lack of quality food, healthcare, exercise, etc.? Considering the mental aspects of well-being, we can examine functioning. What coping skills are available, what are the life experiences and circumstances, and are behavioral or emotional issues present? Social well-being points to the instrument's ability to contribute to the orchestra's sound, whether it is coordinated or harmonious. What are the support systems available, hobbies, interests, or level of community engagement? Lastly, spiritual well-being reflects how the instrument gains energy and dynamics. Is there a belief in a higher power, engagement in meditation or prayer, and renewal activities integrated into a lifestyle? (Lomas & VanderWeele, 2022, p. 7).

As we can see, all dimensions are interrelated and interdependent; if a person is not functioning well or lacks healthcare, this likely will contribute to poor well-being outcomes. This multidimensional view of well-being is a crucial aspect of the health system, which will require restructuring to ensure that the healthcare environment assists workers and patients to thrive. See Figure 10.2 for a visual of the well-being orchestra.

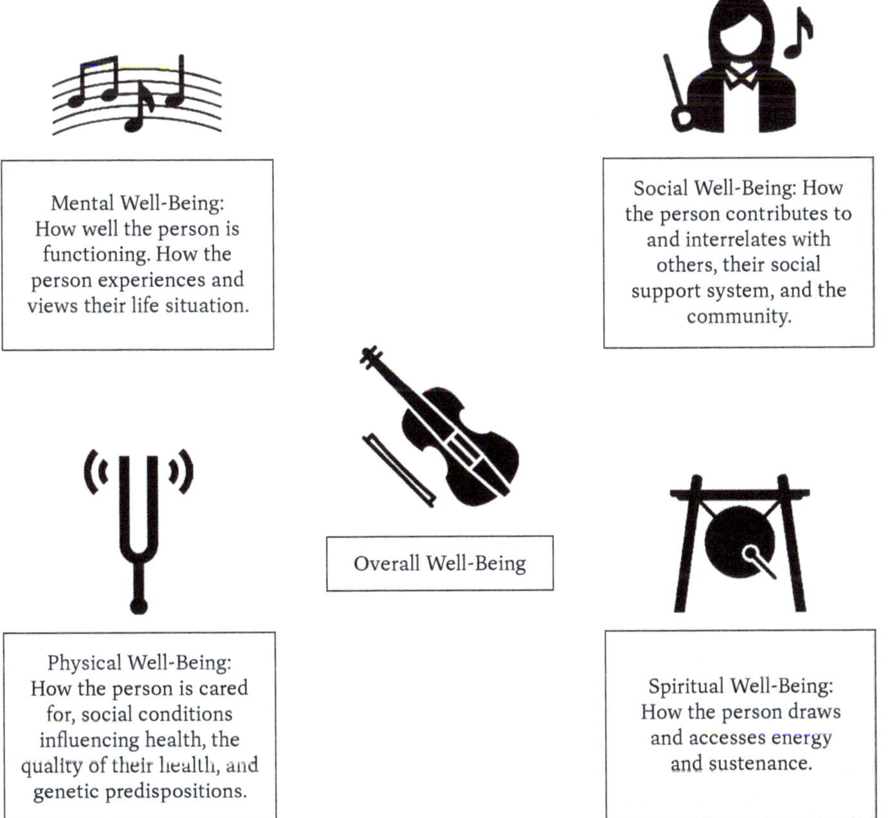

FIGURE 10.2 Well-Being Orchestra

Proactive Care Coordination

The introduction of **proactive care coordination** services will assist in supporting both the well-being of patients and the healthcare workforce. Care coordination has been shown to positively impact the quality of life, perceptions of care, satisfaction of healthcare received, communication, and resource management and to meet better the needs of those with chronic or complex needs (Palusak et al., 2022). Proactive care coordination is an approach to care coordination practice that focuses on proactively identifying and addressing care coordination needs—rather than awaiting poor outcomes or the need for urgent care coordination—by utilizing tools such as risk identification, patient engagement, and health system thinking.

Through risk stratification and identification, populations of patients can be offered care coordination services once the risk is identified, rather than waiting for untoward outcomes or significant coordination needs. This will assist not only with better patient well-being outcomes but also increase workforce satisfaction with decreased fatigue, decreased workload, and increased meaningfulness of work (Ward, 2023; Young, 2022a).

Actively seeking out those who may need support in lifestyle changes or management of chronic illnesses or who may need further education and information to become active and engaged in their self-management of health is a system thinking level change. This will call for more systems-level changes, such as prioritizing reimbursement for this type of intervention and developing evidence-based methods and policies to direct the integration of proactive care coordination across the continuum of care. Proactive care coordination is a healthcare trend that will gain traction and likely become essential to organizational procedures and health system redesign.

Social Media Healthcare Influencers

Social media is everywhere today and can be a powerful influencer on beliefs, thoughts, behaviors, and lifestyles. Several people are healthcare social influencers who engage in promoting specific health behaviors and influencing health awareness and education. Social media healthcare influencers can impact health behaviors and knowledge negatively or positively and are known for their ability to affect health (Powell & Pring, 2024). The importance of addressing the social media influence on health behaviors is apparent, requiring the health system to understand and engage in innovative digital health platforms for education delivery that address the social media influence on health (Smit et al., 2022).

With the rise of health technology innovation and the development of education, health interventions, and support programs delivered digitally, more information concerning how social media influencers affect health and healthcare practices is needed to inform policy, regulations, and health system structure (Smit et al., 2022). Improving health by organizations partnering with social media healthcare influencers to promote preventative health or lifestyle changes may become more commonplace. However, this will require vetting of the social media influencer to ensure that misinformation is not disseminated and that any regulations or guidelines needed are followed (Schwarz, 2024). The use of social media influencers in health promotion and education is a key aspect of the transformation of the healthcare system to a consumer-oriented approach. But this will also necessitate nurses to be aware of the potential benefits and limitations of using social media healthcare influencers and any apps, programs, or health behaviors they are promoting.

Health System Culture

As the healthcare delivery system transitions from an acute care, intensive intervention approach to a decentralized system of preventative, equitable, and accessible care, we will see more care move into the community or home setting. This may be through the increase of telemedicine and digital health delivery systems, integrated care delivery networks, or innovative access points of care, such as grocery stores with cash pricing for services, pharmacy lockers, or other nonmedical settings that leverage technology and delivery systems like Google or Amazon (Zimlichman et al., 2021).

We will also see more specialization among nurses and other healthcare providers. Nurses will continue to grow in specialization, filling roles previously filled by physicians or other providers, and new roles in the healthcare workforce will develop (Zimlichman et al., 2021). Interprofessional team practice and collaboration will continue to become critical aspects of healthcare delivery, utilizing the specialty and expert knowledge of the multiple professionals represented and giving voice to the patient as the expert on themselves.

The Future of Healthcare

Of clinicians surveyed, 99% agree or somewhat agree that the future of healthcare will involve patient and healthcare teams linked through digital solutions, that healthcare and treatment will be delivered outside of traditional clinical settings, such as the patient's home, and that the healthcare system will expand to include a variety of healthcare workers, some of which may not be present today (GE Healthcare, 2023, p. 10).

There will be a continuing focus on developing patient and provider trust in the health system and confidence that it will meet patient healthcare needs. Currently, patients report a lack of confidence and trust in the healthcare system, believing they may not receive the care they need or will be met by uncompassionate and unempathetic healthcare providers (GE Healthcare, 2023). This transition to a trusting person and relationship-centered care perspective will require nurses to embrace collaborative care delivery, understand their role in the interprofessional team, and decrease fragmented care. Additionally, nurses will need to comprehend the transforming health system, grasping the need for flexible access points to meet patient needs, not focusing solely on delivery of intensive, disease-focused healthcare. Furthermore, nurses will be required to engage in informatics and be digitally literate to make personalized, data-driven care decisions that meet the patients' holistic care needs.

Healthcare Technology Integration and Advances

Healthcare technology will continue to grow in application, meeting data integration needs and enhancing clinical decision-making. Solutions will be found to seamlessly integrate hardware and software to improve communication and information exchange. This will continue to support the transformation of the healthcare culture to a consumer-oriented system, which will require nurses to learn how to build and leverage relationship-centered care and integrate patient data appropriately into clinical decision-making. This will also mean that nurses must understand how to assess for health and digital literacy and its role in integrating technology into healthcare delivery. Nurses themselves will need to have significant digital literacy, be able to apply and utilize technology appropriately, and understand the benefits and limitations of technology (Mesko, 2018).

Currently, approximately 97% of data collected in healthcare is unused (GE Healthcare, 2023). Healthcare technology innovation and advancement will assist with using and integrating big data analytics into policy, legislation, and population-level interventions. The enhanced use and management of big data will help with data-driven predictive and preventative care, as through data analytics, health conditions may be detected and treated more quickly for improved health outcomes. This will require nurses to understand the critical nature and ethical concerns of the secondary use of patient information (using data for purposes other than originally intended) and the regulatory and compliance issues associated with this data.

This will lead to the development of new nursing roles related to health technology and digital data management. An example of a new nurse role might be partnering with artificial intelligence (AI) engineers to develop nursing prompts or requests to guide AI nursing care solutions to promote better health outcomes. "Healthcare organizations are headed for greater optimization of technologies, greater interoperability, increased use of artificial intelligence, and ability to exchange the necessary information among providers, payers, regulatory agencies, and patients" (Sherifi et al., 2021, p. 8).

Ethical Considerations

Ethics is central to nursing practice and is an area that can affect care coordination and the health system. When the nurse is coordinating care, there are often multiple healthcare team members with different priorities or views of what the outcome should look like. Additionally, the patient themselves may at times present situations that are ethically challenging related to factors influencing their health or life circumstances or experiences. Moreover, the process and goals of care coordination practice may, at times, be in ethical conflict with the patient's desired outcomes or recommended care. It is crucial that nurses consider the variety of ethical situations that may present themselves and gain an awareness of their role in navigating these potential challenges to coordinated care delivery.

Self-Determination and Patient Choice

Patient self-determination is a foundational ethic of nursing and healthcare. It is recognized that all people have the right to determine what actions will be taken involving them, to receive information that assists them in making informed decisions, to be assisted in weighing the benefits, burdens, and options of treatments, and to have the choice of no treatment (ANA, 2015, p. 2). This is also supported by the Centers for Medicare and Medicaid Services (CMS), which requires that all beneficiaries be given an informed choice concerning post-acute discharge providers (Dietz, 2019). This concept is also a foundational aspect of person-centered care, the integration of the patient in the interprofessional team, and the cultural shift to the patient as a driver of their care. Yet some ethical dilemmas can present themselves as the care coordinating nurse supports the patient in self-determination and choice.

Privacy

One prominent area of concern is that of privacy. As patients enter the healthcare setting, they are often asked to divulge sensitive aspects of their life, health, and finances so the interprofessional team can provide quality and holistic care. This can lead to oversharing, which, in some cases, can cause the patient stress or distress related to reliving a situation or explaining a circumstance (Hansson & Fröding, 2020). Obtaining healthcare does not negate a person's right to choose to disclose or not disclose information (ANA, 2015). Nurses must be cognizant of nonverbal and verbal communication, expressing that the patient is uncomfortable with the request and validating to the patient that it is their choice to share information or not. Nurses may provide education as to why a particular piece of information is relevant to the patient's care, but the nurse must respect their right not to share information if that is their choice.

Role Blurring

Another issue can be the blurring of the nurse's role. Because patients often bring various issues that need coordination and addressing other than a specific health condition, including financial or housing insecurity, domestic or intimate partner violence, or linguistic or cultural considerations, the nurse may find themselves dealing with areas they are unfamiliar with or are uncomfortable addressing. This can also lead the nurse to feel that it is appropriate to advise on these areas, which can lead to something referred to as "**reverse quackery**" (Hansson & Fröding, 2020). This is defined as the nurse overextending their role to provide a service or type of care without possessing the necessary qualifications.

For example, let's say a nurse is caring for a patient who is due to have foot amputation surgery, and the patient is noticeably upset at the prospect. In this case, the nurse tells the patient it is okay to be angry and encourages them to "scream it out" to release their anger and face the foot amputation head-on. What is wrong with this scenario? At times, screaming can release endorphins and contribute to released stress, but has this nurse done a thorough assessment of this patient's coping mechanisms, whether the patient is currently receiving counseling, what has led to the foot amputation, and if this type of stress-releasing experience fits into their personal or emotional constructs? Is the nurse qualified to make this type of assessment and diagnosis and prescribe the intervention of screaming it out?

We find that here the nurse has blurred roles and is not embracing the patient's right to self-determination and choice. The patient may feel they have no choice but to engage in this behavior as they trust the nurse and feel they should do what they are told, or they may feel uncomfortable confronting the nurse concerning not wanting to participate in the behavior. They may already be addressing their foot amputation by seeing a professional counselor who has worked with the patient on ways to deal with their upcoming surgery, which does not include screaming it out. It would be better, in this case, to ask for a social worker to visit with the patient before their surgery, to ask the patient if they would like to have the hospital chaplain or other support person come to see them, or to use their nursing presence and therapeutic communication skills to offer support and resources to the patient as needed and requested by the patient.

Decision-Making

This example falls into another ethical issue with patient self-determination and choice related to the decision-making process. In informed decision-making and person-centered care practices, the patient is to be offered options and educated appropriately concerning benefits and burdens regarding the options so that they can make an informed choice concerning their health. However, at times, patients may not have decision-making capacity or may have a reduced ability to engage in informed decision-making, such as lower health literacy or a current highly emotional or stressful situation (Hansson & Fröding, 2020). In this case, the nurse has a responsibility to ensure that information and education are provided at an appropriate literacy level, to revisit the decision at a time that is less emotional or stressful, or to include family members, caregivers, or support system members in the decision-making process as appropriate, rather than becoming the decision-maker themselves.

Decision-Making and Family Involvement

Family involvement in decision-making is common and often valued and desired by the patient (Menon et al., 2020). However, this can also cause potential ethical issues regarding self-determination and choice. In this situation, the nurse has a crucial role and responsibility in supporting patient self-determination and navigating through conflicts or emotional situations related to family involvement in decision-making (Menon et al., 2020). For example, some family members may not want to share medical information with a patient, or they may not want the nurse to discuss options and choices with the patient but only with the family members. In this situation, the nurse will need to clarify with the patient, without family members present, if this is their desire. If it is not, they will need to act as an advocate for the patient with their family, ensuring the patient can express their opinions and that their choices are being followed.

Resource Management

A key aspect of care coordination and value-based healthcare is the appropriate use of healthcare resources and the management of costs. Healthcare organizations must manage costs, show value in the care delivered, and meet the regulations and guidelines that payers and national organizations and systems put forth. When considering the management of resources and costs, there is an obvious ethical issue concerning resource allocation and who approves the use of resources. In the current system, payers and regulatory bodies can approve or deny the use of specific resources. We can consider the issue of utilization review and whether a patient should be admitted, inpatient or outpatient. Sometimes, a provider may feel the patient needs an inpatient admission, but according to the utilization management software, the patient does not meet the criteria. Or a physical therapist may recommend a subacute rehabilitation (SAR) placement post-acute care. Still, the payer may determine that the patient does not qualify or does not need placement in a SAR and will only authorize home health physical therapy. This, at times, can lead to ethical issues in which the nurse care coordinator will need to advocate with the payer to ensure the patient is getting the most appropriate care needed.

Additionally, the Quintuple Aim and value-based reimbursement strategies require healthcare organizations to ensure that the resources are equitable and accessible and contribute to better outcomes. The basic tenets of resource management are that it should create cost-effectiveness and that the resources should be used to maximize health outcomes. Whether the processes, policies, and HIT systems utilized further health equity and accessibility or create unintended consequences may need consideration. Policies and processes may need to be changed to ensure health equity and accessibility with better outcomes while resources are being managed and quality care and support are provided (NIH, 2023). Ultimately, if we are not managing resources effectively, fewer people can benefit from the resources. Nurses also have an ethical obligation to engage in a primary commitment to those who receive healthcare services, and at times they may need to engage in advocacy and foster appropriate policy and procedure development at an organizational, local, state, or national level for effective, efficient, and proper resource management that contributes to health equity and accessibility (ANA, 2015).

Refused Discharges

One such resource management and self-determination issue is that of a refused discharge. Sometimes a patient may refuse to discharge from a setting. They may not feel prepared to return home or may find solace in receiving care in an acute care facility. They may need help to understand the financial implications of this decision or how it may cost them significantly. This is a common ethical situation, as the care coordinating nurse must manage resources, support reimbursement of the organization, and advocate for and provide appropriate education to the patient so they may engage in informed and shared decision-making.

Many social issues can relate to a successful transition of care, such as food scarcity, caregiver burden, or other problems that make the patient feel unsafe or vulnerable. As such, they do not want to leave the setting they are in. The care coordinating nurse must leverage relationship- and person-centered care to discover challenges, barriers, or fears. Any identified challenges or fears will need to be addressed through resource connections, appropriate referrals, and further education if required. The problem may also be that they do not understand where they are going or what type of care they will receive if they go to another level of care, and they need further information and education (Young, 2022b).

Furthermore, the care coordinating nurse must provide appropriate education concerning the goals of the healthcare organization about the discharge or transition in care and if there are financial implications to refusal. The nurse must work to create a solution that will meet the patient's goals, as well as the goals of the healthcare organization. Some payers, such as Medicare, have appeals processes and forms that must be followed and completed to ensure patient rights are respected and the transition in care is appropriate. The care coordinating nurse must also know these processes and inform patients of their rights and responsibilities regarding discharge or transition refusals.

Healthcare Has Changed, Leaving the Patient Uniformed: A Hospitalist Perspective

The Centers for Medicare and Medicaid Services, as well as other payers, have developed intricate systems to determine appropriate admission diagnosis for acute care, as well as length of stay guidelines, but may have failed to inform the public adequately of these changes, the reason they have been made, and how they may affect care. Dr. L., a hospitalist, expressed frustration with this aspect of "healthcare transformation," indicating that

> Many older patients grew up with hospital stays for a week or more not being an unusual occurrence, and believing this was needed for good outcomes. This has created a disconnect, as many older patients had their children stay for a week in the hospital for a tonsillectomy or stayed themselves 2 weeks post-delivery of their children and do not understand why they cannot stay an additional day or until they feel comfortable returning home. Healthcare has transformed but has not educated the public about the how or why, which can lead to unsatisfied patients.

The Future of Care Coordination

It is clear that care coordination across the continuum is here to stay. The health system and patients need integrated care, effective cross-setting communication, and care coordination practices to ensure better outcomes and enhance the well-being of nurses and patients. This calls for the nurse to be a key ally in care coordination advocacy, advancement, and integration into the health system and nursing discipline. The future of care coordination begins with nursing education and professional development, embracing the need for this valuable skill and knowledge set in nursing practice, and translating the multitude of ways that coordinated care can contribute to a value-based health system, nurse and patient satisfaction, and better outcomes for all. This may require currently practicing nurses, nurse educators, and nursing students to engage in continuous learning practices concerning their knowledge base of care coordination and its critical role in the health system.

As regulations, legislation, policies, guidelines, and technology continually change and transform, it will require nurses to keep current on best practices of care coordination, areas of legislative advocacy needed, advances in health technology and AI, and areas of improvement concerning collaborative and integrated care in their places of work and communities. Nurses have a vital role in the advancement and development of care coordination in the health system, and they give voice to the critical need for nurses to contribute to and develop care coordination roles and practices.

The Nurse's Role as Care Coordinator

Many healthcare workers may fill the role of care coordinators, such as the community health worker, cultural mediator, or a person who has the title of care coordinator but is not a nurse. This can lead to confusion among patients and providers and contribute to a lack of clarity on the importance and foundation of care coordination practice, as well as needed licensure and proper reimbursement strategies for care coordination integration into the health system (Huber, 2018). Nurses must understand and advocate for the nursing role in care coordination practice. A specific part of the nursing process calls for the nurse to effectively coordinate care through collaboration with other interprofessional team members and the patient. In addition, the nurse is called to provide advocacy and communication that facilitates seamless care transitions and empowers patients to navigate the health system (ANA, 2021). This is no small role and requires the critical analysis, compassion, and trusting relationship nurses bring to the health system.

Additionally, there is a growing provider shortage, and advanced practice nurse practitioners (NPs) have become integral to person-centered, accessible, and quality healthcare (Amer, 2013). Approximately 70% of NPs practice in primary care, and over 80% see Medicare and Medicaid patients, with many NPs holding hospital and long-term care privileges (American Association of Nurse Practitioners, 2024). All levels of nurses have a leading role in care coordination practice to meet quality outcomes, effectively manage resources, and demonstrate integrated person- and relationship-centered care. Nurses must embrace this role and advocate for the discipline to be an essential part of care coordination models, processes, policies, and delivery across the health system. This calls for all nurses to be educated in foundational care coordination practices and common barriers of coordinated care, and gain a systems-level understanding of the value of care coordination being integrated across the health system.

Nursing Education and Professional Development

Nurse educators, whether in a pre-licensure capacity or from a professional development function, have a critical role in integrating care coordination practices into all nursing care delivered. All practicing nurses must understand the complex health system and how the forces of value-based healthcare, national legislation, and the inherent need to provide better, safe, quality, cost-effective, and holistic healthcare are driving the need for care coordination knowledge, skills, and attitudes to be integrated into nursing practice. Care coordination competency areas related to interprofessional collaborative practice, continuous quality improvement, transitions in care, person-centered care, quality and safe healthcare, policy advocacy, and ethical application must be infused into all nursing education and training programs.

It has been identified that there may be a knowledge gap among nursing faculty and professional development educators concerning the value of the nurses' role in care coordination and continuity of care, as well as the practice of care coordination (Swan et al., 2019). Incorporating care coordination competencies across the curriculum and into organizational orientations and training must be embraced by all nursing educators. The inherent value of care coordination necessitates that this value be communicated to nursing students and practicing nurses so that they may develop a vision for how care coordination and continuity of care will be incorporated into their nursing practice, advancing the Quintuple Aim and assisting in the healthcare transformation journey.

Example Competency Model Application

Many nurse educators may be unsure how to integrate care coordination content. However, a variety of competency frameworks can be used as a reference, such as the COLLABORATE© model. In this model, nurses can be trained and learn to apply 11 competencies to various other aspects of nursing practice. See Table 10.1 for a detailed examination of this model and how it can be applied to all nursing practice and education, no matter the setting and whether or not care coordination is the focus of the nursing role. It is apparent that care coordination practices, competencies, and content easily apply to all settings and across the continuum of care. Care coordination competencies and the application of these should be infused into ongoing training and courses to ensure the nursing workforce is prepared to meet the needs of value-based healthcare transformation and person-centered care.

Nursing Faculty Barriers

"You know, I think one barrier is just the lack of knowledge from the academic side of it. The other barrier is not having a focus on anything other than inpatient ... how do we get the word out that we really do need to pay attention to what's happening in healthcare delivery" (Swan et al., 2019, p. 83).

TABLE 10.1 The COLLABORATE© Competency Model Application

Acronym	Competency	Application to Nursing Practice	Example Application to Nursing Education and Professional Development
All competencies in this model are appropriate for care coordination, resource management, or continuum of care courses or training or can be connected to the care coordination aspect of the nursing process in any course or training.			
C	Critical Thinking	This is the foundation of all nursing practice. Nurses must be able to critically assess, analyze, and synthesize data gained with knowledge held to direct appropriate nursing practice decisions.	This competency can be integrated into all nursing or professional development courses or parts of training.
O	Outcome Driven	Outcomes identification is a key step in the nursing process. Furthermore, outcomes are the basis of evidence-based practice development, as well as any continuous quality improvement process.	This competency can be introduced in nursing professionalism, research, and leadership courses or training, as well as training in documentation.
L	Lifelong Learning	An attitude concerning the value of lifelong learning is essential for any professional development and to meet care coordination and healthcare needs through continuing education and advanced degrees. This includes understanding the value of working interprofessionally to integrate various ways of knowing.	This competency could be integrated into courses and trainings concerning preparation for advanced learning, healthcare innovations, interprofessional practice, and communication skills.
L	Leadership	Leadership includes the ability to practice inteprofessionally and to advance the discipline of nursing through a clear view of how the profession of nursing contributes to a better healthcare system.	This competency could be integrated into a professional concepts, leadership, health systems science, management, or policy courses or trainings.

A	Advocacy	A key ethical standard of nursing practice and essential for empowering patients to be as activated and engaged in their care as possible. Advocacy is manifested in all settings and with a variety of audiences, the patient, interprofessional teams, or the organization/system.	The competency is appropriate in courses or trainings such as foundational medical/surgical or specialty care courses, professional concepts, leadership, research, and person-centered care.
B	Big-Picture Orientation	This is health systems science and thinking. Understanding the multiple ways of viewing health, how policy and legislation affects healthcare delivery, and the nurse's role in assisting with healthcare transformation.	The competency is appropriate in practically all courses or training, such as health systems thinking, leadership, policy, quality and safety, informatics, and service recovery.
O	Organized	This competency directs nurses to be efficient and effective and complements the organized approach of the nursing process.	This competency is appropriate in all courses or trainings, as the ability to be organized is key to safe and quality patient care as well as interprofessional practice and person-centered care.
R	Resource Awareness	Resource awareness is a critical aspect of value-based healthcare and patient outcomes. This includes understanding policy and regulations that direct payment structures, the value of population-level data and intervention, and the resource needs of patients within the settings they work.	This competency would be appropriate for courses or trainings in leadership, management, health systems, policy, organizational systems and processes, and orientations.
A	Anticipatory	An essential competency for proactive healthcare delivery and value-based healthcare. This competency includes being self-directed and reflective of any biases or assumptions that may interfere with nursing practice. This also includes looking ahead at potential barriers or challenges and proactively addressing them through interprofessional practice including the patient.	This competency is appropriate for any course or training as proactive care is a foundational feature of all nursing practice.

(Continued)

TABLE 10.1 ***(Continued)***

T	Transdisciplinary	This competency embraces the value of the variety of disciplines needed to meet patient needs across the continuum of care. It includes the nurse having a clear understanding of the role of each interprofessional team member and the value their alternate ways of knowing can bring to person-centered care.	This competency is appropriate for any course or training as interprofessional practice is a foundational feature of all nursing practice
E	Ethical–Legal	All nursing practice has an ethical application directed by the nursing code of ethics. Nurses must be aware of national and state regulations and standards of practice, organizational policies, and actions to be taken if engaged in an ethical dilemma or one that requires moral courage.	This competency is appropriate for any course or training as ethical practice is a foundational feature of all nursing practice

(Treiger & Fink-Samnick, 2013, p. 133)

Collaborative and Integrated Care

For the nursing workforce to meet patients' needs and implement care coordination practice across the continuum of care, there is a need for a renewed focus on cross-setting, cross-discipline, and cross-organization collaboration and integration (Taylor, 2023). Quality and value-added collaboration has the most significant potential to improve confidence and trust in the health system (GE Healthcare, 2023). Nurses will need expertise in collaborative practice and an understanding of integrated care to assist in managing resources and costs and meeting patient's holistic health and wellness needs. Collaborative and integrated care will require forming and supporting interprofessional teams across healthcare settings, community services, and resources in which patients and their families/support systems have a voice concerning the healthcare delivered (Braithwaite et al., 2018). As patients continue to embrace their role in their own health, becoming more activated and engaged, they will demand person-centered, integrated, and collaborative care in which they are key players in the interprofessional team. This will assist in addressing patient care needs with an integrated approach, including healthcare services and needed social and community resource services.

We will likely also see the call for and the development of more partnerships across settings and services, such as what is called for in H.R. 773, the "Homelessness and Behavioral Health Care Coordination Act of 2023" (H.R. 773, 2023–2024). It will be crucial that these collaborative partnerships have the voice of the local community and healthcare system to meet the community's needs, resources, and challenges (Taylor, 2023). This will involve a continued focus on infrastructure, systems thinking, and capacity building.

The reality of the current healthcare system situation, with high costs and poor outcomes, has created a climate in which collaborative care coordination is a necessity in how healthcare is delivered. Nurse expertise in the practice of collaborative care coordination will assist with the trend of decentralizing healthcare into homes and communities, engaging with and delivering digital health solutions, and ensuring that health technologies meet regulatory requirements while protecting patient rights and meeting their health and well-being needs throughout the ongoing healthcare transformation. Nurses will be called to bring the voice of the patient and the discipline to the creation and implementation of all aspects of healthcare transformation, which will require the persistent application of collaborative and integrated practice knowledge, skills, and attitudes.

Artificial Intelligence

Artificial intelligence (AI) is being integrated into all aspects of society along with the health system. Machine learning, a subset of AI, has already been available in healthcare for several years in the forms of health information technology (HIT) and big data analytics.

AI and machine learning are often used interchangeably, yet it is important to understand the differences. AI is a technology that can "think" like a human, performing tasks that normally require human thought, perception, and intelligence, such as decision-making or identifying patterns (Treiger, 2023). It is the brainpower of the technology. Machine learning is what most nurses in healthcare may think of when they hear the term AI. **Machine learning** is the process in technology that can identify patterns, engage in predictive modeling, use data for decision-making, and learn from data with negligible or limited human instructions or intervention. It is the method of AI brainpower. Nurses must also understand the use and application of artificial intelligence (AI) and machine learning. This will not only be needed for nursing practice but also to assess barriers to patient use of AI technologies and to provide education and training if needed.

AI and machine learning are significant tools for care coordination. An example of this includes the ability of technology to transmit real-time health data, such as overnight weight gain for a patient with congestive heart failure, and then alert the patient as to the best solution (e.g., take an additional diuretic pill, call their primary care doctor, go to the emergency room), while also sending an alert to the patient's primary care clinic. This example of AI and machine learning would lead to the appropriate use of healthcare resources, timely treatment, enhanced communication, and improved health outcomes (Kumar et al., 2022). Furthermore, the integration of AI into technologies like remote patient monitoring devices allows for individualized and person-center health recommendations, enhancing patient engagement and activation (Wang et al., 2023).

AI and machine learning can also assist in automating the care coordination process by analyzing patient variables and generating a risk-stratified list of the patient population, prioritizing care coordination interventions based on risk levels (Treiger, 2023). In this way, the care coordination nurse can use data-driven decision-making, focus their time and care delivery on those most needing care coordination interventions, and create personalized care coordination plans (Swift, 2023). Automating aspects of the care coordination process through AI also supports decreased patient information fragmentation, reduces repetitive tasks, and improves communication. See Figure 10.3 for a visual of how AI can support the nurse care coordinator.

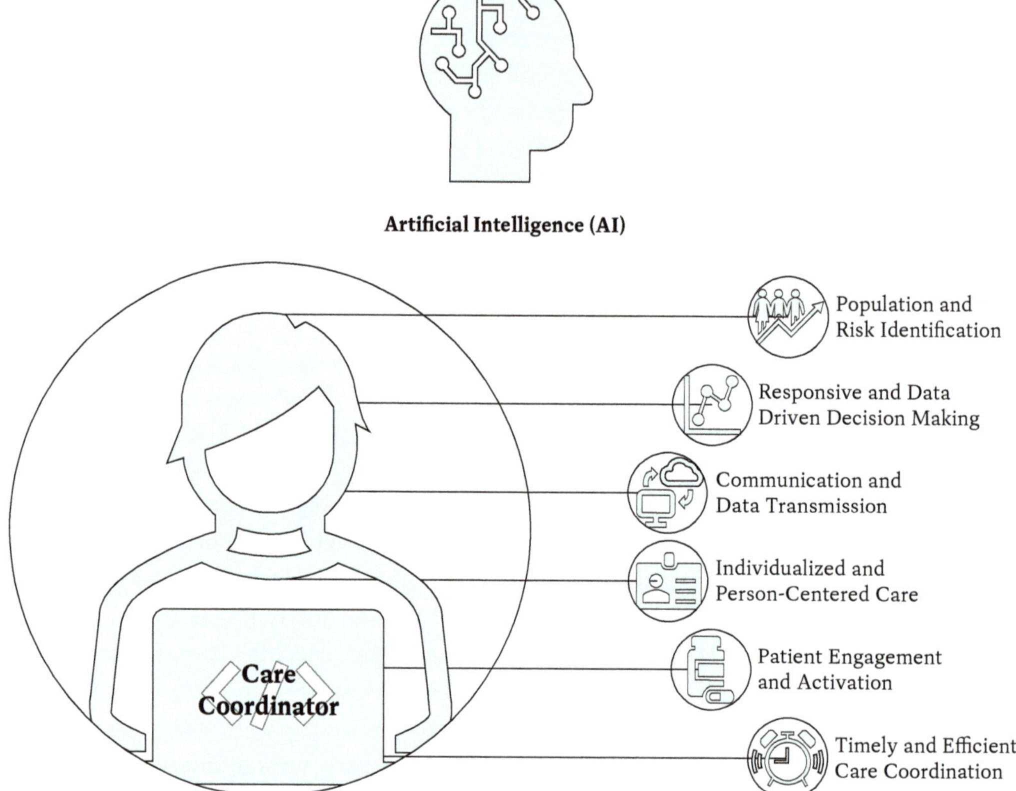

FIGURE 10.3 Example Artificial Intelligence (AI) Support of Care Coordination

There are concerns about integrating AI and machine learning because the decisions generated are only as good as the data utilized. If the data or parameters input into an AI model are biased or incomplete, this will direct the decision made by AI (Oram, 2022). Additionally, there is skepticism and a lack of trust on the part of the healthcare workforce and patients regarding the use of AI to direct healthcare decisions, and this must be addressed through transparency on the use of AI as well as providing education as to the function and purpose of AI in healthcare (GE Healthcare, 2023). Another aspect of AI use that needs further consideration is the fact that AI cannot be and should not be universally applied. It must be applied intelligently, considering potential unintended consequences or outcomes and addressing them through processes, workflows, and policies (Yaraghi, 2024).

CHAPTER SUMMARY

The future of care coordination has a foundation of nurses trained in communication, collaboration, and health technologies, focusing on working as an interprofessional team in a decentralized healthcare delivery setting, with coordinated care at the core. Advanced and integrated health technologies will allow for the seamless sharing of information and support quality, safe, accessible healthcare in conjunction with care-coordinating nurses with high levels of digital literacy. For this future to be realized, it will be required for the care coordination nurse to engage in health systems science and thinking and integrate aspects of various biological and social sciences to deliver quality healthcare to meet whole-person needs.

Nurses must also understand and engage in advocacy leadership to ensure that regulations and legislation meet patients' needs, contributing to coordinated and integrated value-based healthcare delivery and not creating unintended consequences that contribute to a lack of coordinated care and poor outcomes. At times, there may be a potential conflict in health care transformation when considering issues such as person-centered care and efficiency or effectiveness, and this will need to be balanced, as it may create tensions among those with conflicting priorities (IOM, 2001). Nurses are uniquely positioned to offer an ethical and person-centered perspective in such situations, advancing the value of care coordination and the trusted role nurses hold in the health system.

As the health system transforms and changes, trends and considerations will influence how nurses do their work. Issues such as the healthcare workforce and patient well-being, the transition from a reactive to a proactive health system, social media influences on health, and the continued advancement of health technologies will create new roles for nurses and new platforms for coordinated care delivery. As nurses embrace the future of care coordination and the integration of new roles and ways of coordinating care, they must also continue to be diligent in ensuring that any ethical concerns in policy, care delivery, or services provided are met with advocacy and education for all parties involved.

The future of care coordination requires the nurse to recognize their essential role in coordinating care across the continuum and the infusion of care coordination content into nursing education and professional development programs. All competencies required for successful care coordination are necessary in all aspects of nursing practice, and comprehending how they translate across practice settings and nursing knowledge skills and attitudes is critical to the future of care coordination. Furthermore, nurses will need to continue to provide expertise in interprofessional practice, be open to other ways of knowing, and remain current on regulatory, policy, and change drivers affecting the health system. Most importantly, it will be necessary for nurses to embrace and communicate the future vision of nurses ensuring coordinated care across settings in many roles, whether assisting in AI prompt creation, legislative advocacy, leading workplace well-being initiatives, or holding the title of nurse care coordinator.

CHAPTER 10 GLOSSARY

Advocacy Leadership: A proactive advocacy approach contributing to health system transformation, dismantling barriers to quality healthcare delivery, and promoting all participants in the health system to achieve their full potential.

Artificial Intelligence (AI): The brainpower of a technology that can "think" like a human, performing tasks that normally require human thought, perception, and intelligence, such as decision-making or identifying patterns.

Biopsychosocial Model: A view of health that includes the connection of biological, psychological, and sociological factors to health.

Healthcare Social Influencers: A person who promotes health behaviors or influences health awareness and education through social media platforms.

Health System Science: The systematic study of the health system to understand how the health system can improve care and care delivery and to inform the development of evidence-based practice, policies, and theoretical approaches concerning health.

Health Systems Thinking: A thinking process applied to the health system that is proactive, looks for patterns and relationships in problem areas, engages stakeholders, and implements systematic problem-solving approaches to health system needs.

Machine Learning: The method of a technology that can identify patterns, engage in predictive modeling, or use data for decision-making and can learn from data with negligible or limited human instructions or intervention.

Nursing Metaparadigm: A view of health that includes the interaction of four factors: the person, their environment, their health, and nursing.

Proactive Care Coordination: An approach to care coordination practice utilizing tools such as risk identification, patient engagement, and health system thinking that focuses on proactively identifying and addressing care coordination needs rather than awaiting poor outcomes or the need for urgent care coordination.

Reverse Quackery: When a nurse overextends their role to provide a service or type of care without possessing the necessary qualifications.

Well-Being: A multidimensional construct of wellness and health that includes objective and subjective aspects of physical, mental, social, and spiritual factors that are interrelated and interdependent.

DISCUSSION QUESTIONS AND ACTIVITIES

Discussion Questions

1. Identify two challenges to the health system meeting the Institute of Medicines (2001) rules for a 21st-century health system. How do you believe legislators should approach meeting these challenges?
2. Discuss the implications of integrating health system science and thinking competencies into nursing practice and how this could improve health outcomes across the continuum of care.

3. Discuss how nurse well-being can support safe and quality healthcare delivery. Identify what you believe is the priority intervention needed on a health system level to address nurse well-being.
4. Describe the nurse's role in advancing care coordination on a health system level. Identify how you will meet these role requirements in your nursing practice.
5. The use of artificial intelligence (AI) in care coordination practice will likely increase in the future. Identify one concern in the use of AI in care coordination practice and how you believe the health system and care coordinating nurse should address this concern.

Activities

1. In teams, create a mental model of care coordination nursing practice as part of the health system. Choose concepts concerning care coordination and the health system and the relationships between these to represent how care coordination fits into the health system. A visual explanation of how you see the various relationships of care coordination working in the health system should be provided and include the following:
   a. Identify the elements of the care coordination nursing practice. Include the main contextual factors and goals related to care coordination (e.g., tools, techniques, attitudes, skills, principles).
   b. Identify the relationships or cause-and-effect links between elements in care coordination practice and the health system. You can use feedback loops, arrows, lines, or whatever communicates the relationships.
   c. Visually identify any gaps, challenges, or barriers to care coordination practice.
   d. Write a brief description of how your mental model of care coordination can contribute to value-based healthcare and health system transformation.
2. Choose a healthcare social media influencer and familiarize yourself with their message and view of health. Once familiarized with your chosen influencer, create a 7 to 10-minute presentation (e.g., PowerPoint, video, in-person) outlining the following:
   a. Who they are, what platform they use, their message, etc.
   b. Vetting the influencer:
      - What are their qualifications?
      - What are their engagement rates? (Engagement = Likes + Comments / Followers × 100)
      - How often does the influencer post?

- Is there alignment with their postings and current healthcare practices? Are they presenting accurate information, misinformation, or a combination of these?
- How do you believe they affect health or healthcare practices through social media postings, and why?

c. Then discuss how you believe social media should be used in care coordination and the health system to advance better outcomes.

d. Finally, outline what type of education you might provide a patient concerning how to determine if they should follow a healthcare social media influencer.

3. Case Study:

A hospital is looking to restructure and redesign its processes for direct inpatient admissions from the community (e.g., the PCP, long-term care facility, etc.). The hospital found through analysis of last year's data that there is usually a 6 to 8-hour delay in direct admissions occurring once the referral was received. This led to physical complications for the patients, which required more intensive healthcare and increasing costs and resource use and decreasing quality benchmark outcomes for this patient population.

After reviewing individual patient data, it was found that the "bed board" office was using inconsistent processes and procedures, causing some admission referrals to have a lengthy back-and-forth communication process to ensure that the patient was appropriate for admission, determining transportation processes to the hospital, and examining the patient's payer source before accepting the patient for admission. An interprofessional committee was created to address the policy and procedure inconsistencies and design an up-to-date process for direct admissions to the hospital. The entire direct admission system, including the hospital and outside community agencies, was examined during the policy redesign and update.

It was found that the most prominent cause of delay in admission was a delay in patient information transfer, as well as the "bed board" office and many community agencies misinterpreting messages sent or delaying response to messages sent. This, in turn, delayed the admitting provider's review of the patient's condition to ensure the patient was admitted to the correct floor in the hospital. Additionally, there was a lack of internal communication from the admitting provider and "bed board" office to the accepting floor nurse, and the nurse often lacked information on essential treatments to be continued, what labs or imaging needed to be followed up on, or the reason for the direct admission. Often, orders were missing and there was no systematic process for a handoff of the patient to the assigned bedside nurse to provide safe and quality care delivery. Furthermore, it was discovered that patient satisfaction scores were decreased among those patients who were directly admitted to the hospital, that there was a lack of systematic referral template for community providers to complete and submit for referral, and that many nurses were expressing they did not want to care for direct admit patients.

Due to these findings, the interprofessional committee developed a new policy and procedure containing a direct admission referral template available on the hospital's website and a methodical checklist delineating each step of the direct admission process, including timelines and types of communication needed and with whom. The checklist outlined what the admitting provider, the "bed board" office, and the accepting bedside nurse were accountable for, as well as a tip sheet for community providers requesting direct admission that would be emailed to the referring provider automatically once a referral was received.

Additionally, the hospital's service recovery team was consulted as they focused on making things right for patients and their families if something went wrong with a hospital stay. A documentation process from the "bed board" office was developed so that in the hospital's EHR, it was easily identified on the demographic page if the patient was a direct admit. In this way, the service recovery team could promptly address any service issues for these patients and collect data on how many and what types of service recoveries were requested for this patient population. The interprofessional committee will evaluate this data and send out anonymous surveys to those involved in direct admissions every 3 months for the next 12 months to determine if these policy and procedure redesigns are working and improving the direct admissions process.

1. Identify the potential long-range implications or consequences if the hospital did not address the delays in admission for patients being directly admitted from the community.
2. What can the bedside nurse do to improve care coordination and interprofessional care practices in this case study?
3. How does this case study represent the use of health systems science and health systems thinking?
4. Describe how the use of health technologies support the redesign and implementation of the interprofessional committee's solutions to this direct admission policy and procedures issue. Are there other ways that health technologies, machine learning, or artificial intelligence (AI) can be used to streamline the direct admission process?

NCLEX Style Questions

1. Which of the following is the best way for nurse care coordinators to influence health policy when working with an interprofessional committee for policy development?

   a. Ensuring they follow the code of ethics
   b. Reviewing and following the policies of the organization in which they work
   c. Identifying competing priorities among team members
   d. Engaging in proactive advocacy to address policy barriers

2. The nurse care coordinator wants to engage in legislative reform and development on the state level and knows that the nurse role supports which of the following? (Select all that apply.)

   a. Conducting a cost-benefit analysis of the legislation implementation

   b. Active legislative lobbying by major healthcare payer organizations

   c. Providing a platform for patient voices in legislation development

   d. Providing expertise and education concerning legislation being considered

3. Which ways can the nurse care coordinator engage in proactive care coordination?

   a. Identifying risks in the patient population

   b. Focusing on the healthy patient population

   c. Using a reactive and priority patient approach

   d. Discontinuing services for non-adherent patients

4. Health system science includes which of the following aspects of the health system? (Select all that apply.)

   a. How healthcare is delivered

   b. How healthcare workers support their discipline

   c. How the health system can improve care

   d. How theory supports the health system

5. The Institute of Medicine developed 10 rules for the transformation of the 21st health system. Which of the following are among the ten rules developed?

   a. Interprofessional practice

   b. Accountability and transparency

   c. Information exchange

   d. All of the above

6. Which of the following aspects of the health system has been affected by the increase in the number of people with chronic or longer-term health conditions?

    a. The increasing cost of private insurance

    b. The increasing need for a fee-for-service model

    c. The increasing number of people choosing holistic care

    d. The increasing use of ethical practice

7. Well-being in patients and the healthcare workforce is multidimensional and includes which of the following aspects?

    a. Physical, emotional, relational, and spiritual

    b. Spiritual, social, biological, psychological

    c. Physical, mental, social, spiritual

    d. Health, environment, nursing, person

    The following two questions relate to this scenario:

    You are a nurse care coordinator working in a community clinic and are meeting with Mr. Fitz, who has newly been diagnosed with Type 2 diabetes.

8. Mr. Fitz is asking you many questions about how to treat diabetes, as he has found a lot on social media about it. He especially likes one healthcare influencer promoting a new apple cider vinegar intervention because he prefers natural treatments to medication. You understand that Mr. Fitz is engaged and active in his health and wants to learn how to self-manage his condition, which is a key aspect of healthcare transformation. What intervention would you offer Mr. Fitz to support his continued involvement in his health?

    a. Tell Mr. Fitz he should only follow the provider's prescribed interventions and not waste his time on social media.

    b. Explain to Mr. Fitz that Type 2 diabetes can rarely be managed without medication and that he should resign himself to the fact that he will need medication for the rest of his life.

    c. Caution, Mr. Fitz about the reliability and validity of some of the information that is on social media and that healthcare influencers provide.

    d. All of the above

9. Mr. Fitz comes in for his 6-week follow-up appointment, and you are discussing how the diabetes management is going for him. Mr. Fitz says he has trouble managing his blood glucose levels but is trying. You know that Mr. Fitz has recently been laid off from his workplace and went through a divorce last year. You wonder if Mr. Fitz has financial difficulties impacting his ability to buy appropriate food for his diabetic condition. You bring the subject up, and Mr. Fitz becomes visibly upset with the topic, stating, "It is none of your business" and he "does just fine." What is your best response to Mr. Fitz?

   a. Explain to Mr. Fitz that you cannot help him if he does not tell you about his situation and whether he is having financial or food insecurity issues.

   b. Validate that it is Mr. Fitz's choice to tell you about his finances and explain that sometimes people with diabetes have difficulty purchasing appropriate foods.

   c. Apologize to Mr. Fitz for upsetting him and let him know you will revisit the topic later.

   d. Ask Mr. Fitz if you can contact his son about this issue because you are aware that he lives just down the street from Mr. Fitz.

10. You are a nurse care coordinator for a visiting nurse community agency. You have been assigned a new family and go on your first visit to find that the mother, Ms. Clarke, has moved from a different state and is now living with her children and her new boyfriend where she is experiencing domestic violence daily. Ms. Clarke tells you that she cannot leave the situation as she would be homeless, without a job or money, and does not know the resources in the area. What would be the best response to this situation?

    a. Tell Ms. Clark that she should be empowered and confront her boyfriend to let him know she will not be abused any longer and then leave the situation immediately.

    b. Provide education on the local emergency hotline for domestic violence and ask Ms. Clark if you can make a referral to the social worker you work with to have them visit with her about potential options in the area.

    c. Call the police and child protective services and report that Ms. Clark is living in a domestic violence situation.

    d. Ask Ms. Clark questions about the frequency and type of domestic violence, ensuring you have a comprehensive assessment and can determine if it is occurring.

11. You are precepting a new graduate nurse and explaining the need to integrate a big-picture perspective into new-hire orientations. The new graduate nurse understands the role of the big-picture orientation and perspective in the health system when they say which of the following:

a. Having a big-picture orientation expands critical thinking and looks at how specific healthcare disciplines can perform better.

b. The big-picture orientation assists in understanding the multiple ways to view health and how policies and legislation can affect healthcare.

c. Big-picture orientation is needed if you are going into leadership or advanced practice nursing.

d. Most student nurses are taught a lot about the need for a big-picture orientation, and this might be repetitive information.

12. Nurse care coordinators will need expertise in collaborative practice and integrated care to assist in which of the following outcomes? (Select all that apply.)

a. Managing resources and costs

b. Meeting patient health and wellness needs

c. Fewer HIPAA violations

d. Appropriate admissions

13. Which aspects of care coordination practice can artificial intelligence technology assist with?

a. Communication and data transmission

b. Patient engagement and activation

c. Responsive and data-driven decision-making

d. All of the above

14. What are some concerns related to using artificial intelligence (AI) in care coordination practice and the health system? (Select all that apply.)

a. Incomplete or inaccurate data input

b. Lack of trust in the use of AI for healthcare decisions

c. The ability for AI to be universally applied

d. Biased decision-making

15. The future of care coordination requires nurses to engage in advocacy leadership to ensure that regulations and legislation *do not* do which of the following:

    a. Create unintended consequences

    b. Support value-based care

    c. Demonstrate resource connections

    d. Contribute to care coordination

REFERENCES

Amer, K. S., (2013). *Quality and safety for transformational nursing: Core competencies.* Pearson.

American Association of Nurse Practitioners. (2024). *NP fact sheet.* https://www.aanp.org/about/all-about-nps/np-fact-sheet

American Medical Association (AMA). (2023). *Teaching health systems science.* https://www.ama-assn.org/education/changemeded-initiative/teaching-health-systems-science

American Nurses Association (ANA). (2015). *Code of ethics for nurses: With interpretive statements.* Author.

American Nurses Association (ANA). (2021). *Nursing: Scope and standards of practice* (4th ed). Author.

Braithwaite, J., Mannion, R., Matsuyama, Y., Shekelle, P. G., Whittaker, S., Al-Adawi, S., Ludlow, K., James, W., Ting, H. P., Herkes, J., McPherson, E., Churruca, K., Lamprell, G., Ellis, L. A., Boyling, C., Warwick, M., Pomare, C., Nicklin, W., & Hughes, C. F. (2018). The future of health systems to 2030: A roadmap for global progress and sustainability. *International Journal for Quality in Health Care: Journal of the International Society for Quality in Health Care, 30*(10), 823–831. https://doi.org/10.1093/intqhc/mzy242

Cancer Research UK. (2021). *Ovarian cancer survival.* https://www.cancerresearchuk.org/about-cancer/ovarian-cancer/survival

Cancer Research UK. (2023). *Survival for cervical cancer.* https://www.cancerresearchuk.org/about-cancer/cervical-cancer/survival

Cook, N. L. (2023). *Patient-centered research is critical to enhancing care coordination.* Patient-Centered Outcomes Research Institute. https://www.pcori.org/leadership-perspective/patient-centered-research-critical-enhancing-care-coordination

Davis, A. J., Fowler, M. D., & Aroskar, M. A. (2010). *Ethical dilemmas & nursing practice* (5th ed.). Pearson

Dietz, C. (2019). New CMS rules put the focus on informed patient choice. *MedCity News.* https://medcitynews.com/2019/12/new-cms-rules-put-the-focus-on-informed-patient-choice/

Fraser, K., Perez, R., & Latour, C. (2018). *CMSA's integrated case management: A manual for case managers by case managers.* Springer Publishing Company.

GE Healthcare. (2023). *Reimagining better health 2023.* https://www.gehealthcare.com/-/jssmedia/gehc/us/images/insights/reimaging-better-health/ge-healthcarereimagining-better-healthstudymay302023jb01690xu.pdf?rev=-1

Hansson, S. O., & Fröding, B. (2020). Ethical conflicts in patient-centered care. *Clinical Ethics, 16*(2). https://doi.org/10.1177/1477750920962356

Hoffman, D. (2022). *Commentary on chronic disease prevention in 2022.* National Association of Chronic Disease Directors. https://chronicdisease.org/wp-content/uploads/2022/04/FS_ChronicDiseaseCommentary2022FINAL.pdf

H.R.773—118th Congress (2023–2024): Homelessness and Behavioral Health Care Coordination Act of 2023. (2023, February 2). https://www.congress.gov/bill/118th-congress/house-bill/773

H.R.6338—118th Congress (2023–2024): Veterans' Cancer Care Coordinator Act of 2023. (2023, November 27). https://www.congress.gov/bill/118th-congress/house-bill/6338

Huber, D. L. (2018). *Leadership & nursing care management* (6th ed.). Elsevier.

Institute of Medicine (IOM). (2001). *Crossing the quality chasm: A new health system for the 21st century.* National Academy Press.

Johnson, J. A., Anderson, D. E., & Rossow, C. G. (2020). *Health systems thinking: A primer.* Jones & Bartlett Learning.

Jónsdóttir, B., Wikman, A., Sundström Poromaa, I., & Stålberg, K. (2023). Advanced gynecological cancer: Quality of life one year after diagnosis. *PloS one, 18*(6), e0287562. https://doi.org/10.1371/journal.pone.0287562

Kumar, S., Qiu, L., Sen, A., & Sinha, A. P. (2022). Putting analytics into action in care coordination research: Emerging issues and potential solutions. *Production and Operations Management, 31*(6), 2714–2738. https://doi.org/10.1111/poms.13771

Lomas, T., & VanderWeele, T. J. (2022). The garden and the orchestra: Generative metaphors for conceptualizing the complexities of well-being. *International Journal of Environmental Research and Public Health, 19*(21), 14544. https://doi.org/10.3390/ijerph192114544

Mason, L., Perez, D., McLemore, A., Monica R., & Dickson E. (2021). *Policy & politics in nursing and health care* (8th Ed.). Elsevier Health Sciences. https://pageburstls.elsevier.com/books/9780323554985

Menon, S., Entwistle, V. A., Campbell, A. V., & van Delden, J. J. M. (2020). Some unresolved ethical challenges in healthcare decision-making: Navigating family involvement. *Asian Bioethics Review, 12*(1), 27–36. https://doi.org/10.1007/s41649-020-00111-9

Mesko, B. (2018). Health IT and digital health: The future of health technology is diverse. *Journal of Clinical and Translational Research, 3*(Suppl 3), 431–434. https://www.ncbi.nlm.nih.gov/pmc/articles/PMC6412600/

National Institute of Health (NIH). (2023). *What is health equity?* https://www.nimhd.nih.gov/resources/understanding-health-disparities/health-equity.html

Nikfarid, L., Hekmat, N., Vedad, A., & Rajabi, A. (2018). The main nursing metaparadigm concepts in human caring theory and Persian mysticism: A comparative study. *Journal of Medical Ethics and History of Medicine, 11,* 6. https://www.ncbi.nlm.nih.gov/pmc/articles/PMC6150916/

Oram, A. (2022). What hinders clinicians from using technology for care coordination? *Healthcare IT* Today. https://www.healthcareittoday.com/2022/01/27/what-hinders-clinicians-from-using-technology-for-coordinated-care/

Palusak, C., Shook, B., Davies, S. C., & Lundine, J. P. (2022). A scoping review to inform care coordination strategies for youth with traumatic brain injuries: Care coordination personnel. *International Journal of Care Coordination, 25*(1), 21–38. doi:10.1177/20534345211070647

Peter G. Peterson Foundation. (2023). *The share of Americans without health insurance in 2022 matched a record low.* https://www.pgpf.org/blog/2023/11/the-share-of-americans-without-health-insurance-in-2022-matched-a-record-low

Porter-O'Grady, T., & Malloch, K. (2018). *Quantum leadership: Creating sustainable value in health care* (5th ed.). Jones & Bartlett Learning.

Powell, J., & Pring, T. (2024). The impact of social media influencers on health outcomes: Systematic review. *Social Science & Medicine, 340,* 1–10. https://doi.org/10.1016/j.socscimed.2023.116472

President's Commission for the Study of Ethical Problems in Medicine and Biomedical and Behavioral Research. (1983). *Summing up: Final report on studies of the ethical and legal problems in medicine and biomedical and behavioral research.* https://www.thaddeuspope.com/images/President_Commission_1983_-_summing_up.pdf

Qin, F. (2020). The debilitating scope of care coordination under HIPAA. *North Carolina Law Review, 98*(6). https://scholarship.law.unc.edu/nclr/vol98/iss6/6/

Schwarz, R. (2024). The intersection of social influencers and healthcare. *Forbes*. https://www.forbes.com/sites/forbescommunicationscouncil/2024/01/03/the-intersection-of-social-influencers-and-healthcare/?sh=1fa5cab7167f

Sherifi, D., Ndanga, M., Hunt, T. T., & Srinivasan, S. (2021). The symbiotic relationship between health information management and health informatics. Opportunities for growth and collaboration. *Perspectives in Health Information Management, 18*(4), 1c. https://www.ncbi.nlm.nih.gov/pmc/articles/PMC8649705/

Shi, L., & Singh, D. (2019). *Essentials of the U.S. health care system* (5th ed.). Jones & Bartlett Learning.

Smit, C. R., Bevelander, K. E., de Leeuw, R. N. H., & Buijzen, M. (2022). Motivating social influencers to engage in health behavior interventions. *Frontiers in Psychology, 13,* 885688. https://doi.org/10.3389/fpsyg.2022.885688

Swan, B. A., Conway-Phillips, R., Haas, S. A., & Peña, L. (2019). Optimizing strategies for care coordination and transition management: Recommendations for nursing education. *Nursing Economics, 37*(2), 77–85. https://www.researchgate.net/publication/332621407_Optimizing_Strategies_for_Care_Coordination_and_Transition_Management_Recommendations_for_Nursing_Education

Swift, T. (2023). Modernizing care management with AI & automation. *Forbes*. https://www.forbes.com/sites/forbestechcouncil/2023/10/16/modernizing-care-management-with-ai--automation/?sh=15b3a4f828e6

Taylor, M. (2023). *The potential of care coordination*. NHS Confederation. https://www.nhsconfed.org/articles/potential-care-coordination

Tikkanen, R., Osborn, R., Mossialos, E., Djordjevic, A., & Wharton, G. A. (2020). *International health care systems profiles: United States*. The Commonwealth Fund. https://www.commonwealthfund.org/international-health-policy-center/countries/united-states

Treiger, T. M. (2023). AI and Case Management: New Tools of Our Trade. *Professional Case Management, 28*(6), 296–298. https://doi.org/10.1097/NCM.0000000000000685

Treiger, T. M., & Fink-Samnick, E. (2013). COLLABORATE©: A Universal competency-based paradigm for professional case management, part I. *Professional Case Management 18*(3), p 122–135. https://doi.org/10.1097/NCM.0b013e31828562c0

Wang, C., He, T., Zhou, H., Zhang, Z., & Lee, C. (2023). Artificial intelligence enhanced sensors—enabling technologies to next-generation healthcare and biomedical platform. *Bioelectronic Medicine*, 9(1), 17. https://doi.org/10.1186/s42234-023-00118-1

Ward, M. (2023). *Anderson Healthcare puts the emphasis on proactive care*. Health Data Management. https://www.healthdatamanagement.com/articles/anderson-healthcare-puts-the-emphasis-on-proactive-care

World Health Organization (WHO). (2024). *Health and well-being*. https://www.who.int/data/gho/data/major-themes/health-and-well-being#:~:text=The%20WHO%20constitution%20states%3A%20%22Health,of%20mental%20disorders%20or%20disabilities.

Yaraghi, N. (2024). *Generative AI in health care: Opportunities, challenges, and policy*. https://www.brookings.edu/articles/generative-ai-in-health-care-opportunities-challenges-and-policy/

Young, M. (2022a). *Focus on Quintuple Aim to address workforce burnout and equity*. Relias Media. https://www.reliasmedia.com/articles/149298-focus-on-quintuple-aim-to-address-workforce-burnout-and-equity

Young, M. (2022b). *Ethicist: Case managers can fairly and ethically handle patient refusal to discharge*. Relias Media. https://www.reliasmedia.com/articles/149294-ethicist-case-managers-can-fairly-and-ethically-handle-patient-refusal-to-discharge

Zimlichman, E., Nicklin, W., Aggarwal, R., & Bates, D. W. (2021). Health care 2030: The coming transformation. *NEJM Catalyst*. https://catalyst.nejm.org/doi/full/10.1056/CAT.20.0569

Credits

Fig. 10.2: Source: T. Lomas & T. J. VanderWeele, "The Garden and the Orchestra: Generative Metaphors for Conceptualizing the Complexities of Well-Being," *International Journal Of Environmental Research and Public Health*, vol. 19, no. 21, 2022.

Fig. 10.2a: Copyright © by Microsoft.

Table 10.1: Teresa M. Treiger and Ellen Fink-Samnick, "A Universal Competency-Based Paradigm for Professional Case Management, Part I," *Professional Case Management* vol. 18, no. 3, p. 133. Copyright © 2013 by Lippincott Williams & Wilkins Inc.

Fig. 10.3a: Copyright © by Microsoft.

CHAPTER 11

Care Coordination Considerations of Special Populations

LEARNING OBJECTIVES

1. Examine the application of trauma-informed care in care coordination practice.
2. Explore health system-level barriers in care coordination practice for special populations.
3. Appreciate the unique characteristics and needs of special populations.
4. Recognize the connection between appropriate care coordination delivery and health outcomes in special populations.

KEY TERMS

- Alzheimer's disease and related dementias (ADRD)
- dementia
- diagnostic overshadowing
- distressed behaviors
- dual-users
- intellectual and developmental disabilities (IDDs)
- person-first language
- re-traumatize
- trauma-informed care (TIC)
- tri-morbidity
- unhoused or houselessness
- veteran

Introduction

While there are common challenges and barriers to effective and efficient care coordination, some populations of patients have unique needs that can impact the care coordination process, creating significant barriers to successful care transitions. These populations also may experience health system-level issues on a more pronounced scale, requiring the nurse to meet and address these challenges proactively. This does not mean that continuity of care cannot be achieved. Nevertheless, it does mean the care coordinating nurse needs specific knowledge, skills, and attitudes to promote meeting overarching goals and rights of care coordination for these patients and address inherent system-level issues such as implicit bias, system complexity, healthcare accessibility, and the need for trauma-informed care (TIC).

Several groups have specific and distinctive care coordination needs. These populations include veterans, persons with Alzheimer's disease and related dementias (ADRD), persons with intellectual or developmental disabilities (IDD), and those who are unhoused. This is not a comprehensive accounting of all populations needing individualized and specific systems-level care coordination efforts and knowledge; however, they are common populations seen in the health system that frequently experience less-than-optimal care coordination. This requires nurses to be aware of the potential for poor outcomes and system-level barriers in these populations and to advocate for and provide effective care coordination across the continuum.

Trauma-Informed Care (TIC) and Care Coordination Practice

A central method of meeting the needs of many of these special populations is utilizing **trauma-informed care (TIC)** in care coordination practice because many of these populations have experienced forms of trauma during their lifetimes. TIC is healthcare delivery based on awareness of the need to understand a person's lived experience and the effect of trauma on health, wellness, and other aspects of life in order to provide effective care. TIC is easily integrated into care coordination practice, as one of the basic foundations of care coordination is providing person-centered care through individualized care planning and supporting the whole person, not the disease or health condition alone. This requires the nurse to understand and consider social determinants of health (SDOH) and the impact of trauma as an SDOH. Trauma is defined as "physically or emotionally harmful or life-threatening with lasting adverse effects on an individual's functioning and mental, physical, social, emotional, or spiritual well-being" (RHIHub, 2018, para. 6).

Trauma as an SDOH is an essential concept for care coordinating nurses to grasp and assess for, as trauma experiences can affect how people view their health, themselves, others, and the health system, along with their sense of trust and safety. Trauma experiences may lead to distrust of healthcare providers and the health system or create physical, mental, or other barriers for the patient's self-management of health or inclination to seek needed care (RHIHub, 2018). Furthermore, the nurse must understand that trauma is what the patient says it is, just like pain or quality of life. It is not the nurse's role to ascertain if the patient should feel a certain way, if the experience was traumatic, or to **re-traumatize** the patient by exposing them to a situation, interaction, environment, or event that causes re-experiencing of trauma symptoms, reactions, or experiences. This requires nurses to provide care that universally promotes safety, trust, and respect for all patients (Fleishman et al., 2019).

The trauma experience can be a one-time event, throughout multiple events, or a set of circumstances (SAMHSA, 2023). None of these types of traumas is more important than another in the sense of the patient's individual experience and how they have integrated the experience into their life, actions, and perspectives. Furthermore, the nurse must understand that trauma can occur on an individual, family, or group level (SAMHSA, 2023) and that some groups or populations of patients may have consistently not received TIC related to health system-level issues and barriers, such as veterans or unhoused populations.

TIC guiding principles include safety, trustworthiness and transparency, peer support, collaboration and mutuality, empowerment, and cultural, historical, and gender issues (SAMHSA, 2023, p. 10). It is not a reach for the care coordinating nurse to engage in TIC in all care coordination encounters because these principles fit well with the principles of care coordination practice, such as proactive advocacy and care planning, evidence-based care, least-restrictive and accessible care, accountability, and integrated, interprofessional, and collaborative care support. If the care coordinating nurse realizes how trauma can affect health and health outcomes, recognizes the signs of trauma (e.g., persistent fatigue, sleep disorders, anxiety, self-injurious behaviors), universally applies TIC with all patients, and avoids re-traumatizing, better outcomes can be met, patient and nurse satisfaction can increase, and continuity of care can be supported (Davidson, 2021). See Table 11.1 for a comparison of TIC principles and care coordination application.

TABLE 11.1 Comparison of TIC Principles and Care Coordination Application

TIC Principles	Care Coordination Application
Safety	Environmental, physical, and psychological safety is provided. Interpersonal interactions avoid repeating traumatic experiences.
Trustworthiness and Transparency	Interventions are performed and decisions made with openness, respect, consistency, and fairness, building, and maintaining trust. Interventions offered are evidence-based, are least restrictive, and respect patient preferences and goals of care.
Peer Support	Support is offered to utilize interprofessional resources. Connection to community support programs is provided, and the patient is allowed to include support people in care planning, goal setting, and decision-making as desired. Gaps and barriers to care and patient needs are monitored, and follow-up is provided.
Collaboration and Mutuality	The patient is part of the interprofessional team, viewed as an expert on themselves, and is a partner in their healthcare. Power differentials or hierarchical relationships are not supported among nurses and patients. Accountability for outcomes and care delivery is shared amongst the interprofessional team.
Empowerment	Strength-based assessments are conducted, and supports and resources are recognized, integrated into the care plan, and built upon. Patient autonomy is supported with relationship and person-centered care and proactive advocacy. Autonomous decision-making and patient engagement and activation is promoted.
Cultural, Historical, and Gender Issues	Nurses are aware of any implicit and explicit biases and actively participate in self-reflective practice to ensure that these are not incorporated into care coordination practice. The patient's lived experience is valued and integrated into care planning, goal setting, and decision-making.

(SAMHSA, 2023, p. 10)

The Veteran Population

Veterans are a vulnerable population in the health system and have specialized needs, as veterans have a higher likelihood of having experienced trauma, environmental hazards, chemical exposure, physical injuries, and other obstacles to their physical and mental health due to their time in service. A **veteran** has served in the active military, naval, or air service and was honorably discharged, served as a reservist or member of the National Guard called to active duty, or is a person disabled from disease or injury incurred in the line of duty or training (U.S. Department of Veterans Affairs, 2019a). There are approximately 18 million veterans in the United States, representing about 6% of the population (Schaeffer, 2023). Additionally, although the number of living veterans is expected to decrease, the number of women, Hispanic, and Black veterans is expected to increase by 2048 (Schaeffer, 2023). Of particular concern in the context of health is that up to 73% of veterans have served during wartime (Schaeffer, 2023). Many veterans have conditions developed through wartime experiences, such as traumatic brain injury, post-traumatic stress disorder (PTSD), substance use disorder (SUD), loss of limbs or other functional abilities, depression, anxiety, difficulty adjusting to civilian life, and socioeconomic issues like houselessness or unemployment.

The Veterans Affairs (VA) Maintaining Internal Systems and Strengthening Integrated Outside Networks Act (MISSION), passed in 2018, allows veterans to seek care outside the VA healthcare system and receive care in the community. This can occur for a variety of reasons, such as the care needed not being available at the VA, living in an area without a VA medical facility, excessive distance or drive time to the nearest VA facility, appointment wait times, or the veteran and their VA provider agreeing it is in the veteran's best interest (U.S. Department of Veterans Affairs, 2019b). This means many veterans are **dual-users**, receiving healthcare and other services from VA and community providers, hospitals, and facilities. It is estimated that approximately 50% of veterans are dual-users (Miller et al., 2019). Many of these veterans have multiple physical and mental health conditions and see several providers in the community setting (Cordasco et al., 2019). Veterans who receive healthcare from the VA and community system need coordinated care to decrease poor outcomes and duplicative services (Miller et al., 2019).

Moreover, about 11% of veterans, or 2 million, are women, and the number of pregnancies in women veterans has increased by more than 80% since 2014 (MyArmyBenefits, 2023; Schaeffer, 2023). Pregnant women veterans have been shown to benefit from care coordination services due to pre-pregnancy physical and mental health conditions and high rates of pregnancy complications (Cordasco et al., 2018). Therefore, the VA has begun to focus on maternity care outcomes and developed a care coordination program to assist veterans in accessing care and resources needed throughout pregnancy and postpartum, even if they give birth at a community facility. The VA will provide its own maternity care coordinators to assist with follow-up, needed consultation, and addressing social determinants of health or risk factors and mental health concerns (MyArmyBenefits, 2023). This means that nurses in community hospitals where deliveries may occur must also be aware of this service to coordinate care between the delivery and VA settings and facilitate continuity of care.

Veterans who live in rural areas also have particular needs related to being dual-users. Often, rural veterans have barriers to care access linked to the distance to the nearest VA facility, lack of specialist providers or provider shortage, and lack of or limited Internet access for telehealth or use of digital health apps and devices (Garvin et al., 2021). Additionally, their VA providers may be unfamiliar with the resources or services in their local rural area for consultations, referrals, and support needs (Garvin et al., 2021). To prevent these gaps in transitions and coordination of care, the nurse will need to perform a comprehensive assessment of needs and resources available as well as alternate healthcare delivery methods for the rural veteran, plan accordingly, and provide education, information, and support for the veteran to receive timely and accessible healthcare (Greenstone et al., 2019).

Veterans who are from historically underrepresented populations that have either been ignored or misrepresented in healthcare, such as the Black and Hispanic populations, often have had poor experiences in the health system (Oregon Heritage, 2018). These veterans may have challenges in accessing healthcare, such as transportation issues. They may feel a lack of trust in the health system or community resources due to the absence of timely responses to needs, difficulty accessing services, or perceived stigma, negative attitudes, or racism (Izquierdo et al., 2018). Additionally, research has shown that Black and Hispanic veterans experience higher wait times for appointments, which likely contributes to perceived stigma and racism (Gurewich et al., 2021). This requires the care coordinating nurse to employ person-centered care strategies, engaging the veteran and collaborating with them to identify barriers to continuity of care, such as financial concerns or lack of consistent or reliable contact information, and also provide education on navigating the health and community resource system effectively (Izquierdo et al., 2018).

Some dual-user veterans have social determinants of health (SDOH) needs that, if not addressed in the community setting, can lead to continued fragmentation of care and poor outcomes. These SDOH issues could be a lack of access to care, financial matters, housing insecurity, or psychosocial stressors or traumatic experiences that contribute to difficulty for the veteran in self-managing their health or coordinating their care (Sjoberg et al., 2022). Often this can occur due to a lack of comprehensive assessment by the care coordinating nurse in the community setting, a lack of access to patient health information, or difficulty in contacting the VA provider to ensure timely follow-up. SDOH issues point to the essential need of the care coordinating nurse to complete a needs assessment, ensure notification of the visit, treatment, discharge plan, or other important health information be sent to and received by the VA provider, and use a structured care coordination handoff, such as IPASSTHEBATON, back to the VA if the community setting will not be continuing to see the patient (Miller et al., 2019).

The veteran population has unique considerations when coordinating care. There are several barriers to coordinating care between community settings and the VA system, including a lack of records exchange and interoperability between the VA and community systems and the potential inability to connect with the veteran, the community, or the VA provider. This can lead to a lack of current or accurate contact information, delayed responses and referrals, and veterans being asked to bring messages or information from the community providers to the VA system or vice versa, which can lead to lack of communication or miscommunication

(Dunkin, 2022; Garvin et al., 2021). This often leaves many veterans coordinating their own care and navigating the complex system between the VA and community providers, contributing to increased stress and lack of TIC for the veteran (Apaydin et al., 2021; Miller et al., 2019).

Care Coordination Considerations

If a veteran does receive care from a community provider, the care will likely be delivered across the episode of care. So it will not be a one-time visit to a community provider or hospital but may include initial consultation, intervention, and follow-up. For example, if a veteran receives a knee replacement at a community facility, they would see the community facility/provider for the initial consultation, pre-operative appointment, surgical intervention, postoperative recovery, follow-up appointments, and therapies (Greenstone et al., 2019). Due to this, care coordinating nurses must understand the unique aspects of the veteran population's care needs and how to engage effectively with the VA system to coordinate care.

VA care has the key foundation of providing a "patient-aligned care team" based on the PACT model, much like the patient-centered medical home. Since the goal is to provide individualized and person-centered care each veteran seen at the VA will be assigned a care team (Spotswood, 2023). The care team will have a specific name, like Team Red or Team Blue, and it is often the team coordinating the patient's care on the VA end (Cordasco et al., 2019). This is an essential piece of information to gather from a veteran because when you coordinate care, you may need to set up follow-up appointments with the veteran's assigned team, and these usually are made directly with the team, not through the overall VA system or facility. Furthermore, the transfer of information is a critical barrier to care coordination for a veteran. Due to other providers outside the VA not using the same electronic health record system (EHR), there can be a delay or gap in information transfer that results in miscommunication or lack of timely follow-up care (Spotswood, 2023). It is essential that the care coordinating nurse proactively address the potential for a delay in information transfer, ensuring that follow-up care is scheduled and timely.

Nurses providing care coordination for veterans should conduct a comprehensive assessment, including SDOH, physical and mental health, medication reconciliation, determining care goals, and establishing if the veteran has applied for or is receiving VA services (Chang et al., 2022). For most VA services, the veteran must apply for benefits, which can be time-consuming. So if the veteran is interested in benefits and has yet to apply for these, the care coordinating nurse can assist with navigating this process. If the veteran receives benefits and services, the care coordinating nurse must work collaboratively with the interprofessional team, including the VA PACT and other VA services the veteran receives.

The VA offers many services, including medical care, mental health care, SUD care, home health care, pharmacy services, various support and care coordination programs, and services for spouses of veterans. As part of the comprehensive assessment, the nurse should ascertain which services the veteran is currently receiving and, if questions or concerns arise, contact their veteran's PACT or VA medical center for more information on current services received or available. Cross-setting communication is of utmost importance when coordinating care

A Care Coordinator's Experience with the VA

I was working on a discharge for a veteran admitted to the hospital for care because the local VA was full. It was a weekend and the patient had been given several new prescriptions to be filled. The patient usually received medications through the VA by mail, but since it was a weekend, the VA pharmacy was closed. I called the local VA medical center and explained that the patient needed the medications filled that day and wanted to avoid paying for the medication at a non-VA pharmacy. I was transferred to the emergency room supervisor, who requested that I fax the prescriptions to them. They would partially fill them until the VA pharmacy opened and could arrange for them to be mailed to the patient. The patient could pick them up in a couple of hours. What a relief for the patient and myself. The VA has many services for veterans, but sometimes, you must advocate and explore to determine what services can be provided to meet your patient's needs.

for veterans, as the VA system and veteran care needs can be complex. The care coordinating nurse must ensure all parties involved in the veteran's care receive essential information, are aware of follow-up care plans, and know who to contact if concerns or questions arise. This will contribute to the continuity of care, increase access to resources and services the veteran is eligible for, decrease duplicative services and care, and facilitate care transitions.

Alzheimer's Disease and Related Dementias (ADRD) Population

Dementia is a term that encompasses many disease processes causing neurocognitive deficits that affect problem-solving abilities, language, and memory. It can result in personality or behavioral changes and affect all aspects of life. It generally is nonreversible, has no cure, and progresses over time. A person may experience dementia due to Alzheimer's disease, Parkinson's disease, a cerebrovascular disease, hippocampal sclerosis, or Lewy Body disease, to name a few. This is why many people refer to the grouping of the most common cause of dementia as **Alzheimer's Disease and Related Dementias or ADRD**. Alzheimer's disease is the most common cause of dementia, accounting for 60% to 80% of dementia diagnoses, while hippocampal sclerosis accounts for 3% to 13%, and vascular dementia for 5% to 10% (Alzheimer's Association, 2023, p. 7). An estimated 6.9 million Americans 65 years or older are living with dementia currently, and by 2060, this number is projected to rise to nearly 14 million (Alzheimer's Association, 2023, pp. 22, 33).

ADRD affects many aspects of a person's life and health, including missing follow-up appointments due to memory issues, experiencing challenges in self-managing health due to problem-solving deficits, and undergoing visual and spatial relationship changes that can contribute to accidents, falls, and impaired driving (Alzheimer's Association, 2023). Additionally, persons with dementia (PWD) eventually require caregivers, and many times these caregivers are family members who may have health issues of their own, experience caregiver strain and burnout, or have financial issues due to the unpaid caregiving needs (Alzheimer's

Association, 2023). Furthermore, as ADRD progresses, many PWD will experience changes in their personality or **distressed behaviors**, which may include aggression, agitation, inappropriate behaviors, or suspicion and may increase when the person is feeling confused or frustrated, or trying to make sense of a situation.

Distressed behaviors can be traumatizing for family members and caregivers, as well as the PWD. Distressed behaviors are estimated to occur in nearly 80% of people living with ADRD (Wolverson et al., 2023). When distressed behaviors occur, the caregiver may bring the PWD to the emergency room because they do not know how to manage the behaviors or they feel the PWD or themselves are in an unsafe situation. Alternatively, they may call the police to assist with the distressing behavioral situation, sometimes leading to the PWD's arrest or the police taking the PWD to the emergency room (Thompson, 2022). These solutions to distressing behaviors can often exacerbate the situation and behaviors, leading to difficulty addressing patient and caregiver needs.

Often the nurse care coordinator in the hospital setting is faced with navigating placement issues for PWD after their arrival in the emergency room. Family members and caregivers may approach the community nurse care coordinator concerning power of attorney issues, support for caregiving, management of distressing behaviors, or education regarding the disease process. These caregiver needs require nurses in all settings to have an overarching knowledge of ADRD, its signs, symptoms, and progression. Additionally, nurses need competency in facilitating care coordination with an interprofessional team, effective and adaptable communication skills, and the ability to recognize signs and symptoms of caregiver burnout or self-neglect and abuse or neglect of the PWD (Josephsen et al., 2023). As the ADRD population is growing and expected to continue to grow, this is no longer an optional area of competency for nurses; rather it is essential for meeting the rights of care coordination, ensuring the PWD receives the right care, in the right setting, at the right time, with the right transition, and with the right resources and education.

Care Coordination Considerations

Care coordinating nurses need to address several areas when working with PWD, but one of the most critical issues is caregiver support. It is not optimum for the caregiver to bring their loved one with ADRD to the emergency room because they feel overwhelmed or for the caregiver themselves to develop physical and mental health conditions due to burnout and the stress experienced through caregiving. Many caregivers experience caregiver burnout syndrome, which has been likened to PTSD, with signs and symptoms of anger, irritability, depression, substance use, and physical, mental, or emotional exhaustion (Alves et al., 2019; BETHESDA, 2020).

Good care coordination with caregiver support as a central component has been shown to reduce emergency room use and delay placement of those with ADRD into memory care or long-term care facilities, therefore supporting the least restrictive and lowest level of care environment and resource management, while promoting quality of life in PWD and their caregiver (Chen et al., 2020). The focus on caregivers for those with ADRD is receiving national recognition as an essential component of care coordination with the Centers for Medicare and Medicaid Services implementing a new demonstration project, the Guiding an Improved Dementia Experience Model (GUIDE), which focuses on maintaining quality of life, reducing caregiver strain, and supporting PWD to remain in their homes through comprehensive care coordination, education, and support services (CMS, 2023).

Supporting PWD in staying in their homes is an important outcome. When a PWD arrives in the emergency room with potential distressing behaviors and the caregiver refuses to take them home, this creates issues in reimbursement and placement and can be traumatizing for the PWD and their caregiver. Most often there is no medical reason for the PWD to be admitted as an inpatient or even outpatient in the hospital setting, yet the hospital cannot discharge the PWD if it is unsafe. Often, these patients are admitted until permanent placement can be found, and at times, this is not reimbursed due to admission requirements not being met.

If the PWD is exhibiting distressing behaviors, which are often exacerbated by being in the hospital setting, many facilities will not accept the patient until the behaviors are managed without the need for a sitter or other intensive intervention. Sometimes a PWD will be referred to a psychiatric hospital to manage the distressing behaviors and then return home or to another permanent placement. However, many psychiatric hospitals will not accept a PWD, as they may not also be equipped to address comorbid medical conditions, not have available beds for this population, or feel those with ADRD are more appropriate for a memory care placement rather than a psychiatric hospital placement (Wolverson et al., 2022). Yet often if the distressing behavior is significant, memory care facilities will not accept the patient either, as they may believe the risk of injury to other residents may be too high. This leaves the care coordinating nurse, the PWD, and their caregivers with little choice regarding placement and limited solutions to problems.

The care coordinating nurse can offer specific interventions to meet the PWD and caregiver needs and to proactively promote the ability of the PWD to stay in their own home with decreased chances of emergency room visits. The first is adaptable communication, which addresses nonverbal and verbal cues, includes discussion concerning disease progression and legal or ethical issues, and provides education and connection concerning support groups and ADRD resources. Engaging in discussions about goals and priorities of care is also essential in determining long-term care goals, providing appropriate referrals—such as to a palliative care or hospice team or other resources—and supporting PWD and their caregivers' safety and health (Jennings et al., 2020; Josephsen et al., 2023).

Lastly, the caregiver needs to be prepared to care for the PWD after the transition in care. Durable medical equipment (DME), medications, and follow-up appointments must be arranged, and the caregiver must be educated on the transition plan, needed follow-up items, which agency is accountable for what, and whom to contact if they have questions. See Figure 11.1 for an example caregiver healthcare transition checklist, which can be reviewed with and provided to the caregiver to ensure they have everything needed for a successful transition. Whether the care coordinating nurse is hospital or community-based, it is imperative that the primary care provider (PCP) is involved as part of the interprofessional team and is aware of the presenting issues so that they can offer ongoing support, resources, and referrals and become the first point of contact for urgent issues, preventing unnecessary use of the emergency room or police services (Jennings et al., 2020).

- Clear explanation of condition, diagnosis, and reason for transition
- Medications Reviewed
    - *Plan in place to pick up medications.*
    - *You understand how to take the medication.*
    - *You understand why it is being given.*
    - *You understand potential side effects or "red flags."*
    - *Interactions with current medications have been reviewed.*
- Barriers to the transition plan or other concerns have been addressed.
- Your needs and goals have been addressed in the transition plan.
- Resources needed have been arranged,
    - *Or you have been given contact information on obtaining the resources needed and are comfortable arranging them.*
- The transition plan has been given to you and your PCP in a documented format.
    - *You are clear on the timeline of the transition.*
    - *You know who will be involved,*
    - *You understand the next steps in the transition or care to be delivered.*
    - *The who, what, when, where, why, and how*
- You understand the next care setting or referral.
    - *What to expect from them,*
    - *If there is anything you need to do to prepare for the transition*
- Equipment is in place before the transition.
    - *Or there is a plan with a timeline for equipment delivery that works for you.*
- Questions are addressed to your satisfaction.
- Follow-up appointments are scheduled, or you are comfortable doing this.
    - *You know when they are and have a way to get to the follow-up appointment.*
    - *If tests are needed, you know when to get them, where, what they are for, and who to contact if you have a question.*
- You know what "red flags" or problems to be aware of and what to do if they occur.
- You know whom to contact if you have general questions, such as your PCP, care coordinator, or patient navigator.

FIGURE 11.1 Caregiver Healthcare Transition Checklist

Intellectual and Developmental Disabilities (IDDs) Population

Intellectual and developmental disabilities (IDDs) are usually present at birth and affect the person's physical, intellectual, or emotional development. IDDs can affect one area or system, or involve multiple physical, cognitive, and behavioral systems and affect functional problem-solving, social, and life skills (NIH, 2021). Examples of IDDs include Down syndrome, Tourette syndrome, autism spectrum disorder, cerebral palsy, and fetal alcohol spectrum disorder. More than 7 million people in the United States are affected by an IDD (RISP, n.d). This population is vulnerable to chronic health conditions like heart disease, diabetes, and dementia (IEC, 2024). This population also experiences a lack of healthcare access and health disparities, with many also not having a primary healthcare provider and not receiving preventative care, leading to poor health outcomes (IEC, 2024; Vi et al., 2023).

Some of these poor outcomes can be linked to a lack of training on the care needs of those with IDD. For example, people with IDD have reported providers only addressing their caregiver or support person, not addressing physical limitations to examinations or interventions related to their IDD, or experiencing **diagnostic overshadowing**, which is the attribution of physical symptoms or concerns to the existing IDD or other conditions rather than a possible health condition. An example of diagnostic overshadowing would be a nonverbal patient with IDD being treated with antianxiety medications for agitation rather than having a thorough assessment performed to determine whether an underlying physical condition may be causing the agitation (Mahoney, 2022). These system-level issues often contribute to a traumatizing healthcare experience for those with IDD. In fact, research has shown that people with IDD were 2.7 times as likely to receive unsafe care and experience harm compared to the general population with hospital admission (Friebel & Maynou, 2022).

Furthermore, those with IDD may not receive appropriate accommodations for communication, may not receive assistance in health system navigation, or may not have their concerns validated and addressed. Many are also dual-eligible, receiving both Medicare and Medicaid, seeing multiple providers, and receiving services from community and home-based services (IEC, 2024). These multiple players in their care can contribute to fragmentation of care and a need for robust care coordination.

Those with IDD have the right to education, information, and engagement in shared decision-making, as all patients do. However, those with IDD frequently will have family, caregivers, guardians, or medical power of attorneys involved in their healthcare decision-making. Engagement of the patient and the family or caregivers in healthcare decisions is essential for person-centered care and transparency, and nurses must ensure that any needed communication accommodations are provided so that the person with IDD and their identified decision-making supports can effectively engage in care planning and shared decision-making. The level of involvement of the person with IDD will vary depending on the decision type and their decision-making abilities. However, the nurse must adapt to the patient and their decision-making support needs and level of functioning. Assessing the patient's understanding of the information and education presented and the goals of care, allowing active participation in the decision-making process, and including the appropriate decision-making support person are essential (Sullivan et al., 2019).

Care Coordination Considerations

Those with IDD are vulnerable to the potential of traumatizing healthcare experiences and poor outcomes. Care coordinating nurses need to proactively and diligently address any potential fragmentation of care issues. The first step in achieving this is to do a strength-based comprehensive assessment of the patient, discovering their available supports and resources and gaps in care or needs (RIC, 2022). Furthermore, education and information must be provided at a literacy level appropriate for the patient, and adaptive communication tools must be used as needed (e.g., personal talkers, picture boards, sign language interpreters) so that the patient understands what interventions are planned and can proactively have their concerns and needs addressed. The care coordinating nurse must try to include the patient in decision-making processes even if the patient has a healthcare power of attorney or guardian who is the decision-maker, unless the patient indicates explicitly that they do not want to be part of the decision-making process or is completely unable to participate due to a severe lack of decision-making capacity (e.g., profound intellectual disability).

Tips for Effective Healthcare for Those with IDD

1. Create and build a relationship with the patient.
2. Address communication barriers.
3. Elicit as much information as possible about strengths, needs, and resources for care plan development.
4. Do not only address caregivers, family members, or other support people with the patient.
5. Speak to the patient, paying attention to any verbal or nonverbal language. Use simple questions and offer clear information about what you will be doing or what will happen.
6. Make sure the patient feels safe and provide reassurance as needed.
7. Rule out physical conditions that may manifest as behavioral changes.
8. Be flexible and adaptable, modifying interventions to meet the patient's limitations.

(Hostetter & Klein, 2018)

Research has shown that nurses may hold negative implicit biases toward those with IDD based on misconceptions about IDD, lack of training or understanding on how to adapt to physical, cognitive, or communication limitations of those with IDD, or general discomfort in working for the IDD population (Derbyshire & Keay, 2024). A common misunderstanding revolves around behaviors that may be used as a method of communication to express pain, environmental discomfort, or some other underlying physical or environmental issue, leading the nurse to ignore critical signs and symptoms of a healthcare issue and the patient not having their needs met. The care coordination nurse must understand this propensity toward implicit bias and provide any needed education on this to other nurses or healthcare workers to ensure that health conditions are appropriately addressed (RIC, 2022). Most importantly, the nurse must collaborate and communicate with the interprofessional team, advocating for person-centered and quality care (IEC, 2024). As written by the CDC, "Disability and functioning are outcomes of interactions between health conditions and the environment" (CDC, 2019, slide 21). This means nurses can positively impact the experiences that those with IDD have in the healthcare environment and promote functioning and interaction with the whole person, not approaching care with biases, viewing the disability as a sickness, or focusing solely on the disability.

The Unhoused Population

The terms **unhoused**, or **houselessness** are being used more frequently to describe people without a permanent physical structure to live in, as these are associated with less stigma, support person-first language, and do not negate or diminish the fact that the person may have strong connections to their community (NIH, 2024). **Person-first** language is vital in delivery care coordination practice as it supports holistic care and focuses on the whole person rather than their disease, disability, or condition, as these are part of the person's lived experience but are not the totality of their personhood. Nevertheless, many agencies still use the terms "homeless" or "homelessness," which is defined as persons who do not have a "fixed, regular, and adequate nighttime residence" and includes categories of homelessness such as trading sex for housing, staying with friends but not being able to stay longer than 14 days, being human trafficked, or leaving home because of physical, emotional, or financial abuse or threats of abuse without safe alternative housing (HUD Exchange, 2019, para. 2).

The U.S. Department of Housing and Urban Development (2022) reported 582,500 unhoused people, with only 60% of this population being in sheltered locations, leaving 40% unsheltered. The highest rates of being unsheltered occurred among gender questioning, American Indian, Alaska Native or Indigenous populations, and Native Hawaiians or other Pacific Islander populations (National Alliance to End Homelessness, 2023, "Who is Unsheltered in 2022"). Additionally, one-third of the population experienced being unhoused with children present (HUD, 2022, p. 2).

Being unhoused has been associated with poor health outcomes and higher rates of chronic disease, as well as oral and dental health issues. Houselessness is also associated with comorbidities of SUD and mental health problems, leading to **tri-morbidity**, where the unhoused individual's physical health is affected by the SUD and mental health issues being experienced and all three are present (Canham et al., 2019). A large portion of the unhoused do not have a PCP and do not receive healthcare consistently, which further exacerbates health issues and causes the main point of healthcare delivery to often be the emergency room for this population (Canham et al., 2019).

Houselessness is a significant SDOH. It is linked with traumatic experiences, with more than 80% of the unhoused reporting a life-altering traumatic experience at some point in their lives (Williams, 2022, para. 1). The stress of being unhoused can also contribute to health issues, such as high blood pressure or diabetes, and contribute to or exacerbate SUD and mental health conditions, such as depression (Bensken et al., 2021). Being unhoused is also associated with decreased treatment completion rates and increased patient-initiated treatment discontinuation, which can worsen health outcomes (Gazzola et al., 2023). Suicidality and houselessness have also been shown to have a strong correlation, with suicidality among those experiencing houselessness estimated to be nine times the rate of the general U.S. population (Bommersbach et al., 2020; Holleran & Poon, 2018). Moreover, even if those who are experiencing houselessness try to access healthcare, many barriers lead to health vulnerability and poor outcomes. These include lack of transportation, lack of childcare, and the inability to receive health education and information due to the lack of a consistent mailing address or phone number (Lee et al., 2023).

It is apparent that the unhoused population has risk factors and needs that the care coordinating nurse must be aware of and implement into their care and transition planning. For example, many people who are unhoused lack health insurance or the ability to pay for medications or follow-up care. This may require the care coordinating nurse to assist the patient in navigating the application process for Medicaid or Medicare funding or accessing local charity or prescription medication funding programs. Treatment plans that include bed rest or follow-up care by home health therapies or nursing must be thoughtfully and interprofessionally approached. Many shelters cannot house patients during the day. If a patient needs bed rest during the day, this must be coordinated with the shelter the patient most often utilizes, assuming they have access to a shelter.

Moreover, shelters often have policies for patients prescribed certain medications, and the patient will need to agree to follow the shelter rules regarding the use, storage, and administration of prescribed medications. If home health services are ordered, the care coordinating nurse must work with the home health agency to ensure they provide care in a shelter setting. Lastly, many shelter systems support the people they serve through their lifespan and health needs, especially those chronically experiencing houselessness.

At times, health conditions will progress to the level that it is unsafe for the person to remain in the shelter, such as with end-of-life care. If this is a potential, the care coordinating nurse will need to proactively work to ensure the patient has applied for all possible health insurance and funding programs so that they will have financial support for placement and care when this time arrives, as well as engaging in goals of care discussions with the patient.

Care Coordination Considerations

One of the most important considerations when coordinating care for those who are unhoused is the trauma and stigma they often experience from their situation. This can often lead people experiencing houselessness to feel a lack of trust in the health system and may cause the patient to fail to disclose pertinent health information. Many situations may contribute to healthcare worker bias toward the unhoused population, one being perceived frequent emergency room visits by those experiencing houselessness to keep warm, access shelter, or obtain food. Unhoused patients may also have difficulty following up with treatment and care planning, which can be frustrating for the nurse or other healthcare worker. However, this requires the care coordinating nurse to understand the lived experience of the unhoused, to engage in collaborative problem-solving, and to work toward proactively addressing continuity of care and the need for shelter or follow-up care (Canham et al., 2019). This may mean the nurse participates in organizational, local, statewide, or national initiatives to address issues that the unhoused experience. The foundation of care coordination practice for the unhoused population must include principles of respect for patient autonomy and practicing "compassion and respect for the inherent dignity, worth, and unique attributes of every person" (ANA, 2015, p. v) with a focus on developing trust and promoting health and TIC.

This requires the nurse to do a comprehensive assessment related to housing needs with every patient to create quality care transition plans. It has been reported that the housing situation is not always assessed, and when houselessness is determined to be an issue, long-term planning concerning housing is often not addressed (Canham et al., 2019). This may not be a one-time assessment, occurring just at admission or intake. If patients are admitted to the hospital or rehabilitation for a more extended period, their housing situation may change. For example, if a patient was admitted following a motor vehicle accident and at admission reported they lived in an apartment with two roommates, but then they had to be hospitalized for two weeks and go to rehabilitation for two more weeks, they may find that they do not have an apartment to return to. The roommates may have had to find another roommate to pay the rent, and not knowing exactly when the patient would return, allowed someone else to rent the patient's room. Alternatively, the patient may have been unable to pay their rent and, when discharged, finds that eviction proceedings have begun, putting them at risk of being unhoused.

Communication and coordination with community agencies and service providers for the unhoused person are also essential. Many unhoused have health and social care needs, which must be addressed simultaneously for good outcomes (Franco et al., 2021). Furthermore, if there is an expectation that a shelter or some other community resource will provide ongoing support or follow-up, the care coordinating nurse must understand any limitations or requirements for these resources. For example, many shelters do not open for housing until specific times of the day, and if the plan is for the patient to go directly to the shelter, this needs to be coordinated with the shelter, or the timing of discharge needs to coincide with shelter availability. Ensuring continuity between required community-based services will also require the care coordinating nurse to facilitate the transfer of pertinent information between the services and health system while meeting HIPAA regulations and organizational policies.

Finally, when coordinating care for those who are unhoused, individualized and person-centered care plans including interprofessional collaboration and expertise are required. Identifying a central go-to person for the unhoused patient to contact with ongoing questions and concerns is also essential, as this person will need to act as a facilitator and liaison across services and settings. This assists with cross-setting communication, promoting healthcare accessibility and essential information sharing so all care providers involved can support positive outcomes. Information and education on self-management of health and follow-ups will need to be provided to the unhoused patient, utilizing teach-back to ensure that the patient understands the plan of care and supporting the empowerment of the patient to become active and engaged in their care and health (Franco et al., 2021). Those who are unhoused tend to have

Medical Respite

Sometimes those who are unhoused have chronic illnesses or conditions that require hospitalization. However, at other times, they are not sick enough to require acute care but not well enough to be discharged to an unhoused situation. Often a shelter setting also cannot provide the support needed for successful recovery. This is where medical respite programs can meet health needs. Medical respite is not available in all communities or states. However, when available, it offers short-term residential care for those who are unhoused to recover and access follow-up care; it addresses the care gap that many of the unhoused experience. These programs follow Standards for Medical Respite Care and operate in various settings, such as shelters, hotel rooms, apartments, or long-term care facilities. Medical respite programs generally provide 24-hour access to a bed, wellness checks by medical staff, appointment transportation services, meals, phone access, or access to other types of communication needed to receive healthcare and care coordination services. Medical respite programs decrease emergency room visits and readmissions, improve outcomes and health, and provide hospital cost savings (Smith, 2023).

multiple and interacting needs, and the care coordinating nurse must recognize this and work in a trusting and respectful relationship with the patient to meet identified needs and goals of care and access resources successfully.

CHAPTER SUMMARY

Several populations of patients experience more significant challenges and barriers to effective and efficient care coordination due to health system-level issues and population characteristics and needs. Care coordinating nurses must be aware of potential additional barriers to continuity of care and work to gain the knowledge, skills, and attitudes needed to facilitate successful care transitions and promote better health outcomes for these populations. Some of these patient populations include veterans, PWD, those with IDD, and the unhoused.

Each of these populations and the general population benefits from implementing TIC into care coordination practice. The principles of TIC complement the guiding principles and rights of care coordination practice and assist in addressing the impact of trauma experiences as an SDOH. Integration of TIC also contributes to building safety, trust, and respect in populations who may have had negative healthcare experiences. Nurses must recognize the signs and symptoms of trauma, apply TIC universally, avoid retraumatizing patients through implicit bias or lack of knowledge, and advocate for health systems that meet holistic patient needs.

Veterans are a large population with significant exposure to trauma and environmental and chemical hazards, with many subpopulations that need additional specialized care coordination interventions, such as women, Black, and Hispanic veterans. The VA system has developed many programs to meet veterans' needs, and the care coordinating nurse must be knowledgeable about VA programs in their area and how veterans can access these resources and supports. This requires the nurse to have an orientation to the VA system structure—where to go for assistance and information—and to ensure that cross-setting communication is effective and essential patient information is transmitted to and received by the VA system for timely and accessible monitoring and follow-up needs.

The ADRD population is growing and is expected to continue to increase. ADRD, as a neurocognitive disorder, affects all aspects of a patient's life and functioning, eventually requiring the involvement of caregivers. PWD often will develop distressing behaviors as part of their disease progression, at times leaving caregivers overwhelmed or unable to navigate the management of the distressing behaviors. This can be a traumatic experience for both the PWD and their caregiver. ADRD caregivers are susceptible to caregiver burnout syndrome, which can manifest in physical, mental, and behavioral health concerns. Due to the combination of ADRD progression, distressing behaviors, and caregiver burnout syndrome, caregivers are sometimes unable to care for the PWD any longer, leading to issues with finding permanent placement. Care coordinating nurses must be cognizant of the potential and proactively address caregiver support needs, integrate adaptable communication, and facilitate interprofessional collaboration and care planning to meet the holistic needs of the PWD and their caregivers and support the PWD goals and priorities of care, including staying in their own home as long as possible, if desired and appropriate.

Those with IDD have also historically experienced health disparities and lack of accessibility, often based on nurses' and other healthcare workers' implicit biases and lack of knowledge concerning IDD. This has contributed to the IDD population experiencing harm and traumatic experiences in the health system, where their physical, cognitive, or communication needs are not met. Furthermore, many times multiple providers and support persons are involved in the care of those with IDD, which can contribute to the fragmentation of care. Nurses must be diligent in addressing any implicit biases they have or see in practice, actively engaging those with IDD in their healthcare decision-making, and approaching care coordination with a strength-based and whole-person perspective rather than focusing on disabilities.

Lastly, the unhoused population has experienced stigma and poor health outcomes, such as higher rates of suicide, SUD, and chronic disease. Those experiencing houselessness cannot always access shelter programs, and even if available, the shelter may be unable to accommodate their healthcare needs. The lack of consistent healthcare, barriers to accessing healthcare (e.g., transportation, finances), and the high frequency of trauma experienced by the unhoused make it a significant SDOH. Nurses must implement TIC while coordinating care for those who are unhoused, performing a complete assessment of the housing situation and revisiting this issue if needed. Furthermore, nurses must implement cross-service communication and coordinate care while integrating community resources and services needed for positive health outcomes.

The care coordinating nurse may interact with and support many special populations in care transitions. The nurse must approach each with TIC and the guiding principles and rights of care coordination as a foundation. They work with each patient to provide coordinated and continuity of care in a safe, respectful, and trustworthy manner and offer TIC and person-centered care that respects patient autonomy and models valuing each person as unique and worthy in every interaction. If these skills and attitudes were consistently implemented in care coordination practice, patient satisfaction could be increased, nurse satisfaction could be increased, better outcomes could be achieved, costs and resources could be well managed, and health equity and accessibility would be promoted.

CHAPTER 11 GLOSSARY

Alzheimer's Disease and Related Dementias (ADRD): A grouping of neurocognitive disorders that refers to the most common causes of dementia, including Alzheimer's, Lewy Body disease, hippocampal sclerosis, and vascular dementia.

Dementia: A term used to describe a group of neurocognitive symptoms that include deficits in problem-solving, language, and memory, can result in personality or behavioral changes, affects all aspects of life, generally is nonreversible, with no cure, and progresses over time.

Diagnostic Overshadowing: Attributing physical symptoms or concerns to the existing IDD or other conditions rather than a possible health condition.

Distressed Behaviors: Personality or behavioral changes that occur in those with dementia and can include aggression, agitation, inappropriate behaviors, or suspicion, often increasing when the person is feeling confused, frustrated, or trying to make sense of a situation.

Dual-users: Veterans that receive healthcare and other services from both VA and community providers, hospitals, and facilities.

Intellectual and developmental disabilities (IDDs): A condition usually present at birth that affects a person's physical, intellectual, or emotional development, can involve one or more systems (e.g., physical, cognitive, and behavioral), and affects functional, social, and life skills.

Person-First Language: Language that focuses on the whole person, viewing the disease, disability, or circumstances as only part of the person and their lived experience, but not the totality of their personhood.

Re-Traumatize: Exposing someone to a situation, interaction, environment, or event, causing them to reexperience trauma symptoms, reactions, or experiences.

Trauma-Informed Care (TIC): Healthcare delivery based on awareness of the need to understand a person's lived experience to provide effective care and the effect of trauma on health, wellness, and other aspects of life.

Tri-Morbidity: Physical health affected by both substance use disorder and mental health issues where all three types of health issues are present in an individual.

Unhoused or Houselessness: A circumstance in which a person is without a permanent physical structure to live in.

Veteran: Someone who has served in the active military, naval, or air service and was honorably discharged, a reservist or member of the National Guard called to active duty, or a person disabled from a disease or injury incurred in the line of duty or training.

DISCUSSION QUESTIONS AND ACTIVITIES

Discussion Questions

1. Consider the concept of trauma-informed care (TIC), and discuss in what ways TIC can be implemented in care coordination practice.
2. Identify one ethical issue concerning care coordination practice with special populations. Discuss how this issue may be addressed or provide a solution to this issue.
3. Consider the health system and system-level barriers to effective care coordination for special populations. Discuss what multilevel factors may support the continuation of these system-level barriers.
4. Discuss how social determinants of health (SDOH), such as trauma or houselessness, can influence care coordination efforts and outcomes.
5. Discuss what could happen to a patient because of implicit bias in nursing care. How might you approach a nurse exhibiting implicit bias toward a special population?

Activities

1. Support Group Observation:

- Choose a support group in your local area related to ADRD or Parkinson's disease. You can go to this link to discover an Alzheimer's support group in your area https://www.alz.org/local_resources/find_your_local_chapter. Or this link for Parkinson's disease https://www.apdaparkinson.org/community/. You may also be able to find a local group through a community hospital, senior center, or other resources.
- Once you find a support group, contact the group leader to obtain permission to attend the meeting, observe the group session. Schedule the date and time so that it is prearranged and they expect you.
  - Only attend the date/time you have prearranged with the group leader or representative.
  - Be on time and plan to stay the entire meeting time so that you are not disrupting the group.
  - Explain why you are there, and give your name if requested by the facilitator or others in the group. Some groups may be anonymous.
  - Share questions and comments with the group facilitator after the group ends.
  - Give participants priority to seating.
  - Maintain absolute confidentiality concerning anything personal or private discussed in the group.
  - Refrain from taking notes during the meeting, which may be uncomfortable for the participants. If you feel you must take notes, ask permission from the group.
- After the observation, address the following in a reflective assignment:
  - Describe the event.
  - Describe how you felt during the experience.
  - Describe what you learned through the experience.
  - Then choose one of the questions below to discuss.
    - In what ways did you see that the support group might assist caregivers or family members in feeling less isolated or distressed?
    - Were coping skills, empowerment, or motivation to self-manage health addressed? If so, how and in what ways?

  - What information about managing the condition, treatment plans, or disease progression was shared?

2. Group Activity

   - In groups, select a vulnerable population (e.g., those with substance use disorder, mental illness, correctional issues, transplants, chronic pain, etc.) and investigate what types of unique needs the population may have, what types of health system-level barriers they may experience, and what considerations the care coordinating nurse needs to take into account to ensure continuity of care.
   - Create a short (5 to 10-minute) presentation to teach your class or colleagues about your selected vulnerable population. Include the following in your presentation:
     - Unique care coordination needs
     - Health system-level barriers
     - Care coordination considerations
   - Provide to your classmates or colleagues a list of local resources that serve your selected vulnerable population.

3. Case Study:

   The nurse care coordinator, working at the local children's hospital, meets with a new family member in their home to determine needs, strengths, and resources and how best to provide coordinated care. The family emigrated several years ago from Costa Rica. They live with extended family in a small 3-bedroom home, and their last child was born with significant disabilities due to a genetic condition. The child is a 3-year-old male named Gael. He is nonverbal, nonambulatory, and has a feeding tube in place. Upon arrival, the nurse care coordinator finds the mother holding her son on the living room floor. His adult sister is just leaving for work. After the sister leaves, the nurse care coordinator begins the assessment process and finds that Gael's mother has limited English ability and cannot read English. As the assessment goes on, the care coordinating nurse finds Gael's vocalizations distracting to the assessment process.

   Gael's mother explains that they take shifts caring for Gael as he needs care 24 hours a day, seven days a week, and is frequently ill with pneumonia or bronchitis. The whole family is involved in caregiving. Gael's mother also informs the nurse that she had a conversation with Gael's specialist, who suggested that when Gael next contracted pneumonia, the family should consider not treating it with medicine and provide "comfortable" care. She asks the nurse care coordinator what "comfortable" care is. The nurse explains comfort care as care focused on managing symptoms and pain, not curing the pneumonia, while letting it run its course. The mother appears upset by this information and asks the nurse if this is OK to do and what the nurse thinks she should do. The care coordinating nurse thinks that Gael has a limited quality of life and will not improve. He provides his mother and family with many caregiving needs, and she considers that maybe the specialist is right. Consider the following questions:

- What is the nurse's responsibility in seeing that ethical healthcare is being delivered? Should self-care ability and views of quality of life be considered in healthcare treatment decisions? If so, in what ways? If not, why not?
- Should Gael's mother be encouraged to follow the advice of the specialist and not pursue continued treatment for any bouts of pneumonia Gael experiences? Why or why not?
- What responsibilities does the nurse care coordinator have in ensuring Gael's mother and family members can participate in shared decision-making concerning goals of care?
- Are there any areas of implicit bias present in this case study? If so, what are they?

NCLEX STYLE QUESTIONS

1. How can the nurse care coordinator demonstrate knowledge, skills, and attitudes that value the unique needs of special populations?

    a. Create a standardized care plan addressing system-level issues.

    b. Use family members or close friends as interpreters for those who speak English as a second language.

    c. Identify and inform the patient or caregiver of ways they will need to change their lifestyle to meet evidence-based practice guidelines for disease management.

    d. Assess and evaluate the patient within the context of their lived experience.

2. The nurse care coordinator can best implement trauma-informed care practices by doing which of the following?

    a. Expose the patient to situations that cause them to reexperience reactions or symptoms of trauma.

    b. Provide care that promotes safety, trust, and respect for all patients.

    c. Acknowledge that trauma is usually a one-time occurrence and can have physical effects.

    d. Assess the patient for their individual trauma experience and how they feel about the experience.

3. Trauma-informed care principles include which of the following?

   a. Safety, Peer Support, Collegiality

   b. Peer Support, Empowerment, Cultural Ideology

   c. Collaboration, Safety, Trustworthiness

   d. Empowerment, Transparency, Group Support

4. A veteran as a dual-user refers to which of the following?

   a. The veteran uses both drugs and alcohol.

   b. The veteran uses both naturopathic and traditional medicine.

   c. The veteran uses both mental health and medical care services.

   d. The veteran uses both community and veterans affairs services.

   Questions 5–6 relate to the following scenario:

   George, a 43-year-old naval veteran, has been admitted to the hospital for hip replacement surgery. George has a history of sleep apnea, post-traumatic stress disorder, and idiopathic ventricular arrhythmia. You are George's care coordinating nurse. The provider has just informed you that George is expected to be discharged to rehabilitation in 2 days. George has health insurance coverage through the Veterans Affairs (VA) and typically receives care at the nearest VA center, approximately 35 miles away.

5. As you plan George's rehabilitation discharge, what care coordination interventions will you need to perform? (Select all that apply.)

   a. Contact the PACT responsible for George's care at the VA and let them know they must arrange rehabilitation.

   b. Determine what services George receives at the VA and ensure the transfer of information concerning what follow-up care will be needed.

   c. Create a discharge packet that George can take to the rehabilitation center with any follow-up needs, and instruct George to go over this with his PACT provider.

   d. Contact the VA to ensure they provide the rehabilitation services needed and that they can accept George.

6. When you call to coordinate follow-up appointments with VA services, you find that George will have to be wait-listed for an appointment with a specialist orthopedic provider at the VA. The VA suggests that a referral be sent to a community orthopedic

provider for continued follow-up since George's follow-up cannot be delayed. You know the ability to do this is due to which of the following acts?

a. The VETERAN Act

b. The COMMUNITY CARE Act

c. The MISSION Act

d. The PACT Act

Questions 7 and 8 relate to the following scenario:

Emma is a 78-year-old female who has been diagnosed with vascular dementia. Her husband, Phil, who is 83 and her primary caregiver, has brought Emma to your clinic after Emma became more agitated, accusing Phil of stealing her jewelry and swearing and yelling at him. Phil is concerned as this is unusual for Emma, and he wants the doctor to make sure she is not sick with something.

7. As you enter the room, you notice Phil is haggard-looking and disheveled, and he has lost weight since you last saw him. As you talk with Phil, he tells you he is exhausted, can barely get out of bed anymore, and feels angry about his life circumstances. You recognize these signs of caregiver burnout syndrome. What interventions should you, as the care coordinating nurse, offer Phil? (Select all that apply.)

    a. Discuss with Phil how vascular dementia may progress.

    b. Connect Phil with support groups and other resources in the community.

    c. Determine Phil and Emma's goals and priorities of care.

    d. All of the above.

8. Phil tells you about Emma's changes in personality and behavior. He is concerned she may have something else wrong with her and says that when she gets very angry and suspicious, he feels he cannot manage her and thinks she may try to hurt him. What symptom of dementia is Emma exhibiting?

    a. Dysfunctional behaviors

    b. Distressed behaviors

    c. Dementia behaviors

    d. Decomposition behaviors

9. You are precepting a new nurse and explaining to them how implicit bias can affect the nursing care of those with intellectual and developmental disabilities (IDD). You know the new nurse understands the negative impact of implicit bias on health outcomes of those with IDD when they say which of the following. (Select all that apply.)

    a. It is important to have the caregiver or support person in the room and primarily address them when speaking, as they will be making healthcare decisions.

    b. Sometimes, when a person with IDD is vocalizing loudly or seems agitated, it is due to the disability. Since they cannot control the behavior, it is best to ignore it and go about my nursing care quickly.

    c. As part of my assessment, I should determine how the person with IDD communicates best and address any barriers to communication.

    d. Since those with IDD may have some physical or cognitive limitations, I should be adaptable and modify how I deliver nursing care if needed.

10. Which of the following supports the use of person-first language in care coordination practice?

    a. Comprehensive assessment of the disease process

    b. Viewing the person holistically, including their lived experience

    c. Focusing on specific aspects of the person's identity

    d. Considering other support people in the person's circle

11. The foundation of care coordination practice when working with the unhoused population includes which of the following?

    a. Understanding that those who are unhoused have mental health issues, and this needs to be addressed.

    b. Directing those who are unhoused to go to urgent care clinics instead of the emergency room to manage resources.

    c. Developing a trusting relationship and providing trauma-informed care.

    d. Conducting a one-time comprehensive assessment concerning housing needs.

12. Medical respite programs are designed to meet the needs of which of the following populations?

    a. Caregivers who are experiencing caregiver burnout syndrome

    b. Unhoused individuals who have illnesses or conditions that need short-term residential care

    c. Pregnant veterans who have tri-morbidity and need continuous monitoring and care coordination

    d. Those with ADRD who do not meet admission criteria but need placement

13. A primary care clinic has not met the quality measure of pneumococcal vaccination, including those over age 65 and those 19 to 65 who are at increased risk for pneumococcal disease. Through the process of risk stratification, the care coordinating nurse has found that most of their patient population with IDD has not been offered the pneumococcal vaccine. The nurse is creating a handout to give to all the nurses in the clinic that outlines how to offer shared decision-making concerning the pneumococcal vaccine to the IDD patient population in order to increase quality measure attainment and health outcomes. Which of the following should be included in the shared decision-making handout?

    a. Instruct the nurse to assess for and provide communication accommodations.

    b. Instruct the nurse to include the family, caregiver, or healthcare decision-maker if appropriate.

    c. Instruct the nurse to elicit active participation of the patient with IDD in the decision-making process.

    d. All of the above.

14. The nurse care coordinator is reviewing a transition checklist with the caregiver of a person with dementia. The nurse knows the caregiver understands the essential aspects of a care transition when they say which of the following. (Select all that apply.)

    a. I should know the red flags or potential side effects of new medications prescribed.

    b. I should expect the provider's office to track lab needs.

    c. I should wait for the physical therapist's office to contact me to schedule an appointment.

    d. I should understand the plan and time line for equipment delivery

15. The mother of a 10-year-old boy diagnosed with Tourette syndrome contacts the pediatric clinic nurse care coordinator to discuss concerns she has about recent increases in head jerking movements and shoulder shrugging. She is wondering if her son may need additional medication or some alternate treatment. Which of the following is the best response by the nurse care coordinator?

    a. I will discuss your concerns with the interprofessional team and get back to you today about their recommendations.

    b. The provider is out on vacation until next week. I will make a note so they can call you when they return.

    c. I have heard that talk therapy sometimes works for those with Tourette syndrome. I will make an appointment with a new talk therapist specializing in Tourette syndrome for you.

    d. I can see how this might be concerning, but head jerking and shoulder shrugging are common in those with Tourette syndrome. Keep track of how often and how long this occurs for a few weeks and call back if it seems to increase.

REFERENCES

Alves, L. C. S., Monteiro, D. Q., Bento, S. R., Hayashi, V. D., Pelegrini, L. N. C., & Vale, F. A. C. (2019). Burnout syndrome in informal caregivers of older adults with dementia: A systematic review. *Dementia & Neuropsychologia, 13*(4), 415–421. https://doi.org/10.1590/1980-57642018dn13-040008

Alzheimer's Association. (2023). *2023 Alzheimer's disease facts and figures.* https://www.alz.org/media/Documents/alzheimers-facts-and-figures.pdf

American Nurses Association (ANA). (2015). *Code of ethics for nurses with interpretive statements.* ANA.

Apaydin, E. A., Rose, D. E., McClean, M. R., Yano, E. M., Shekelle, P. G., Nelson, K. M., & Stockdale, S. E. (2021). Association between care coordination tasks with non-VA community care and VA PCP burnout: An analysis of a national, cross-sectional survey. *BMC Health Services Research, 21*(1), 809. https://doi.org/10.1186/s12913-021-06769-7

Bensken, W. P., Krieger, N. I., Berg, K. A., Einstadter, D., Dalton, J. E., & Perzynski, A. T. (2021). Health status and chronic disease burden of the homeless population: An analysis of two decades of multi-institutional electronic medical records. *Journal of Health Care for the Poor and Underserved, 32*(3), 1619–1634. https://doi.org/10.1353/hpu.2021.0153

BETHESDA. (2020). *Caregiver Stress Syndrome: You're not alone.* https://bethesdahealth.org/blog/2020/03/19/caregiver-stress-syndrome-youre-not-alone/

Bommersbach, T. J., Stefanovics, E. A., Rhee, T. G., Tsai, J., & Rosenheck, R. A. (2020). Suicide attempts and homelessness: Timing of attempts among recently homeless, past homeless, and never homeless adults. *Psychiatric Services (Washington, D.C.), 71*(12), 1225–1231. https://doi.org/10.1176/appi.ps.202000073

Canham, S. L., Davidson, S., Custodio, K., Mauboules, C., Good, C., Wister, A. V., & Bosma, H. (2019). Health supports needed for homeless persons transitioning from hospitals. *Health & Social Care in the Community, 27*(3), 531–545. https://doi.org/10.1111/hsc.12599

Centers for Disease Control and Prevention (CDC). (2019). *CDC public health grand rounds: Addressing gaps in health care for individuals with intellectual disabilities* [Slides]. https://www.cdc.gov/grand-rounds/pp/2019/20191015-intellectual-disabilities-H.pdf

Centers for Medicare and Medicaid Services (CMS). (2023). *Guiding an Improved Dementia Experience (GUIDE) Model*. https://www.cms.gov/priorities/innovation/innovation-models/guide

Chang, E. T., Newberry, S., Rubenstein, L. V., Motala, A., Booth, M. J., & Shekelle, P. G. (2022). Quality measures for patients at risk of adverse outcomes in the Veterans Health Administration: Expert panel recommendations. *JAMA Network Open, 5*(8), e2224938. https://doi.org/10.1001/jamanetworkopen.2022.24938

Chen, B., Cheng, X., Streetman-Loy, B., Hudson, M. F., Jindal, D., & Hair, N. (2020). Effect of care coordination on patients with Alzheimer disease and their caregivers. *The American Journal of Managed Care, 26*(11), e369–e375. https://doi.org/10.37765/ajmc.2020.88532

Cordasco, K. M., Hynes, D. M., Mattocks, K. M., Bastian, L. A., Bosworth, H. B., & Atkins, D. (2019). Improving care coordination for veterans within VA and across healthcare systems. *Journal of General Internal Medicine, 34*(Suppl 1), 1–3. https://doi.org/10.1007/s11606-019-04999-4

Cordasco, K. M., Katzburg, J. R., Katon, J. G., Zephyrin, L. C., Chrystal, J. G., & Yano, E. M. (2018). Care coordination for pregnant veterans: VA's Maternity Care Coordinator Telephone Care Program. *Translational Behavioral Medicine, 8*(3), 419–428. https://doi.org/10.1093/tbm/ibx081

Davidson, B. (2021). *Coordination of care is trauma-informed care*. Comprehensive Healthcare. https://comphc.org/coordination-of-care-is-trauma-informed-care/

Derbyshire, D. W., & Keay, T. (2024). "But what do you really think?" Nurses' contrasting explicit and implicit attitudes towards people with disabilities using the implicit association test. *Journal of Clinical Nursing*, 00, 1–12. https://doi.org/10.1111/jocn.17097

Dunkin, M.A. (2022). *Community care coordination puts strain on VA staff, finances*. U.S. Medicine: The Voice of Federal Medicine. https://www.usmedicine.com/agencies/military-health-system/community-care-coordination-puts-strain-on-va-staff-finances/

Fleishman, J., Kamsky, H., & Sundborg, S. (2019). Trauma-informed nursing practice. *OJIN: The Online Journal of Issues in Nursing, 24*(2). https://doi.org/10.3912/OJIN.Vol24No02Man03

Franco, A., Meldrum, J., & Ngaruiya, C. (2021). Identifying homeless population needs in the emergency department using community-based participatory research. *BMC Health Services Research,* **21**(428). https://doi.org/10.1186/s12913-021-06426-z

Friebel, R., & Maynou, L. (2022). Assessing the dangers of a hospital stay for patients with developmental disabilities in England, 2017–19. *Health Affairs, 41*(10), 1486–1495. https://doi.org/10.1377/hlthaff.2022.00493

Garvin, L. A., Pugatch, M., Gurewich, D., Pendergast, J. N., & Miller, C. J. (2021). Interorganizational care coordination of rural veterans by Veterans Affairs and community care programs: A systematic review. *Medical Care, 59*(Suppl 3), S259–S269. https://doi.org/10.1097/MLR.0000000000001542

Gazzola, M. G., Carmichael, I. D., Christian, N. J., Zheng, X., Madden, L. M., & Barry, D. T. (2023). A national study of homelessness, social determinants of health, and treatment engagement among outpatient medication for opioid use disorder-seeking individuals in the United States. *Substance Abuse, 44*(1–2), 62–72. https://doi.org/10.1177/08897077231167291

Greenstone, C. L., Peppiatt, J., Cunningham, K., Hosenfeld, C., Lucatorto, M., Rubin, M., & Weede, A. (2019). Standardizing care coordination within the Department of Veterans Affairs. *Journal of General Internal Medicine, 34*(Suppl 1), 4–6. https://doi.org/10.1007/s11606-019-04997-6

Gurewich, D., Shwartz, M., Beilstein-Wedel, E., Davila, H., & Rosen, A. K. (2021). Did access to care improve since passage of the Veterans Choice Act?: Differences between rural and urban veterans. *Medical care, 59*(Suppl 3), S270–S278. https://doi.org/10.1097/MLR.0000000000001490

Holleran, L., & Poon, G. (2018). Dying in the shadows: Suicide among the homeless. *Harvard Public Health Review, 20*, 1–5. https://www.jstor.org/stable/48515221

Hostetter, M., & Klein, S. (2018). *Creating better systems of care for adults with disabilities: Lessons for policy and practice*. The Commonwealth Fund. https://www.commonwealthfund.org/sites/default/files/2018-09/Hostetter_better_care_adults_disabilities_cs_0.pdf

HUD Exchange. (2019). *HUD's Definition of homelessness: Resources and guidance*. https://www.hudexchange.info/news/huds-definition-of-homelessness-resources-and-guidance/

Institute for Exceptional Care (IEC). (2024). *A national roadmap for disability inclusive healthcare*. https://cdn.userway.org/auto-remediations/pdf/3836916/original/IEC_Full-National-Roadmap-for-Disability-Inclusive-Healthcare_31024.pdf

Izquierdo, A., Ong, M., Jones, F., Jones, L., Ganz, D., & Rubenstein, L. (2018). Engaging African American veterans with health care access challenges in community partnered care coordination initiative: A qualitative needs assessment. *Ethnicity & Disease, 28*(2). 475–484. https://www.researchgate.net/publication/327491433_Engaging_African_American_Veterans_with_Health_Care_Access_Challenges_in_a_Community_Partnered_Care_Coordination_Initiative_A_Qualitative_Needs_Assessment

Jennings, L. A., Hollands, S., Keeler, E., Wenger, N. S., & Reuben, D. B. (2020). The effects of dementia care co-management on acute care, hospice, and long-term care utilization. *Journal of the American Geriatrics Society, 68*(11), 2500–2507. https://doi.org/10.1111/jgs.16667

Josephsen, J., Ketelsen, K., Weaver, M., & Scheuffele, H. (2023). Dementia Care Competency Model for Higher Education: A Pilot Study. *International Journal of Environmental Research and Public Health, 20*(4), 3173. https://doi.org/10.3390/ijerph20043173

Lee, J. J., Jagasia, E., & Wilson, P. R. (2023). Addressing health disparities of individuals experiencing homelessness in the U.S. with community institutional partnerships: An integrative review. *Journal of Advanced Nursing*, 79, 1678–1690. https://doi.org/10.1111/jan.15591

Mahoney, S. (2022). *Caring for adults with intellectual and developmental disabilities.* Association of American Medical Colleges (AAMCNews). https://www.aamc.org/news/caring-adults-intellectual-and-developmental-disabilities

Miller, L. B., Sjoberg, H., Mayberry, A., McCreight, M. S., Ayele, R. A., & Battaglia, C. (2019). The advanced care coordination program: A protocol for improving transitions of care for dual-use veterans from community emergency departments back to the Veterans Health Administration (VA) primary care. *BMC Health Services Research 19*, 734. https://doi.org/10.1186/s12913-019-4582-3

MyArmyBenefits. (2023). *VA expands maternity care coordination for Veterans.* https://myarmybenefits.us.army.mil/News/VA-expands-maternity-care-coordination-for-Veterans

National Alliance to End Homelessness. (2023). *State of homelessness: 2023 edition.* https://endhomelessness.org/homelessness-in-america/homelessness-statistics/state-of-homelessness/#homelessness-in-2022

National Institute of Health (NIH). (2021). *About intellectual and developmental disabilities (IDDs).* https://www.nichd.nih.gov/health/topics/idds/conditioninfo

National Institute of Health (NIH). (2024). *Person-first and destigmatizing language.* https://www.nih.gov/nih-style-guide/person-first-destigmatizing-language

Oregon Heritage. (2018). Researching historically marginalized communities. *Oregon Heritage Bulletin, 34*, 1–5. https://www.oregon.gov/oprd/OH/Documents/HB34_Researching_Historically_Marganized_Communities.pdf

Residential Information Systems Project (RISP). (n.d). *People with IDD in the United States.* University of Minnesota, RISP, Research and Training Center on Community Living, Institute on Community Integration. https://publications.ici.umn.edu/risp/infographics/people-with-idd-in-the-united-states-and-the-proportion-who-receive-services#:~:text=There%20were%207.39%20million%20people,in%20addition%20to%20case%20management.

Resources for Integrated Care (RIC). (2022). *Strategies for delivering person-centered care for individuals with I/DD* [Slides]. https://www.resourcesforintegratedcare.com/wp-content/uploads/2022/08/Strategies-for-Delivering-Person-Centered-Care-for-Individuals-with-IDD-Slides.pdf

RHIHub. (2018). *Adopting a whole person mindset.* https://www.ruralhealthinfo.org/toolkits/care-coordination/3/whole-person

Schaeffer, K. (2023). *The changing face of America's veteran population.* Pew Research Center. https://www.pewresearch.org/short-reads/2023/11/08/the-changing-face-of-americas-veteran-population/

Sjoberg, H., Liu, W., Rohs, C., Ayele, R. A., McCreight, M., Mayberry, A., & Battaglia, C. (2022). Optimizing care coordination to address social determinants of health needs for dual-use veterans. *BMC Health Services Research, 22*(1), 59. https://doi.org/10.1186/s12913-021-07408-x

Smith, Y. (2023). *How medical respite provides support to people experiencing homelessness.* National Alliance to End Homelessness. https://endhomelessness.org/blog/how-medical-respite-provides-support-to-people-experiencing-homelessness/

Spotswood, S. (2023). *Care integration: Is VA trying to reinvent something that already exists?* U.S. Medicine: The Voice of Federal Medicine. https://www.usmedicine.com/treatment/care-integration-is-va-trying-to-reinvent-something-that-already-existed/

Substance Abuse and Mental Health Services Administration (SAMHSA). (2023). *Substance Abuse and Mental Health Services Administration: Practical guide for implementing a trauma-informed approach.* SAMHSA Publication

No. PEP23-06-05-005. National Mental Health and Substance Use Policy Laboratory. Substance Abuse and Mental Health Services Administration. https://store.samhsa.gov/sites/default/files/pep23-06-05-005.pdf

Sullivan, W. F., Heng, J., McNeil, K., Bach, M., Henze, M., Perry, A., & Vogt, J. (2019). Promoting health care decision-making capabilities of adults with intellectual and developmental disabilities. *Canadian family physician Medecin de famille canadien*, *65*(Suppl 1), S27–S29. https://www.ncbi.nlm.nih.gov/pmc/articles/PMC6501714/

Thompson, C. (2022, November 22). As police arrest more seniors, those with dementia face deadly consequences. *USA Today*. https://www.usatoday.com/in-depth/news/investigations/2022/11/22/police-arrests-elderly-unique-risks-dementia-alzheimers/10455567002/

U.S. Department of Housing and Urban Development (HUD). (2022). *The 2022 annual homelessness assessment report (AHAR) to congress*. https://www.huduser.gov/portal/sites/default/files/pdf/2022-AHAR-Part-1.pdf

U.S. Department of Veterans Affairs. (2019a). *Determining veteran status*. https://www.va.gov/OSDBU/docs/Determining-Veteran-Status.pdf

U.S. Department of Veterans Affairs. (2019b). *Veteran community care: General information* [Fact Sheet]. https://www.va.gov/COMMUNITYCARE/docs/pubfiles/factsheets/VHA-FS_MISSION-Act.pdf

Vi, L., Jiwa, M. I., Lunsky, Y., & Thakur, A. (2023). A systematic review of intellectual and developmental disability curriculum in international pre-graduate health professional education. *BMC Medical Education*, *23*(1), 329. https://doi.org/10.1186/s12909-023-04259-4

Williams, J. (2022, September 1). *"I Have No One": Understanding homelessness and trauma. Psychiatric Times*. https://www.psychiatrictimes.com/view/i-have-no-one-understanding-homelessness-and-trauma

Wolverson, E., Dunning, R., Crowther, G., Russell, G., & Underwood, B. R. (2022). The characteristics and outcomes of people with dementia in inpatient mental health care: A review. *Clinical Gerontologist*. https://doi.org/10.1080/07317115.2022.2104145

Wolverson, E. L., Harrison Dening, K., Dunning, R., Crowther, G., Russell, G., & Underwood, B. R. (2023). Family experiences of inpatient mental health care for people with dementia. *Frontiers in Psychiatry*, *14*, 1093894. https://doi.org/10.3389/fpsyt.2023.1093894

Glossary of Acronyms

A

AAACN—American Academy of Ambulatory Care Nursing

AAAHC—Accreditation Association for Ambulatory Health Care

AACN—American Association of Colleges of Nursing

AAHC—American Accreditation Healthcare Commission

ACHC—Accreditation Commission for Health Care

ACM—Accredited Case Manager

ACMA—American Case Management Association

ACO/ACOs—Accountable Care Organization/Organizations

ACO REACH—Accountable Care Organization Realizing Equity, Access, and Community Health

ADLs—Activities of Daily Living

ADPIE—Assessment, Diagnosis, Planning, Implementation, and Evaluation

ADOPIE—Assessment, Diagnosis, Outcomes Identification, Planning, Implementation, and Evaluation

ADRD—Alzheimer's disease and related dementias

AHA—American Hospital Association

AHC—Accountable Health Community

AHRQ—Agency for Healthcare Research and Quality

AI—Artificial Intelligence

ALF—Assisted Living Facility

AMAP—American Medical Accreditation Program

ANA—American Nursing Association

APC—Ambulatory Payment Classifications

B

BPCI Advanced—Bundled Payments for Care Improvement Advanced

C

CABG—Coronary Artery Bypass Surgery

CAD—Coronary Artery Disease

CAH—Critical Access Hospital

CAHPS®—Consumer Assessment of Healthcare Providers and Systems

CARF—Commission on Accreditation of Rehabilitation Facilities

CBR—Cost-Based Reimbursement

CCM—Certified Case Manager

CCMC—Commission for Case Manager Certification

CDC—Centers for Disease Control and Prevention

CEHRT—Certified Electronic Health Record Technology

CER—Comparative Effectiveness Research

CHAP—Community Health Accreditation Partner

CHEMS—Community Health Emergency Medical Services

CHF—Congestive Heart Failure

CHIP—Children's Health Insurance Program

CHW—Community Health Worker

CIHQ—Center for Improvement in Healthcare Quality

CIRI—Clinical Information Reconciliation and Incorporation

CMI—Case Mix Index

CMS—Centers for Medicare and Medicaid Services

CMSA—Case Management Society of America

CoCM—Collaborative Care Model

CODE—Courage, Obligations to Honor, Danger Management, and Expression and Action

CoP—Conditions of Participation

COPD—Chronic Obstructive Pulmonary Disease

CPOE—Computerized Physician Order Entry

CPT®—Current Procedural Terminology

CQI—Continuous Quality Improvement

CSSC—Council for Six Sigma Certification

CVICU—Cardiovascular Intensive Care Unit

D

DME—Durable Medical Equipment

DPOA—Durable Power of Attorney

DRG—Diagnostic-Related Group

E

EBP—Evidence-Based Practice

ED—Emergency Department

EHR—Electronic Health Record

e.g.—Latin *exempli gratia*, meaning for example

EMS—Emergency Medical Services

EMT—Emergency Medical Technicians

ER—Emergency Room

ESRD—End Stage Renal Disease

F

FECC—Family Experiences with Care Coordination

FQHC—Federally Qualified Health Center

G

GUIDE—Guiding an Improved Dementia Experience Model

H

HBPC—Home-Based Primary Care

HC—Hospice Care

HCAHPS—Hospital Consumer Assessment of Healthcare Providers and Systems

HCPCS—Healthcare Common Procedure Coding System

HEDIS—Healthcare Effectiveness Data and Information Sets

HHA—Home Health Aide

HHS—Health and Human Services

HIE—Health Information Exchange

HIPAA—Health Insurance Portability and Accountability Act

HIT—Health Information Technology

HITECH—Health Information Technology for Economic and Clinical Health Act

HMO—Health Maintenance Organization

HRSA—Health Resources and Services Administration

HRSN/HRSNs—Health-Related Social Need/Needs

I

IADL—Instrumental Activities of Daily Living

ICARE—Integrity, Compassion, Accountability, Respect, and Empathy

ICD-10—International Classification of Diseases Tenth Revision

ICU—Intensive Care Unit

IDD—Intellectual or Developmental Disabilities

IDEAL—Include, Discuss, Educate, Assess, Listen

IOM—Institute of Medicine

IPASSTHEBATON—Introduction, Patient, Assessment, Situation, Safety Concerns, THE, Background, Actions, Timing, Ownership, Next

IPFQR—Inpatient Psychiatric Facility Quality Reporting Form

IRF—Inpatient Rehabilitation Facility

J

JCAHO—The Joint Commission/Joint Commission on the Accreditation of Healthcare Organizations

JIT—Just In Time

L

LOS—Length of Stay

LPN—Licensed Professional Nurse

LTACH—Long-Term Acute Care Hospital

LTC—Long-Term Care

M

MA—Medical Assistant

MDS—Minimum Data Set

MH—Mental Health

MI—Motivational Interviewing

MISSION—Maintaining Internal Systems and Strengthening Integrated Outside Networks

MS—Multiple Sclerosis

N

NACHC—National Association of Community Health Centers

NANDA—North American Nursing Diagnosis Association

NBCM—National Board for Case Management

NCI—National Cancer Institute

NCQA—National Committee for Quality Assurance

NHIN—Nationwide Health Information Network

NIAHO—National Integrated Accreditation for Healthcare Organizations

NIH—National Institute of Health

NORFA—National Outpatient Rehabilitation Facility Accreditation

NP—Nurse Practitioner

NQF—National Quality Forum

NTOCC—National Transitions of Care Coalition

O

OARS—Open-Ended Questions, Affirmation, Reflective Listening, and Summary

OASIS—Outcome and Assessment Information Set

ONC—Office of the National Coordinator for Health Information Technology

OT—Occupational Therapy/Therapist

P

PACT—Patient Aligned Care Team

PAM®—Patient Activation Measure®

PASRR—Preadmission Screening and Resident Review

PC—Palliative Care

PCMH—Patient-Centered Medical Home, also known as Advanced Primary Care

PCORI—Patient-Centered Outcomes Research Institute

PCP—Primary Care Provider

PCS—Personal Care Services

PHI—Protected Health Information

PHQ-9—Patient Health Questionnaire version 9

PMPM—Per Member Per Month

POS—Point of Service

PPO—Preferred Provider Organization

PT—Physical Therapy/Therapist

PTSD—Post-Traumatic Stress Disorder

PWD—Person with Dementia

Q

QHINs™—Qualified Health Information Networks™

R

RCC—Relationship-Centered Care

REH—Rural Emergency Hospital

RN—Registered Nurse

ROM—Range of Motion

RPM—Remote Patient Monitoring

RW—Relative Weight

S

SAMHSA—Substance Abuse and Mental Health Services Association

SAR—Sub-Acute Rehabilitation

SDM—Shared Decision-Making

SDOH—Social Determinants of Health

SIOH—Social Influencers of Health

SNF—Skilled Nursing Facility

SUD—Substance Use Disorder

SW—Social Worker

T

TCPs—Transitional Care Programs

TEFCA—Trusted Exchange Framework and Common Agreement℠

TIC—Trauma Informed Care

TPS—Total Performance Score

U

UM—Utilization Management or Utilization Manager

URAC—Utilization Review Accreditation Commission

V

VA—Veterans Affairs

VBP—Value-Based Purchasing

W

WHO—World Health Organization

Answers to NCLEX Style Questions

Chapter 1

1. a, c [Answer available in "Introduction" section]
2. Care coordination is the primary but critical function of organizing and managing patient care across the care continuum through information sharing and person-centered-care practices. [Answer available in the "Care Coordination Overview" section.]
3. c [Answer available in "Care Coordination Across Settings" section]
4. Population care coordination includes health promotion and disease prevention activities. [Answer available in the "Population Care Coordination" section]
5. a [Answer available in the "Population Care Coordination" section]
6. b [Answer available in the "Transition Management" section]
7. d [Answer available in the "Transition Management" section]
8. a, c, d [Answer available in the "Care/Case Management" section]
9. Right for the patient, right care, right setting, right time, right resource, right transition, and right education. [Answer available in Figure 1.4: The Seven Rights of Care Coordination]
10. d [Answer available in the "Resource and Utilization Management" section]
11. c [Answer available in Figure 1.5: The Evolution of the Quintuple Aim]
12. a, c [Answer available in the "Case Management Society of America (CMSA) and Commission for Case Manager Certification (CCMC) Collaboration" section]
13. d [Answer available in the "American Nursing Association (ANA)" section]
14. a [Answer available in the "American Association of Colleges of Nursing (AACN)" section]
15. d [Answer available in Figure 1.3: The Health Triune]

Chapter 2

1. d [Answer available in "Cross-Setting Communication" section]
2. b [Answer available "Cross-Setting Communication" section]

3. d [Answer available in "Connection with Community Resources" section]
4. c [Answer available in "Person-Centered Care and Relationship-Centered Care" section]
5. c [Answer available in "Interprofessional Care Coordination" section]
6. b, c [Answer available in "Advocacy" section]
7. d [Answer available in "Moral Courage in Nursing" text box]
8. d [Answer available in Figure 2.4: The Relationship Between Assessment and Critical Analysis in Care Coordination]
9. a [Answer available in the "Functional Abilities" text box]
10. c [Answer available in the "Key Tips to Managing Challenging Conversations" text box]
11. c [Answer available in "Connection with Community Resources" section]
12. a, b, c [Answer available in "Interprofessional Collaboration" section]
13. c [Answer available in Figure 2.6: Example Application of the Donabedian Model to Care Coordination Practice Monitoring]
14. b [Answer available in "Evaluation" section]
15. b, c [Answer available in Figure 2.2: Foundational Care Coordination Competencies and Sub-Competencies]

Chapter 3

1. b [Answer available in "Planning" section]
2. b [Answer available in "Health Teaching and Health Promotion" section]
3. d [Answer available in "Diagnosis" section]
4. a [Answer available in "Practice Focus: Assessing risk" section]
5. b [Answer available in "Health Teaching and Health Promotion" section]
6. d [Answer available in "Introduction" section]
7. b [Answer available in "Guiding Principles of Care Coordination" figure]
8. c [Answer available in "Diagnosis" section]
9. a [Answer available in "Outcomes Identification" section]
10. d [Answer available in "Coordination of Care" section]
11. d [Answer available in "Gap Analysis" section]
12. a [Answer available in "Practice Focus: Preparing for Transitions in Care" section]
13. b [Answer available in "Practice Focus: Preparing for Transitions in Care" section]
14. b, c [Answer available in "Practice Focus: Monitoring Coordination of Care" section]
15. a [Answer available in chapter glossary]

Chapter 4

1. b [Answer available in "Patient Engagement" section]
2. d [Answer available in "Health Literacy" section]
3. d [Answer available in "Caring Practices and Patient Engagement Model" text box]
4. a [Answer available in "10 Elements of Competence for Using Teach-Back Effectively" text box]
5. b, c, d [Answer available in "Health Self-Management" section]
6. c [Answer available in "Core Health Self-Management Skills" text box]
7. b [Answer available in "Trajectory Framework of Health Self-Management" figure]
8. a, c [Answer available in "Patient Engagement" section]
9. c [Answer available in "Activation Language" section]
10. a, b [Answer available in "The Nurse's Role" section]
11. c [Answer available in "The Patient's Role" section]
12. d [Answer available in "Health Literacy" section]
13. b [Answer available in "Organization Health Literacy" section]
14. b [Answer available in "The Nurse's Role" section]
15. b [Answer available in "Motivational Interviewing and Stages of Change" section]

Chapter 5

1. c [Answer available in "Introduction" section]
2. d [Answer available in "Introduction" section]
3. d [Answer available in "The Continuum of Care" section]
4. a [Answer available in "Unique Considerations of the Acute Care Hospital" section]
5. c [answer available in "The Continuum of Care" section]
6. a [Answer available in "Unique Considerations of Inpatient Rehabilitation" section]
7. b [Answer available in "Levels of Care" section]
8. d [Answer available in "Long-Term Acute Care Hospitals (LTACH)" section]
9. b [Answer available in "Personal Care Services" section]
10. a [Answer available in "Unique Considerations of Home Health Services" section]
11. a, d [Answer available in "Unique Considerations of the Psychiatric Hospital" section]
12. d [Answer available in "Factors Affecting the Decision to Admit to Psychiatric Hospitalization" text box]

13. b [Answer available in "Psychiatric Hospitals" section]
14. a, b [Answer available in "Palliative and Hospice Care" section]
15. a, c [Answer available in "Unique Considerations of Palliative and Hospice Care" section]

Chapter 6

1. a, b [answer available in "Introduction" section]
2. a [answer available in "Introduction" section]
3. a, b, c [answer available in "Quality Healthcare and Care Coordination" section]
4. Continuity of care—Quality

   Improved follow-up—Quality

   Decreased emergency room visits—Resource

   Prevention of delays in care—Quality

   Prevention of admission to acute care—Resource

   [Answer available in "Quality and Resource Use Outcomes of Nurse Case Management" text box]
5. b [Linking to transportation resources in the community is required so that appointments are not missed. Answer available in "Quality Healthcare and Care Coordination" section]
6. c [Performing a comprehensive assessment is the best way to determine the patient's needs and health goals and how smoking cessation may fit into them. Answer available in "Quality Healthcare and Care Coordination" section]
7. c [Answer available in the "Meaningful Quality Measures" section]
8. d [Answer available in "Value-Based Healthcare Quality Measures" section]
9. c [Answer available in "Value-Based Healthcare Quality Measures" section]
10. c [Answer available in the "Meaningful Quality Measures" section]
11. a, b [Answer available in the "Continuous Quality Improvement (CQI) Model: Lean" section]
12. d [Answer available in "Continuous Quality Improvement (CQI) Model: Lean" section]
13. a [Answer available in "Continuous Quality Improvement (CQI) Model: Lean" section]
14. Meaningful measures 2.0 is an initiative to promote value in healthcare by focusing on high-impact quality areas that are meaningful to patients and are person-centered. [Answer available in chapter glossary]
15. a, b, d [Answer available throughout chapter]

Chapter 7

1. a, b [Answer available in "Transitional Care Programs (TCPs)" section]
2. c [Answer available in "Telehealth/Telemedicine/Virtual Healthcare" section]
3. a, d [Answer available in Table 7.1 "Example Healthcare System Change Drivers" table]
4. b, d [Answer available in "Collaborative Care Model (CoCM)" section]
5. c [Answer available in "Advanced Primary Care: The Patient-Centered Medical Home (PCMH)" section]
6. b, d [Answer available in "Advanced Primary Care: The Patient-Centered Medical Home (PCMH)" section]
7. c [Answer available in the "Federally Qualified Health Center (FQHC)" section]
8. d [Answer available in "Home-Based Primary Care (HBPC): House Calls" section]
9. d [Answer available in the "Home-Based Primary Care (HBPC): House Calls" section]
10. a, b [Answer available in the "Home-Based Primary Care (HBPC): House Calls" section]
11. a [Answer available in "Telehealth/Telemedicine/Virtual Healthcare" section]
12. d [Answer available in "Accountable Health Communities (AHC)" section]
13. a, b [Answer available in "Accountable Health Communities (AHC)" section]
14. c [Answer available in chapter glossary]
15. a [Answer available in Figure 7.1: Patient-Centered Medical Home (PCMH) Model]

Chapter 8

1. d [Answer available in "Introduction" section]
2. d [Answer available in "Quality Measures and Value-Based Healthcare Payment Models" section]
3. Value = quality divided by cost. [See Figure 8.3]
4. d [Answer available in "Accountable Care Organizations (ACO)" section]
5. d [Answer available in "Hospital Value-Based Purchasing" section]
6. a [Answer available in "Capitated Payment Model" section]
7. Medicare Part A: Requires the person to work and pay Medicare taxes for at least 10 years or be eligible through their spouse for the premium free option.

   Medicare Part B: Reimburses for outpatient healthcare needs, outpatient hospital services, physician services, home healthcare services, and durable medical equipment.

   Medicare Part C: Often is based on an HMO or PPO model of care delivery and may be referred to as a Medicare Advantage Plan.

Medicare Part D: Has a "donut hole" where the beneficiary potentially will experience a temporary limit on what the plan will cover for prescription medications.

Medigap Plan: An optional private insurance plan that can assist in covering copayment and deductible costs.

[Answer available in "Medicare" section]

8. c [Answer available in "Quality Measures and Value-Based Healthcare Payment Models" section]
9. a, b, d [Answer available in "Coding Considerations" section]
10. a [Answer available in "Medicare Part A" section]
11. a, c [Answer available in "Medicaid" section]
12. c [Answer available in "Medicaid" section]
13. d [Answer available in "Uninsured" section]
14. d [Answer available in "Uninsured" section]
15. c [Answer available in "The No Surprises Act" section]

Chapter 9

1. c [Answer available in "Health Information Technology for Economic and Clinical Health (HITECH) Act" section]
2. b [Answer available in chapter glossary, Digital Inclusion definiton]
3. c [Answer available in chapter glossary, Informatic definition]
4. c [Answer available in Figure 9.2: Nursing Informatics Process]
5. b, c [Answer available in "Digital Health" section]
6. d [Answer available in Figure 9.3: The Symbiosis of HIT, Informatics, and Digital Health]
7. d [Answer available in "Health Information Technology for Economic and Clinical Health (HITECH) HITECH Act" section]
8. a [Answer available in "Health Information Technology for Economic and Clinical Health (HITECH) Act" section]
9. d [Answer available in "Health Insurance Portability and Accountability Act (HIPAA)" section]
10. d [Answer available in "Health Insurance Portability and Accountability Act (HIPAA)" and "Provider Patient Privacy Concerns" sections]
11. c [Answer available in "Data Management Considerations" section]
12. c [Answer available in "Infrastructure Considerations" section]
13. b [Answer available in "Nurse-Patient Relationship" section]

14. d [Answer available in "Nurse-Patient Relationship" section]
15. d [Answer available in "Ethical, Equity, and Accessibility Considerations" section]

Chapter 10

1. d [Answer available in "The Role of the Nurse in Advancing Care Coordination in Legislation" section]
2. c, d [Answer available in "The Role of the Nurse in Advancing Care Coordination in Legislation" section]
3. a [Answer available in "Proactive Care Coordination" section]
4. a, c [Answer available in "Health Systems Thinking" section]
5. d [Answer available in "Health System Science" section]
6. a [Answer available in "Legislative Trends and Issues" section]
7. c [Answer available in Figure 10.2: Well-Being Orchestra]
8. c [Answer available in "Social Media Healthcare Influencers" section]
9. b [Answer available in "Privacy" section]
10. b [Answer available in "Role Blurring" section]
11. b [Answer available Table 10.1 "The COLLABORATE© Competency Model Application"]
12. a, b [Answer available in "Collaborative and Integrated Care" section]
13. d [Answer available in Figure 10.3: Example Artificial Intelligence (AI) Support of Care Coordination]
14. a, b, d [Answer available in "Artificial Intelligence" section]
15. a [Answer available in "Chapter Summary" section]

Chapter 11

1. d [Answer available in "The Unhoused Population" section]
2. b [Answer available in "Trauma-Informed Care (TIC) and Care Coordination Practice" section]
3. c [Answer available in "Trauma-Informed Care (TIC) and Care Coordination Practice" section]
4. d [Answer available in "The Veteran Population" section]
5. b, d [Answer available in "The Veteran Population" section]
6. c [Answer available in "The Veteran Population" Section]
7. d [Answer available in "Alzheimer's Disease and Related Dementias (ADRD) Population" section]

8. b [Answer available in “Alzheimer’s Disease and Related Dementias (ADRD) Population” section]
9. c, d [Answer available in “Intellectual and Developmental Disability (IDDs) Population” section]
10. b [Answer available in “The Unhoused Population” section]
11. c [Answer available in “The Unhoused Population” section]
12. b [Answer available in “Medical Respite” text box]
13. d [Answer available in “Intellectual and Developmental Disability (IDDs) Population” section]
14. a, d [Answer available in Figure 1.1: Caregiver Healthcare Transition Checklist”]
15. a [Answer available in “Intellectual and Developmental Disability (IDDs) Population” section]

Index

D

www.ingramcontent.com/pod-product-compliance
Ingram Content Group UK Ltd.
Pitfield, Milton Keynes, MK11 3LW, UK
UKHW050139280726
14058UKWH00006B/723